Essentials of Medical Geology

Essentials of Medical Geology

Editor: Paolo Sander

STATES
ACADEMIC PRESS
www.statesacademicpress.com

www.statesacademicpress.com

STATES
ACADEMIC PRESS

Cataloging-in-Publication Data

Essentials of medical geology / edited by Paolo Sander.
p. cm.
Includes bibliographical references and index.
ISBN 978-1-63989-793-3
1. Medical geography. 2. Geology--Health aspects. 3. Environmental health.
4. Public health. 5. Environmental geology. I. Sander, Paolo.
RA792 .E87 2023
614.42--dc23

States Academic Press,
109 South 5th Street,
Brooklyn, NY 11249, USA

ISBN 978-1-63989-793-3 (Hardback)

Contents

Preface

The Earth is primarily composed of minerals and rocks. These components are the source of all chemical elements that have an effect on human and animal populations. Medical geology is an emerging interdisciplinary scientific field that studies the interrelation between natural geological factors and their impact on human and animal health. There are various geologic processes in which humans are exposed to chemical elements of the Earth. Some of the geologic processes are erosion, transportation and deposition, and the action of wind, water and ice. Volcanic eruption is also a major source that can release huge quantities of harmful chemicals such as arsenic, beryllium, cadmium, mercury, lead, radon, and uranium into the atmosphere. The field of medical geology is complex and requires a multidisciplinary approach to find the right balance and intake of elements in order to improve and maintain health. This book provides comprehensive insights into the field of medical geology. Students, professional researchers, policymakers and the general public will find it full of crucial and unexplored concepts.

Various studies have approached the subject by analyzing it with a single perspective, but the present book provides diverse methodologies and techniques to address this field. This book contains theories and applications needed for understanding the subject from different perspectives. The aim is to keep the readers informed about the progresses in the field; therefore, the contributions were carefully examined to compile novel researches by specialists from across the globe.

Indeed, the job of the editor is the most crucial and challenging in compiling all chapters into a single book. In the end, I would extend my sincere thanks to the chapter authors for their profound work. I am also thankful for the support provided by my family and colleagues during the compilation of this book.

Editor

1

Unraveling Health Risk and Speciation of Arsenic from Groundwater in Rural Areas of Punjab, Pakistan

Muhammad Bilal Shakoor [1], Nabeel Khan Niazi [1,2,*], Irshad Bibi [1,2], Mohammad Mahmudur Rahman [3,4,5], Ravi Naidu [4,5], Zhaomin Dong [4,5], Muhammad Shahid [6] and Muhammad Arshad [1]

1 Institute of Soil and Environmental Sciences, University of Agriculture Faisalabad, Faisalabad 38040, Pakistan; E-Mails: bilalshakoor88@gmail.com (M.B.S.); irshad.niazi81@gmail.com (I.B.); arshad_ises@yahoo.com (M.A.)

2 Southern Cross GeoScience, Southern Cross University, Lismore 2480, NSW, Australia

3 Centre for Environmental Risk Assessment and Remediation (CERAR), Mawson Lakes Campus, University of South Australia, SA 5095, Australia; E-Mail: mohammad.rahman@unisa.edu.au

4 Global Centre for Environmental Remediation (GCER), Faculty of Science and Information Technology, The University of Newcastle, University Drive, Callaghan, NSW 2308, Australia; E-Mails: ravi.naidu@newcastle.edu.au (R.N.); morrow.dong@newcastle.edu.au (Z.D.)

5 Cooperative Research Centre for Contamination Assessment and Remediation of the Environment (CRC CARE), P.O. Box 486, Salisbury South, SA 5106, Australia

6 Department of Environmental Sciences, COMSATS Institute of Information Technology, Vehari 61100, Pakistan; E-Mail: muhammadshahid@ciitvehari.edu.pk

* Author to whom correspondence should be addressed; E-Mail: nabeelkniazi@gmail.com or nabeel.niazi@uaf.edu.pk

Academic Editor: Paul B. Tchounwou

Abstract: This study determined the total and speciated arsenic (As) concentrations and other health-related water quality parameters for unraveling the health risk of As from drinking water to humans. Groundwater samples (n = 62) were collected from three previously unexplored rural areas (Chichawatni, Vehari, Rahim Yar Khan) of Punjab in Pakistan. The mean and median As concentrations in groundwater were 37.9 and 12.7 $\mu g \cdot L^{-1}$ (range = 1.5–201 $\mu g \cdot L^{-1}$). Fifty three percent groundwater samples showed higher As value than WHO safe limit of 10 $\mu g \cdot L^{-1}$. Speciation of As in groundwater samples (n = 13) showed the presence of inorganic As only; arsenite (As(III)) constituted 13%–67% of total As and arsenate (As(V)) ranged from 33% to 100%. For As health risk assessment, the hazard quotient and cancer risk values were 11–18 and 46–600 times higher than the recommended values of US-EPA (*i.e.*, 1.00 and 10^{-6}, respectively). In addition to As, various water quality parameters (e.g., electrical conductivity, Na, Ca, Cl^-, NO_3^-, SO_4^{2-}, Fe, Mn, Pb) also enhanced the health risk. The results show that consumption of As-contaminated groundwater poses an emerging health threat to the communities in the study area, and hence needs urgent remedial and management measures.

Keywords: arsenic; groundwater; speciation; health risk; cancer; contamination; toxicity

---

1. Introduction

Contamination of groundwater aquifers with arsenic (As) is a global health issue because As is a toxic element and has been classified as a Group A human carcinogen [1]. Arsenic is a metalloid and a member of Group VA of the periodic table. It has an atomic number of 33, atomic weight of 74.9216 g·mol^{-1} and an electronic configuration of $[Ar]^{18}\ 4s^2\ 3d^{10}\ 4p^3$ [2]. In aquatic environments, As is mainly found in arsenite (As(III), as AsO_3^{3-}) and arsenate (As(V), as AsO_4^{3-}) oxyanionic forms; the redox potential and pH play an important role in determining the chemical forms of As. At high pH and under reducing conditions, As(III) is the predominant species, while As(V) is the major species in an oxidizing environment, at low pH [3]. The dissociation constant (pK) values for As(V) range from 2.20 to 11.53, while for As(III) pK values range between 9.22 and 13.40. The toxicity of As depends on its chemical species. Inorganic forms of As (As(III), As(V)) are more toxic than the organo-As forms (e.g., monomethyl arsenate (MMAA)) [4].

Arsenic is released into the aquatic environments through the natural processes (such as weathering reactions, volcanic emissions) and anthropogenic activities for instance, petroleum refining, use of wood preservatives, leather tanning operation, agricultural use of pesticides and herbicides [5–7].

Arsenic contamination of groundwater (up to 5000 μg·L^{-1}) has been reported worldwide in over 105 countries [8]. It has been estimated that over 200 million people in the world are at the health risk of As poisoning due to ingestion of As-rich water. Arsenic affected countries (with their corresponding maximum permissible limits) include the USA (10 μg·L^{-1}), Canada (10 μg·L^{-1}), Poland (10 μg·L^{-1}), Japan (10 μg ·L^{-1}), Australia (10 μg·L^{-1}), Taiwan (10 μg·L^{-1}), Vietnam (10 μg·L^{-1}), Brazil (50 μg·L^{-1}), Hungary (50 μg·L^{-1}), Mexico (50 μg·L^{-1}), Argentina (50 μg·L^{-1}), Nepal (50 μg·L^{-1}), Laos (50 μg·L^{-1}), Myanmar (50 μg·L^{-1}), Cambodia (50 μg·L^{-1}), China (50 μg·L^{-1}), Chile (50 μg·L^{-1}), Bangladesh (50 μg·L^{-1}), India (50 μg·L^{-1}) and Pakistan (50 μg·L^{-1}) (Table S1, Supplementary Material) [9,10]. Given the highly toxic nature of As and widespread As contamination, the World Health Organization (WHO) has set an As safe limit of 10 μg·L^{-1} in drinking water [11].

Bangladesh and several states in India where people rely on As-contaminated groundwater for drinking, cooking and also to irrigate food crops such as rice and vegetables have seen the worst As induced poisoning of the century [12,13]. In Bangladesh, 59 out of 64 districts that have been investigated display As levels above the WHO safe limit of 10 μg·L^{-1} [14]. The maximum As levels in

South 24 Parganas (India) and Noakhali (Bangladesh) were observed to be 3700 $\mu g \cdot L^{-1}$ and 4730 $\mu g \cdot L^{-1}$, respectively [15,16]. According to an estimate, about 80 million people in Bangladesh alone and 43 million people in (West Bengal) India have been exposed to health risks from As-contaminated drinking water [17].

The people exposed to chronic As poisoning through drinking water can show dermatological symptoms such as keratosis (dry, rough, papular skin lesions) and melanosis (change pigmentation) [4,18]. Arsenic toxicity may also result in neurological, reproductive, cardiovascular, hepatic, hematological, respiratory and diabetic effects in humans. Chronic exposure to high level of As is linked to the increased risk of carcinogenicity such as lung, bladder, liver, skin and kidney cancers [4].

Arsenic health risk can be calculated from As-contaminated water and food, the two major exposure routes of As in humans [19]. From food, health risk assessment can be measured in terms of estimated daily intake (EDI) by evaluating the exposure dose of As due to the consumption of food crops. However, health risk assessment based on consumption of As-contaminated water is highly significant due to the direct, intense and continuous human exposure to As. Arsenic concentration in drinking water is used to calculate potential health risk assessment (chronic and carcinogenic effects) such as, average daily dose (ADD), hazard quotient (HQ), and carcinogenic risk (CR) [20–23]. Hazard quotient and CR are considered to be present if the values are HQ > 1.00 and CR > 10^{-6} [24].

Arsenic health risk assessment was previously estimated based on total As in water or in food crops in Pakistan. In the Khyber Pakhtunkhwah province of Pakistan, the As health risk assessment was calculated by Muhammad *et al.* [25], who reported HQ values >1 in the study area. Arain *et al.* [26] calculated the ADD of As in the food to be 9–12 $\mu g \cdot kg^{-1}$ day^{-1} in Sindh and Punjab provinces (only in urban areas of Lahore and Kasur). Sultana *et al.* [27] documented that 87% water samples in Lahore exceeded the typical HQ values of 1.00 (HQ = 2.3–48.6) in Punjab.

In Pakistan, a study in Muzaffargarh district demonstrated that the natural (oxidation of As-rich minerals) as well as anthropogenic sources (use of fertilizers) resulted in a release of As in groundwater up to 906 $\mu g \cdot L^{-1}$ [28]. A few more studies investigating groundwater As concentration have been carried out in Lahore and Kasur (As levels up to 1900 $\mu g \cdot L^{-1}$) districts of Punjab [27,29–32]; in Jamshoro (As up to 106 $\mu g \cdot L^{-1}$) [33] and Tharparkar (As up to 2580 $\mu g \cdot L^{-1}$) districts of Sindh [34,35]. To the best of our knowledge, aqueous phase speciation of As (As(III) and As(V)) has not been determined by using advanced hyphenated techniques such as ion chromatography (IC) coupled with inductively coupled plasma mass spectrometry (ICP-MS) in the previously unexplored study area of Punjab, Pakistan (as we examined in this study).

To our understanding, investigating the speciated and total As contents and assessing the human health risk from intake of As-contaminated water are the critically-important and existing gaps to resolve the emerging issue of As-contamination in Punjab (Pakistan). The primary and specific objectives of the present study were to: (i) determine the total As content and species of As in groundwater from three previously unexplored areas of Punjab (Pakistan); (ii) evaluate the concentration of various water quality parameters such as major cations, anions and trace metals, and (iii) estimate the health risk of As by calculating ADD, HQ and CR values for As-contaminated drinking water by US-EPA model and bootstrap method.

2. Experimental Section

2.1. Topography

The study was conducted in three rural areas (Chichawatni, Vehari, Rahim Yar Khan) in Punjab, Pakistan. Chichawatni is a city in Sahiwal district of Punjab, Pakistan. It is situated 30°53′33″ N and 72°70′00″ E (Figure 1a). It lies approximately 45 km away from Sahiwal and its population is approximately 120,000 [36]. This city has a semi-arid alluvium plain area with the exception of a few belts of ravines and uneven land formed by gully erosion along the lower Bari Doab and its distributaries. The River Ravi flows on its north-west and the River Sutlej (Figure 1a) on its south [36].

Vehari is situated between 30°04′19″ N and 72°35′28″ E (Figure 1b) with a population of 7,000,000. Literally, Vehari means low lying riverine settlement. It is situated on right bank of the River Sutlej in the heart of Nili Bar which is between Ravi, Bias and Sutlej Rivers (Figure 1b). Vehari consists of alluvium plain area with fertile land which is irrigated with the fertile water of Chenab and Ravi Rivers [37].

Rahim Yar Khan is situated in the alluvium plain between Indus River in the west and Cholistan desert in the east. The city lies between 28°42′00″ N and 70°30′00″ E (Figure 1c) with the population of 240,000. This city is divided into three main physical features: (i) riverine area. (ii) canal irrigated area, and (iii) desert area (Cholistan). The riverine area of Rahim Yar Khan lies close to the Indus River mainly falling in the river bed [38].

2.2. Groundwater Sampling

Groundwater samples (n = 62) were collected from hand-pumps, electric pumps and tube wells at depths of 9–107 m (Table 1) around three rural areas (Chichawatni, Vehari and Rahim Yar Khan) of Punjab in Pakistan. All pumps/wells were flushed for 5 min to obtain fresh groundwater prior to collect water sample. The groundwater samples (100 mL each) were taken in triplicate in three separate plastic bottles having airtight caps. One water sample was acidified on-site by adding 2–3 drops of concentrated nitric acid (HNO_3) to stabilize As and metal ions and reduce their precipitation [39]. The acidified water samples were used to analyse total As, iron (Fe), manganese (Mn), nickel (Ni), lead (Pb), cadmium (Cd), copper (Cu), silicon (Si), cobalt (Co), aluminum (Al), zinc (Zn), boron (B), chromium (Cr), phosphorus (P), sulfur (S) and major cations including calcium (Ca), magnesium (Mg), potassium (K) and sodium (Na). The second water sample was kept non-acidified to analyse various anions including carbonates (CO_3^{2-}), bicarbonates (HCO_3^-), chloride (Cl^-), nitrate (NO_3^-), sulfate (SO_4^{2-}), phosphate (PO_4^{3-}) and fluoride (F^-). For As speciation (Table 2), the third sample was preserved with 0.025 M ethylenediaminetetraacetic acid (EDTA) [40]. Samples were kept in insulated cooler containing ice, transported to the laboratory and stored at 4 °C, then transported to Centre for Environmental Risk Assessment and Remediation (CERAR) laboratory, University of South Australia, Australia by FedEx courier with dry ice under strict quarantine regulations and stored at 4 °C prior to various chemical analyses.

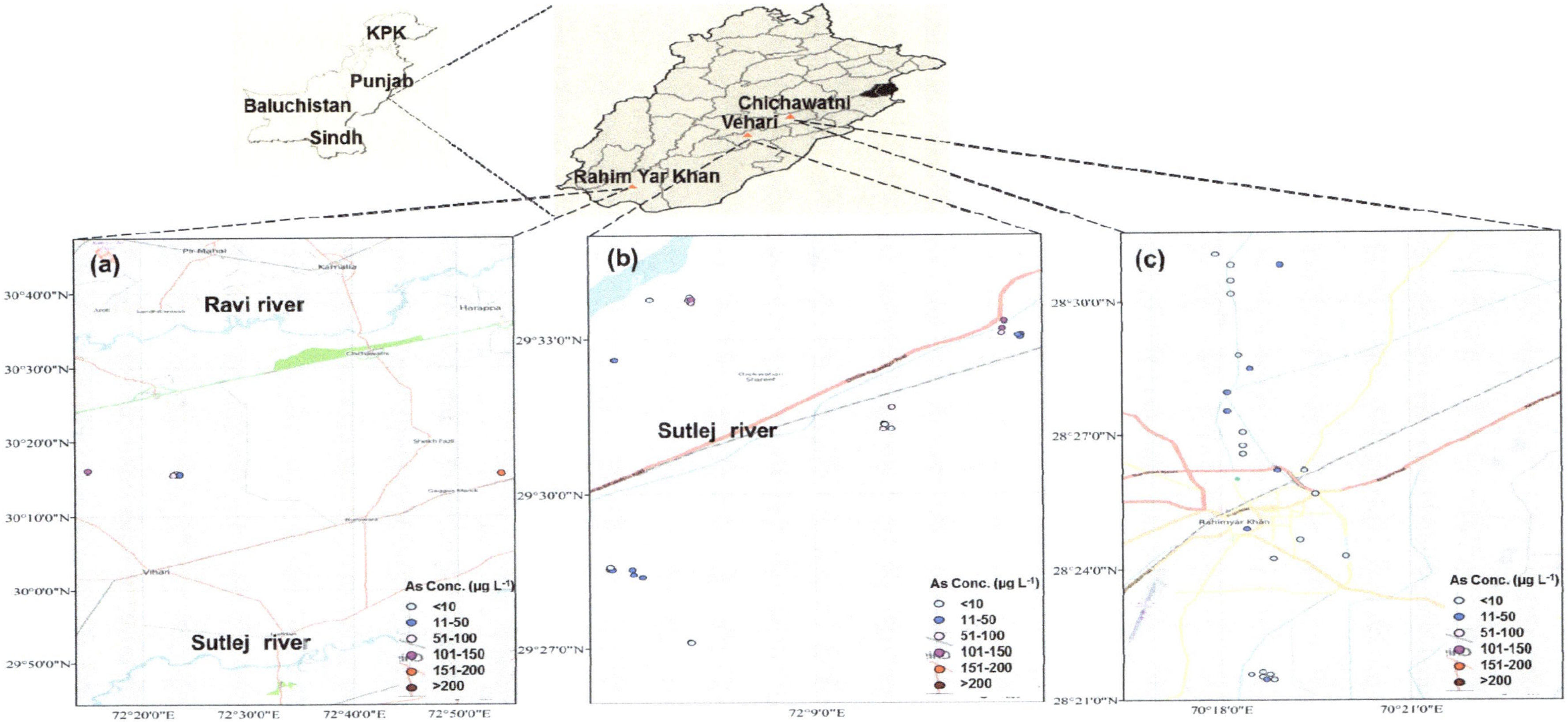

Figure 1. Map of the study area showing locations of groundwater sampling for As ($\mu g \cdot L^{-1}$) in Punjab, Pakistan; (**a**) Chichawatni; (**b**) Vehari; (**c**) Rahim Yar Khan.

2.3. Analytical Methods

The electrical conductivity (EC) and pH of water samples were measured *in situ* by using an EC meter (Model 470, Jenway, Stone, Staffordshire, U.K.) and a pH meter (Model 370, Jenway), respectively (Table 1). Total dissolved solids (TDS) were measured by using a TDS meter (Model 3000c, Ohaus, Parsippany, NJ, USA). An inductively coupled plasma mass spectrometer (ICP-MS; Model 7500ce, Agilent, Santa Clara, CA, USA) with an octopole reaction system (ORS) was used for multi-elements analysis (total As, Al, Cr, Ca, Mg, Na, Fe, P, K, Ni, Pb, Mn, Cd, Cu, Si, Co, Zn, B, S) (Table 3). For anions (NO_3^-, SO_4^{2-}, F^-, Cl^-, PO_4^{3-}) analyses in water samples, ion chromatography (IC, Model ICS 2000, Dionex, Carlsbad, CA, USA) was used. Arsenic speciation was done by using an IC-ICP-MS. Other anions such as CO_3^{2-} and HCO_3^- were determined by acid titration (H_2SO_4) using phenolphthalein, and methyl orange as indicators [41]. Calcium hardness, Mg hardness and total hardness as $CaCO_3$ were calculated following the methodology described by Spellman [42].

2.4. Quality Control

A standard reference material (SRM) from the National Institute of Standard and Technology (NIST, Gaithersburg, MD, USA) such as SRM 1640 (trace elements in natural water) was used to check accuracy of the analytical results for As. The concentration of As in SRM 1640 was estimated by following the same analysis procedure as for the groundwater samples. The certified concentration of As in NIST SRM 1640 was 26.67 ± 0.41 μg·L^{-1}. From our ICP-MS results, the mean As concentration of NIST SRM 1640 was detected as 27.32 ± 0.65 μg·L^{-1} ($n = 8$) with a recovery of 104.21%.

2.5. Water Consumption Patterns of People in the Study Area

In the study area, average water intake rates were 2.1 and 1.9 L per day for adult males and females, respectively (data not shown). The average daily water intake in our study was almost similar to the findings of Sultana *et al.* [27], Brahman *et al.* [43] and Kazi *et al.* [44], who reported 2 L·day^{-1} of average drinking water intake in Punjab (Lahore and Kasur) and Sindh (Nagarparkar and Manchar lake) provinces of Pakistan. However, in the current study the average daily water intake rate was less than the results of Rahman *et al.* [45] in Bangladesh (3.2 and 2.7 L·day^{-1} for adult males and females, respectively) and Mondal *et al.* [46] in West Bengal, India (3.1 and 2.6 L·day^{-1} for adult males and females, respectively).

2.6. Human Health Risk Assessment

2.6.1. Exposure Assessment

The human health risk assessment model derived by US-EPA Equations (1–3) was used to evaluate the toxic effects of As present in drinking water on the health of people in three study locations [47]. The health risk assessment was done to estimate the probability of individuals being exposed to As poisoning from drinking water. For this purpose, average daily dose (ADD) of As due to the intake of As-contaminated drinking water was calculated by the Equation (1):

$$ADD = \frac{C \times IR \times ED \times EF}{BW \times AT} \quad (1)$$

where:

C = Concentration of As in water (mg·L^{-1})

IR = Water ingestion rate (L·day^{-1})

ED = Exposure duration (assumed 67 years to make a comparison with previous studies from Pakistan and other countries)

EF = Exposure frequency (365 days year^{-1})

BW = Body weight (72 kg) [27]

AT= Average life time (24,455 days)

2.6.2. Human Health Risk Assessment

Chronic and carcinogenic risk levels were also determined in individuals of the study area. The hazard quotient (HQ) was computed by the Equation (2) [47]:

$$HQ = \frac{ADD}{RfD} \quad (2)$$

where RfD represents oral reference dose (0.0003 mg·kg^{-1}·day^{-1}) for As calculated by US-EPA [24]. Cancer risk (CR) was calculated by using the Equation (3):

$$CR = \frac{ADD}{CSF} \quad (3)$$

where CSF is the cancer slope factor for As which is 1.5 mg·kg^{-1}·day^{-1}, according to US-EPA [24].

2.7. Carcinogenic and Non-Carcinogenic Risk

Considering the potential cancer risk from As-contaminated groundwater (used as drinking water in the study area, the cancer probability for As is also calculated as described in our earlier study for Bangladesh and India [23] Equation (4):

$$R_i = 1/5000 \times \sum_{j=1}^{5000} C_{ij} \times k_j \quad (4)$$

where the subscript i represents the sampling regions, $C \times j$ is the average concentration of As in groundwater that was estimated by the bootstrap method, j is the sampling time in the bootstrap method, and k_j is the random number of sampling from the distribution for cancer slope of As for drinking water. The cancer slope (5 × 10^{-5} per µg·L^{-1}, with the range of 3 × 10^{-5} per µg·L^{-1} to 7 × 10^{-5} per µg·L^{-1}) recommended by US-EPA was used in this study [48]. In this study, the non-carcinogenic risk was also estimated by using the bootstrap (re-sampling) method as described for cancer risk. The value of 3 × 10^{-4} mg·kg^{-1} was recommended as reference dose.

2.8. Statistical Analysis

Basic descriptive statistical analyses were done by using JMP version 9.0 software and the maps were prepared using the Arc GIS 9.2 computer package [45].

3. Results and Discussion

3.1. Total and Speciated As Contents

Figure 1 shows the distribution of As concentrations in groundwater and locations of the study area. Arsenic concentration ranged 1.5–201 $\mu g \cdot L^{-1}$ (Table 1; Figure S1, Supplementary Material) in groundwater samples of the study area. Sixty two percent groundwater samples showed As levels 15–19 times (Table S2, Supplementary Material) higher than the safe limit (10 $\mu g \cdot L^{-1}$) set by the WHO, US-EPA and Health Canada (HC) (Table S3, Supplementary Material). In Chichawatni (CW), 100% samples, in Vehari (Vh) 66% and in Rahim Yar Khan (RYK) 20% samples contained 2–19 times higher As concentrations as compared with the safe limits set by the WHO, US-EPA and HC (Table S3, Supplementary Material). Groundwater samples of CW (88%) and Vh (60%) showed 2–4 times greater As concentration than Pakistan-Environmental Protection Agency (Pak-EPA) permissible limit for As (50 $\mu g \cdot L^{-1}$).

Arsenic speciation data of the selected groundwater (n = 13) samples (*i.e.*, having maximum total As concentration) in CW, Vh and RYK showed that As(III) constituted 13% to 67% of total As and As(V) ranged from 33% to 100% (Table 2). High proportion of As(V) in groundwater samples indicated that the subsurface sediments and aquifers would have been oxidized over time due to continuous pumping of groundwater [30]. Also, presence of high HCO_3^- (>250 $mg \cdot L^{-1}$) and SO_4^{2-} (>1400 $mg \cdot L^{-1}$) concentrations supports oxidation of sediments and aquifers [3]. Enrichment of groundwater with As may arise by oxidation of As containing minerals such as arsenopyrite (FeAsS) thus discharging soluble As, SO_4^{2-} and ferric iron (Fe(III)) or by the reduction of iron oxides resulting in the release of ferrous iron (Fe(II)), As(III) and As(V) in the groundwater [49,50]. Further research is warranted to determine the exact mechanism of As release in the groundwater of the study area.

The maximum As concentration in groundwater was higher than the maximum As concentration (96 $\mu g \cdot L^{-1}$) reported by Arain *et al.* [26] and Baig *et al.* [33] (106 $\mu g \cdot L^{-1}$) in Jamshoro (Sindh) groundwater. Nevertheless, this study first time assessed the nature of As species present in the groundwater of Punjab, which could be used to better characterize the risks posed by consuming As-contaminated water in the previously unexplored study area.

Figure 2 demonstrates the mean As concentrations found in this study and the earlier studies in order to compare the extent of groundwater As contamination. Mean As concentrations found in our study were higher than the As concentrations reported previously in Pakistan [30], Indonesia [51] and Vietnam [52], but less than the concentrations documented in Cambodia, Bangladesh and India [23,52].

Table 1. Summary statistics of anions and hydrochemical water quality parameters in groundwater samples collected from three rural areas of Punjab, Pakistan.

Parameter	Chichawatni (CW, $n = 8$)				Vehari (Vh, $n = 28$)				Rahim Yar Khan (RYK, $n = 26$)			
	Mean	Median	Range	S.D (±)	Mean	Median	Range	S.D (±)	Mean	Median	Range	S.D (±)
As ($\mu g \cdot L^{-1}$)	95	90	23–201	60.52	41.5	22.12	1.5–144	45.61	9.2	6	1.66–31	8
pH	6.84	7.4	2.83–7.98	1.65	7.36	7.52	3.01–8.06	0.87	7.6	7.7	6.9–8.35	0.4
EC ($dS \cdot cm^{-1}$)	0.17	0.16	0.14–0.3	0.05	0.1	0.08	0.03–0.5	0.08	0.08	0.06	0.02–0.34	0.07
Ca hardness	168	157	91–277	61	152	145	73–230	45.6	152	90	35–569	130
Mg hardness	148	152	80–188	39	115.5	105	12–260	54	138	109	36–339	93.5
Total hardness	316	330	171–461	91	268	254	85–474	90	291	207	72–908	213
TDS	1.77	1.65	1.44–2.82	0.46	1	0.8	0.3–5	0.83	0.8	0.7	0.23–3.35	0.7
SAR	5.6	7	0.006–9	2.8	2.5	2.2	0.35–6.4	1.3	4.6	2.9	0.7–16	4
CO_3^{2-} ($mg \cdot L^{-1}$)	26.4	26.4	19–36	5.9	25.5	19.2	7.2–108	23.5	33.6	28.8	7.2–85.2	20.2
HCO_3^- ($mg \cdot L^{-1}$)	104.62	75.6	52.5–215	63.7	95	72.59	33–277	63	56.2	50.6	9.8–133	26.8
NO_3^- ($mg \cdot L^{-1}$)	1189	1110.6	632.5–2229	490	1395	1457	0–2365	581	2250.1	2275.3	0–5370	1309.9
SO_4^{2-} ($mg \cdot L^{-1}$)	1002	935.5	751–1447	240.7	277	223.95	0–752	170	261.3	180.2	20.4–1082	252.9
Cl^- ($mg \cdot L^{-1}$)	194	183.5	69–381	100	92	88.75	7–218	50.5	244.2	156.6	39–902	220.2
F ($mg \cdot L^{-1}$)	0	0	0	0	0.004	0	0–0.09	0.02	0.002	0	0–0.045	0.009

As, Arsenic; EC, electrical conductivity; Ca, Calcium; Mg, Magnesium; TDS, Total dissolved solids; SAR, Sodium Adsorption Ratio; CO_3^{2-}, Carbonates; HCO_3^-, Bicarbonates; NO_3^-, Nitrate; SO_4^{2-}, Sulfate; Cl^-, Chloride; F, Fluoride; S.D (±), Standard Deviation.

Table 2. Speciated As contents in selected groundwater samples (n = 13) collected from three rural areas of Punjab, Pakistan.

Sample Name	As(III) (%)	As(V) (%)
CW1	29	71
CW2	40	60
CW3	33	67
CW4	48	52
CW5	46	54
CW8	55	45
Vh21	0	100
Vh22	43	57
Vh28	0	100
Vh34	17	83
RYK42	67	33
RYK55	34	66
RYK56	13	87

CW, Chichawatni; Vh, Vehari; RYK, Rahim Yar Khan; As(III), arsenite; As(V), arsenate.

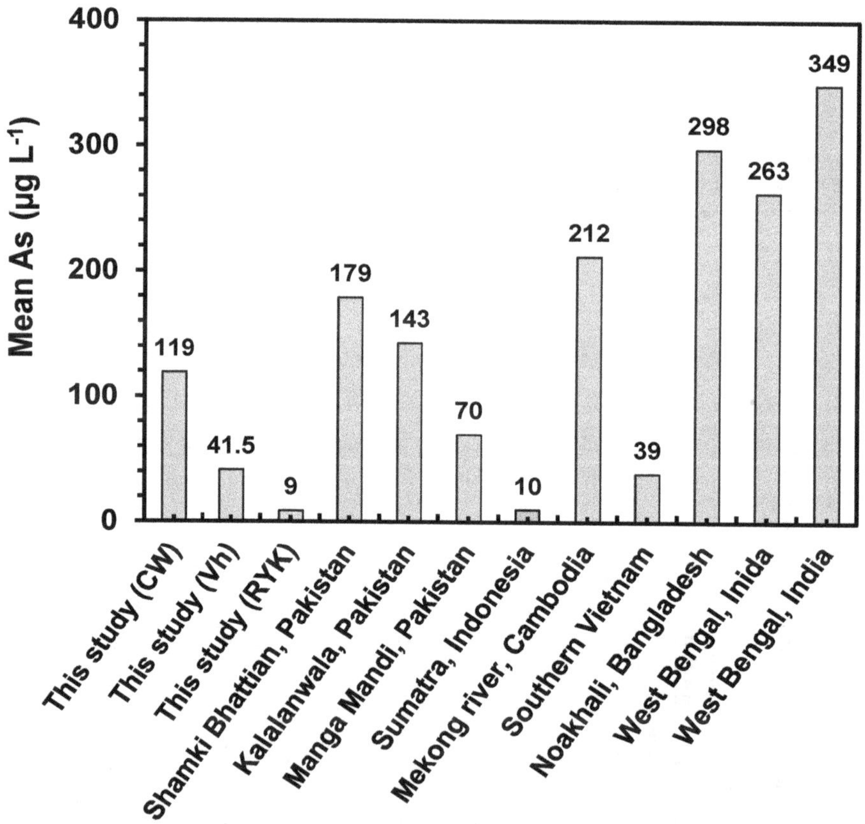

Figure 2. Comparative mean As concentrations ($\mu g \cdot L^{-1}$) in groundwater recorded in this study with other studies conducted in Pakistan (Sultana *et al.* [24]), Indonesia (Wnikle *et al.* [46]), Cambodia (Buschmann *et al.* [47]), Vietnam (Buschmann *et al.* [47]), Bangladesh and India (Rahman *et al.* [18]).

3.2. Groundwater Composition/Chemistry

The pH and EC values of groundwater samples are shown in Table S2, Supplementary Material. The mean values of pH were 7.4, 7.52 and 7.60 in groundwater samples of CW, Vh and RYK, respectively (Table 1). The pH of all the groundwater samples was within the range of permissible limit (6.5–8.5) set by WHO (Supplementary Table S3, Supplementary Material). The data showed that groundwater was slightly alkaline and the dissolved carbonates were predominantly in the form of bicarbonates (HCO_3^-) [53].

In all groundwater samples, EC values ranged from 0.14 to 0.5 $dS{\cdot}cm^{-1}$ (Table 1) in the study area, which were 125-fold higher than the WHO permissible limit (0.004 $dS{\cdot}cm^{-1}$). The maximum EC value (0.5 $dS{\cdot}cm^{-1}$) was found in the water sample from a hand pump in Vh. The excessive level of soluble salts in groundwater of the area could possibly be due to the dissolution of carbonate minerals such as aragonite [$CaCO_3$], calcite [$CaCO_3$], dolomite [$CaMg(CO_3)_2$] and siderite ($FeCO_3$) from indigenous soil and bed rock [54].

Calcium hardness (35–569 $mg{\cdot}L^{-1}$), Mg hardness (12–339 $mg{\cdot}L^{-1}$) and total hardness (72–908 $mg{\cdot}L^{-1}$) as $CaCO_3$ are shown in Table 1. The total hardness values of groundwater samples indicated that groundwater of the study area is very hard water having concentrations >180 $mg{\cdot}L^{-1}$ (*i.e.*, indication value of very hard water) [42] in most of the groundwater samples. Total dissolved solids (TDS) ranged from 0.23 to 3.35 $mg{\cdot}L^{-1}$ (Table 1) and found within the safe limit of WHO (1000 $mg{\cdot}L^{-1}$) [23]. Sodium adsorption ratio (SAR) values of groundwater samples ranged from 0.006 to 16 (Table 1). In most of the groundwater samples of study area, SAR values were greater than its permissible limit [55].

Groundwater concentrations of major cations in the study area are presented in Table 3. The results showed that in the study area, 42%, 4%, 11% and 38% groundwater samples contained higher sodium (Na), calcium (Ca), magnesium (Mg) and potassium (K) levels, respectively, compared to Pak-EPA, WHO and HC safe limits for these elements (Table S3; Supplementary Material). The data regarding major anions is presented in Table 1. Chloride (Cl^-), nitrate (NO_3^-) and sulfate (SO_4^{2-}) concentrations exceeded the Pak-EPA, WHO, US-EPA and HC safe limit (Supplementary Table S3, Supplementary Material) in 20%, 63% and 99% of groundwater samples, respectively, in the study area.

3.3. Trace Elements

Iron was found to be less than the safe limit (0.3 $mg{\cdot}L^{-1}$) set by WHO, US-EPA and HC in most of the groundwater samples of the study area (Table 3; Table S2, Supplementary Material). However, 1 sample in CW, 3 samples in Vh and 5 samples in RYK showed higher concentrations of Fe than WHO, US-EPA and HC permissible limits (Supplementary Material Table S3,). Low Fe concentration in the groundwater samples might be due to the high positive redox potential which indicates the oxidizing conditions thus prohibits Fe dissolution as reported by Farooqi *et al.* [30] and Rasool *et al.* [56] in different areas of east (Lahore) and south (Mailsi) Punjab, Pakistan. Furthermore, presence of high SO_4^{2-} concentration in the groundwater of the study area also supports our earlier argument (oxidized environment).

Lead (Pb) concentration was also higher than the WHO safe limit (Table S4, Supplementary Material) in the groundwater samples of CW (67%), Vh (67%) and RYK (81%) (Table 3).

Groundwater Pb contamination might be the result of leaching from plumbing system and transportation [57]. After ingestion, Pb tends to accumulate in the skeleton, brain, kidneys leading to subencephalopathic, neurological and behavioral disorders [58,59]. Manganese (Mn) concentration ranged from 0.004 to 0.8 $mg \cdot L^{-1}$, however, only six groundwater samples exceeded the previous WHO safe limit (0.4 $mg \cdot L^{-1}$) [23] and three exceeded the current Pak-EPA safe limit (0.5 $mg \cdot L^{-1}$) [60] of Mn in the study area. High levels of Mn can cause intelligence quotient (IQ) and nervous system damage in children. In addition, concentrations of F, Cd, Cu, Cr, Ni, Al, B and Zn (Tables 1 and 2) were found within the safe limit set by Pak-EPA, WHO, US-EPA and HC (Table S3, Supplementary Material) in the groundwater samples of CW, Vh and RYK.

The correlation results of major cations showed significant and positive relationship for Fe–Al ($r = 0.90$, $p < 0.05$), Ca–Mg ($r = 0.80$, $p < 0.05$), Ca–Na ($r = 0.70$, $p < 0.05$) and Na–Mg ($r = 0.72$, $p < 0.05$). This may indicate that these correlated major cations have a common origin of release in the groundwater systems which could be due to geogenic sources from dissolution of their minerals [49].

3.4. *Health Risk Assessment of As Via Drinking Water*

3.4.1. Potential Health Risk Assessment

Residents were interviewed about age, livelihood, literacy rate, health status and drinking water in the study area (data not shown). It was noted that most of the individuals had insufficient income, low literacy rate and lacked access to basic living facilities resulting in poor health conditions. People of the study area cannot afford safe and healthy bottled water, hence, they use hand-pump, electric pump and tube well water as the most common sources of drinking and cooking water. Therefore, these available sources of drinking water in the study area were analyzed for the potential health risk assessment through exposure assessment and risk assessment.

3.4.2. Exposure Assessment and Cancer Risk Assessment

Table 4 demonstrates the health risk assessment of As in terms of ADD, HQ, and CR for the people who were exposed to the intake of As-rich groundwater. In the study area, ADD ranged from 3.6×10^{-5} to 5.6×10^{-3} $mg \cdot kg^{-1} \cdot day^{-1}$. The results indicate that ADD values were comparable to those calculated in Bangladesh (5.00×10^{-2}–5.00×10^{-1} $mg \cdot kg^{-1} \cdot day^{-1}$), Turkey ($2.3 \times 10^{-5}$–$5.21 \times 10^{-3}$ $mg \cdot kg^{-1} \cdot day^{-1}$) and Vietnam ($1.1 \times 10^{-3}$–$4.3 \times 10^{-3}$ $mg \cdot kg^{-1} \cdot day^{-1}$) drinking water [20,22,61]. The ADD values in this study was greater than others reported by Muhammad *et al.* [25] (0–5.56×10^{-7} $mg \cdot kg^{-1} \cdot day^{-1}$) and Farooqi *et al.* [29] (1.1×10^{-4}–3.7×10^{-3} $mg \cdot kg^{-1} \cdot day^{-1}$) in Khyber Pakhtunkhwah and Punjab (Pakistan). In this study As speciation (As(III/V)) data confirms that groundwater is highly contaminated with inorganic As and people are exposed to inorganic As species through intake of drinking water.

The results (Table 4) elaborate that HQ ranged from 0.12 to 18.53 with 75% samples in CW, 61% samples in Vh and 27% samples in RYK exceeded the typical toxic risk index 1.00 [27]. The maximum toxic risk index (HQ = 18.54) was noted in CW. The potential CR values ranged from 5.4×10^{-5} to 8.3×10^{-3} (Table 4) in the area under investigation. In CW the potential CR values ranged from 9×10^{-4} to 8×10^{-3}, in Vh 5.54×10^{-5}–6×10^{-3} and in RYK it was 6.9×10^{-5}–2×10^{-3}.

Table 3. Summary statistics of major cations and trace metals in groundwater samples collected from three rural areas of Punjab, Pakistan.

Parameter	Chichawatni (CW, $n = 8$)				Vehari (Vh, $n = 28$)				Rahim Yar Khan (RYK, $n = 26$)			
	Mean	Median	Range	S.D (±)	Mean	Median	Range	S.D (±)	Mean	Median	Range	S.D (±)
Fe ($mg \cdot L^{-1}$)	0.19	0.14	0.11–0.6	0.15	0.27	0.13	0.1–2	0.42	0.2	0.2	0.01–0.6	0.1
Cr ($mg \cdot L^{-1}$)	0.001	0.0009	0.0003–0.002	0.0004	0.0007	0.0006	0–0.001	0.0003	0.0008	0.001	0.0003–0.002	0.0003
Si ($mg \cdot L^{-1}$)	8.21	8.3	6.4–10	1.1	8.5	8.64	5–10.3	1.2	9	8.8	3.9–17.5	2.8
P ($mg \cdot L^{-1}$)	0.01	0.007	0–0.04	0.02	0.0007	0	0–0.007	0.001	0.006	0	0–0.07	0.01
B ($mg \cdot L^{-1}$)	0.5	0.55	0.13–0.7	0.2	0.2	0.17	0.04–0.5	0.1	0.3	0.2	0.06–1.4	0.3
Al ($mg \cdot L^{-1}$)	0.004	0.001	0.00008–0.02	0.009	0.004	0.0006	0–0.03	0.001	0.0002	0.0001	0–0.001	0.0003
Ca ($mg \cdot L^{-1}$)	67	62.8	36–111	24.4	61	58	29.3–92	18.3	61.1	35.8	14.1–228	51.9
Mg ($mg \cdot L^{-1}$)	36	37	19.5–46	9.5	28	25.5	3–63	13	33.5	26.5	9–82	22.7
Na ($mg \cdot L^{-1}$)	308.5	364	0.3–398	132.5	117.7	110	10.2–271.5	58	246.9	125.9	27–1242	305.8
K ($mg \cdot L^{-1}$)	16.6	14.37	10.5–36	8	16	9	1.51–85.2	20.4	12.8	9.2	3.6–31	8.3
Pb ($mg \cdot L^{-1}$)	0.003	0.002	0.0008–0.006	0.002	0.003	0.002	0.0005–0.01	0.003	0.004	0.002	0.0008–0.02	0.004
Cd ($mg \cdot L^{-1}$)	0.0002	0.0001	0.00002–0.0004	0.0001	0.00005	0.00003	0–0.0002	0.00006	0.0001	0.00004	0–0.0006	0.0001
Cu ($mg \cdot L^{-1}$)	0.01	0.02	0.004–0.04	0.01	0.02	0.009	0.001–0.2	0.04	0.03	0.02	0.002–0.2	0.04
Co ($mg \cdot L^{-1}$)	0.0005	0.0005	0.0002–0.0008	0.0001	0.0006	0.0004	0.0001–0.002	0.0006	0.0004	0.0003	0–0.002	0.0003
Ni ($mg \cdot L^{-1}$)	0.006	0.005	0.002–0.01	0.002	0.005	0.004	0.001–0.009	0.001	0.006	0.006	0.002–0.02	0.004
Zn ($mg \cdot L^{-1}$)	0.2	0.11	0.02–0.4	0.12	0.15	0.05	0.01–2	0.4	0.3	0.2	0.05–1.5	0.3
Mn ($mg \cdot L^{-1}$)	0.22	0.2	0.05–0.5	0.12	0.24	0.24	0.02–0.8	0.2	0.1	0.1	0.004–0.25	0.1
S ($mg \cdot L^{-1}$)	176.5	177.5	106–226	39	53.55	49	6.3–128.3	31	137.4	59	13.7–827	192.1

Fe, Iron; Cr, Chromium; Si, Silicon; P, Phosphorus; B, Boron; Al, Aluminum; Ca, Calcium; Mg, Magnesium; Na, Sodium; K, Potassium; Pb, Lead; Cd, Cadmium; Cu, Copper; Co, Cobalt; Ni, Nickel; Zn, Zinc; Mn, Manganese; S, Sulfur; S.D (±), Standard Deviation.

Table 4. Summary of average daily dose, hazard quotient and carcinogenic risk of As in groundwater samples collected from three rural areas of Punjab, Pakistan.

Parameter		Chichawati (CW, $n = 8$)	Vehari (Vh, $n = 28$)	Rahim Yar Khan (RYK, $n = 26$)
As ($\mu g \cdot L^{-1}$)	Mean	119	41.5	9.2
	Median	118	22.12	6
	Range	23–201	1.33–144	1.66–31
	SD (±)	60.52	45.61	8
Average daily dose ($mg^{-1} \cdot kg^{-1} \cdot day^{-1}$)	Mean	3.3×10^{-3}	1.1×10^{-2}	2.5×10^{-4}
	Median	3×10^{-3}	6.2×10^{-4}	1.6×10^{-4}
	Range	6×10^{-4}–5.6×10^{-3}	3.69×10^{-5}–4×10^{-3}	4.62×10^{-5}–8×10^{-4}
	± S.D	0.0017	0.0013	0.0003
Hazard quotient	Mean	11.01	3.84	0.85
	Median	10.88	2.05	0.55
	Range	2.16–18.58	0.13–13.36	0.15–2.87
	± S.D	5.61	4.23	0.74
Carcinogenic risk	Mean	0.005	0.0017	0.0004
	Median	0.005	0.0009	0.0003
	Range	9×10^{-4}–8.3×10^{-3}	5.54×10^{-5}–6×10^{-3}	6.9×10^{-5}–2×10^{-3}
	± S.D	0.0025	0.002	0.0003

n, No. of samples; As, Arsenic; S.D, Standard Deviation.

The CR values were higher than the US-EPA limit (10^{-6}) suggesting that the people in the study area were at high carcinogenic risk. Therefore, constant monitoring of As level in groundwater is needed in order to assess if any potential health risk from consumption of As-rich water exists, thereby protecting individuals from drinking of As-contaminated water that might be harmful to their health.

3.5. Carcinogenic and Non-Carcinogenic Risks

In this study, a normal distribution was assumed for the cancer slope, and 95% confidence interval (CI) was estimated as the same range provided by US-EPA. Thus, the mean and standard deviation were estimated to be 5×10^{-5} per $\mu g \cdot L^{-1}$ and 1.03×10^{-5} per $\mu g \cdot L^{-1}$, respectively. Considering the variability for the exposure population, the estimated cancer risks for CW, Vh and RYK were 0.6% (95% CI: 0.4%–0.8%), 0.21% (95% CI: 0.13%–0.29%), 0.046% (95% CI: 0.032%–0.062%), respectively. The mean cancer risk was 46–600 times higher than a cancer risk of 10^{-6}, which is the default acceptable level. When plus the uncertainties, the 95% CI for the three regions were estimated to be 0.31%–0.94%, 0.10%–0.34%, 0.025%–0.072%. The estimated risk presented here indicated a very high cancer risk due to the As exposure from groundwater in this region. The standard deviation's ratio between variability and uncertainty was estimated to be 0.80%–0.92%. The HQs were estimated to be 11.36 (95% CI: 7.54–15.14), 3.95 (95% CI: 2.46–5.60) and 0.87 (95% CI: 0.61–1.18) for CW, Vh and RYK, respectively (water consumption of 2 L and body weight of 70 kg were assumed for adult). The HQs in CW and Vh were higher than 1.00, which mean that all the exposures were higher than the reference dose value [48].

Both the US-EPA model and bootstrap method demonstrated that carcinogenic and non-carcinogenic risks were found to be 46–600 and 11–18 times higher than the safe limits of 10^{-6} and 1.00, respectively, in the study area. But bootstrap method showed higher cancer risk values than the US-EPA model.

4. Conclusions

The results showed that 62% groundwater samples collected from various sites of CW, Vh and RYK were unfit for drinking purpose. High values of EC, Cl^-, NO_3^-, SO_4^{2-}, Fe, Mn and Pb were observed in many water samples and thus do not fall under the permissible limits for these parameters. Nevertheless, parameters like CO_3^{2-}, F, Al, B, Cd, Cu, Cr, Ni and Zn were within the safe limit in all samples of study area. High concentration of As was detected in groundwater of study area. Both the US-EPA model and bootstrap method provided high carcinogenic and non-carcinogenic As risks to the individuals of the study area. The ADD and HQ were in the order of CW > Vh > RYK with the maximum HQ value of 18.54 reported in CW. The CR values were significantly (46–600 times) higher than its default acceptable level (10^{-6}), thus exposing people to chronic As carcinogenicity. Higher cancer risk values were obtained by bootstrap method compared to US-EPA model. Our results demonstrated that (53%) groundwater samples contained toxic inorganic species of As(III/V) which are posing serious health risk to the people due to the intake of As-rich groundwater—the only source of drinking water in the study area. Given the health risk associated with extent of groundwater As contamination, government of Pakistan should reduce current (50 $\mu g \cdot L^{-1}$) safe limit of As to 10 $\mu g \cdot L^{-1}$, so that people of Punjab should be protected from mass poisoning of As. Additionally, in the study area future research should be focused on assessing the health risk of As in food and fodder crops that human and animals consume for their daily diet and how As can be transferred from water to crops.

Acknowledgments

The authors are thankful to the Grand Challenges Canada–Stars in Global Health (GCC Grant No. S5 0433-01) and International Foundation for Science (IFS Grant No. W/5698-1) for providing financial support and the University of Agriculture Faisalabad. We acknowledge financial support from the Cooperative Research Centre for Contamination Assessment and Remediation of the Environment (CRC-CARE project 3.1.3.11/12), Australia. Thanks to Zahid Mahmood (Institute of Soil and Environmental Sciences, University of Agriculture Faisalabad) and Naeem Shahid (Department of Environmental Sciences, COMSATS Institute of Information Technology, Vehari) for helping us in groundwater sampling.

Author Contributions

Muhammad Bilal Shakoor, Nabeel Khan Niazi, Irshad Bibi conceived and designed the study; Muhammad Bilal Shakoor performed all the groundwater sampling and analyses; Muhammad Bilal Shakoor prepared the paper; Nabeel Khan Niazi, Irshad Bibi, Muhammad Shahid, Mohammad Mahmudur Rahman, Zhaomin Dong, Ravi Naidu and Muhammad Arshad read and edited the paper; Mohammad Mahmudur Rahman and Ravi Naidu provided analytical facilities.

References

1. IARC. Some drinking-water disinfectants and contaminants, including arsenic. *IARC Monogr. Eval. Carcinog. Risks Hum.* **2004**, *84*, 1–477.
2. Gräfe, M.; Sparks, D.L. Solid phase speciation of arsenic. In *Managing Arsenic in the Environment: From Soil to Human Health*; CSIRO publishing: Victoria, Australia, 2006; Volume 3–31.
3. Smedley, P.; Kinniburgh, D. A review of the source, behaviour and distribution of arsenic in natural waters. *Appl. Geochem.* **2002**, *17*, 517–568.
4. Rahman, M.M.; Ng, J.C.; Naidu, R. Chronic exposure of arsenic via drinking water and its adverse health impacts on humans. *Environ. Geochem. Health* **2009**, *31*, 189–200.
5. Gecol, H.; Ergican, E.; Fuchs, A. Molecular level separation of arsenic (V) from water using cationic surfactant micelles and ultrafiltration membrane. *J. Memb. Sci.* **2004**, *241*, 105–119.
6. Zaw, M.; Emett, M.T. Arsenic removal from water using advanced oxidation processes. *Toxicol. Lett.* **2002**, *133*, 113–118.
7. Niazi, N.K.; Singh, B.; van Zwieten, L.; Kachenko, A.G. Phytoremediation of an arsenic-contaminated site using *Pteris vittata* L. and *Pityrogramma calomelanos* var. austroamericana: A long-term study. *Environ. Sci. Pollut. Res.* **2012**, *19*, 3506–3515.

8. Ravenscroft, P.; Brammer, H.; Richards, K. *Arsenic Pollution: A Global Synthesis*; John Wiley & Sons: Oxford, UK, 2009; Volume 28.
9. Rahman, M.M.; Naidu, R.; Bhattacharya, P. Arsenic contamination in groundwater in the Southeast Asia region. *Environ. Geochem. Health* **2009**, *31*, 9–21.
10. Naidu, R.; Smith, E.; Owens, G.; Bhattacharya, P.; Nadebum, P. Arsenic around the world—An overview. In *Managing Arsenic in the Environment: From Soil to Human Health*; CSIRO publishing: Victoria, Australia, 2006; Volume 3–31.
11. WHO. *Guidelines for Drinking Water Quality*; World Health Organisarion: Geneva, Switzerland, 1996.
12. Nickson, R.; McArthur, J.; Burgess, W.; Ahmed, K.M.; Ravenscroft, P.; Rahman, M. Arsenic poisoning of Bangladesh groundwater. *Nature* **1998**, *395*, 338–338.
13. Niazi, N.K.; Singh, B.; Minasny, B. Mid-infrared spectroscopy and partial least-squares regression to estimate soil arsenic at a highly variable arsenic-contaminated site. *Int. J. Environ. Sci. Technol.* **2015**, *12*, 1965–1974.
14. Chakraborti, D.; Rahman, M.M.; Das, B.; Murrill, M.; Dey, S.; Mukherjee, S.C.; Dhar, R.K.; Biswas, B.K.; Chowdhury, U.K.; Roy, S. Status of groundwater arsenic contamination in Bangladesh: A 14-year study report. *Water Res.* **2010**, *44*, 5789–5802.
15. Chakraborti, D.; Rahman, M.M.; Das, B.; Nayak, B.; Pal, A.; Sengupta, M.K.; Hossain, M.A.; Ahamed, S.; Sahu, M.; Saha, K.C. Groundwater arsenic contamination in Ganga-Meghna-Brahmaputra plain, its health effects and an approach for mitigation. *Environ. Earth Sci.* **2013**, *70*, 1993–2008.
16. Brammer, H.; Ravenscroft, P. Arsenic in groundwater: A threat to sustainable agriculture in South and South-east Asia. *Environ. Int.* **2009**, *35*, 647–654.
17. Sharma, P.; Goel, G.; Ashekuzzaman, S.M.; Saini, G.; Singh, R. Groundwater Arsenic in South-East Asia: Extent, Effects and Solutions. *Asian J. Water Environ. Pollut.* **2014**, *11*, 1–11.
18. Wasserman, G.A.; Liu, X.; Parvez, F.; Ahsan, H.; Factor-Litvak, P.; van Geen, A.; Slavkovich, V.; Lolacono, N.J.; Cheng, Z.; Hussain, I. Water arsenic exposure and children's intellectual function in Araihazar, Bangladesh. *Environ. Health Persp.* **2004**, *112*, 1329–1333.
19. Niazi, N.K.; Bishop, T.F.; Singh, B. Evaluation of spatial variability of soil arsenic adjacent to a disused cattle-dip site, using model-based geostatistics. *Environ. Sci. Technol.* **2011**, *45*, 10463–10470.
20. Caylak, E. Health risk assessment for arsenic in water sources of Cankiri Province of Turkey. *CLEAN-Soil Air Water* **2012**, *40*, 728–734.
21. Kavcar, P.N.; Sofuoglu, A.; Sofuoglu, S.C. A health risk assessment for exposure to trace metals via drinking water ingestion pathway. *Int. J. Hyg. Environ. Health* **2009**, *212*, 216–227.
22. Nguyen, V.A.; Bang, S.; Viet, P.H.; Kim, K.-W. Contamination of groundwater and risk assessment for arsenic exposure in Ha Nam province, Vietnam. *Environ. Int.* **2009**, *35*, 466–472.
23. Rahman, M.M.; Dong, Z.; Naidu, R. Concentrations of arsenic and other elements in groundwater of Bangladesh and West Bengal, India: Potential cancer risk. *Chemosphere* **2015**, *139*, 54–64.
24. USEPA. *Guidelines for Carcinogen Risk Assessment*; EPA/630/P-03/001F; Risk Assessment Forum: Washington, DC, USA, 2005.
25. Muhammad, S.; Shah, M.T.; Khan, S. Arsenic health risk assessment in drinking water and source apportionment using multivariate statistical techniques in Kohistan region, northern Pakistan. *Food Chem. Toxicol.* **2010**, *48*, 2855–2864.

26. Arain, M.B.; Kazi, T.G.; Baig, J.A.; Jamali, M.K.; Afridi, H.I.; Shah, A.Q.; Jalbani, N.; Sarfraz, R.A. Determination of arsenic levels in lake water, sediment, and foodstuff from selected area of Sindh, Pakistan: Estimation of daily dietary intake. *Food Chem. Toxicol.* **2009**, *47*, 242–248.
27. Sultana, J.; Farooqi, A.; Ali, U. Arsenic concentration variability, health risk assessment, and source identification using multivariate analysis in selected villages of public water system, Lahore, Pakistan. *Environ. Monit. Asess.* **2014**, *186*, 1241–1251.
28. Nickson, R.T.; McArthur, J.M.; Shrestha, B.; Kyaw-Myint, T.O.; Lowry, D. Arsenic and other drinking water quality issues, Muzaffargarh District, Pakistan. *Appl. Geochem.* **2005**, *20*, 55–68.
29. Farooqi, A.; Masuda, H.; Firdous, N. Toxic fluoride and arsenic contaminated groundwater in the Lahore and Kasur districts, Punjab, Pakistan and possible contaminant sources. *Environ. Pollut.* **2007**, *145*, 839–849.
30. Farooqi, A.; Masuda, H.; Kusakabe, M.; Naseem, M.; Firdous, N. Distribution of highly arsenic and fluoride contaminated groundwater from east Punjab, Pakistan, and the controlling role of anthropogenic pollutants in the natural hydrological cycle. *Geochem. J.* **2007**, *41*, 213–234.
31. Farooqi, A.; Masuda, H.; Siddiqui, R.; Naseem, M. Sources of arsenic and fluoride in highly contaminated soils causing groundwater contamination in Punjab, Pakistan. *Arch. Environ. Cont. Toxicol.* **2009**, *56*, 693–706.
32. Sadun, A.A. Mitochondrial optic neuropathies. *J. Neurol. Neurosurg. Psychiatry* **2002**, *72*, 423–425.
33. Baig, J.A.; Kazi, T.G.; Arain, M.B.; Afridi, H.I.; Kandhro, G.A.; Sarfraz, R.A.; Jamal, M.K.; Shah, A.Q. Evaluation of arsenic and other physico-chemical parameters of surface and ground water of Jamshoro, Pakistan. *J. Haz. Mat.* **2009**, *166*, 662–669.
34. Kumar, P.J.S.; James, E.J. Physicochemical parameters and their sources in groundwater in the Thirupathur region, Tamil Nadu, South India. *Appl. Water Sci.* **2013**, *3*, 219–228.
35. Brahman, K.D.; Kazi, T.G.; Afridi, H.I.; Naseem, S.; Arain, S.S.; Ullah, N. Evaluation of high levels of fluoride, arsenic species and other physicochemical parameters in underground water of two sub districts of Tharparkar, Pakistan: A multivariate study. *Water Res.* **2013**, *47*, 1005–1020.
36. Basharat, M. Spatial and Temporal Appraisal of Groundwater Depth and Quality in LBDC Command-Issues and Options. *Pak. J. Engg. Appl. Sci.* **2012**, *11*, 14–29.
37. Pakistan-Punjab Municipal Service Improvement Project: Resettlement Action Plan. Available online: http://documents.shihang.org/curated/zh/2010/03/14102002/pakistan-punjab-municipal-services-improvement-project-resettlement-action-plan (accessed on 5 June 2015).
38. Khan, F.M. Participatory appraisal and scanning surveillance based contagious diseases risk profile of district Rahim Yar Khan (Pakistan). *Pak. Vet. J.* **2010**, *30*, 198–202.
39. Khan, S.; Shahnaz, M.; Jehan, N.; Rehman, S.; Shah, M.T.; Din, I. Drinking water quality and human health risk in Charsadda district, Pakistan. *J. Clean. Prod.* **2013**, *60*, 93–101.
40. Bednar, A.J.; Garbarino, J.R.; Ranville, J.F.; Wildeman, T.R. Preserving the distribution of inorganic arsenic species in groundwater and acid mine drainage samples. *Environ. Sci. Technol.* **2002**, *36*, 2213–2218.
41. Reitemeier, R. Semimicroanalysis of saline soil solutions. *Indust. Eng. Chem. Analyt. Ed.* **1943**, *15*, 393–402.
42. Spellman, F.R. *Handbook of Water and Wastewater Treatment Plant Operations*; CRC Press: New York, NY, USA, 2013.

43. Brahman, K.D.; Kazi, T.G.; Baig, J.A.; Afridi, H.I.; Khan, A.; Arain, S.S.; Arain, M.B. Fluoride and arsenic exposure through water and grain crops in Nagarparkar, Pakistan. *Chemosphere* **2014**, *100*, 182–189.
44. Kazi, T.G.; Arain, M.B.; Baig, J.A.; Jamali, M.K.; Afridi, H.I.; Jalbani, N.; Sarfraz, R.A.; Shah, A.Q.; Niaz, A. The correlation of arsenic levels in drinking water with the biological samples of skin disorders. *Sci. Total Environ.* **2009**, *407*, 1019–1026.
45. Rahman, M.; Asaduzzaman, M.; Naidu, R. Arsenic Exposure from Rice and Water Sources in the Noakhali District of Bangladesh. *Water Qual. Expo. Health* **2011**, *3*, 1–10.
46. Mondal, D.; Banerjee, M.; Kundu, M.; Banerjee, N.; Bhattacharya, U.; Giri, A.K.; Ganguli, B.; Roy, S.S.; Polya, D.A. Comparison of drinking water, raw rice and cooking of rice as arsenic exposure routes in three contrasting areas of West Bengal, India. *Environ. Geochem. Health* **2010**, *32*, 463–477.
47. USEPA Arsenic, inorganic. United States Environmental Protection Agency, Integrated Risk Information System (IRIS), (CASRN 7440-38-2). 1998. Available online: http://www.epa.gov/iris/subst/0278.htm (accessed on 12 February 2015).
48. IRIS. Arsenic, Integrated Risk Information System. U.S. Environmental Protection Agency: Washington, DC, USA, 2007. Available online: http://www.epa.gov/iris/subst/index.html (accessed on 12 February 2015).
49. Basu, A.; Saha, D.; Saha, R.; Ghosh, T.; Saha, B. A review on sources, toxicity and remediation technologies for removing arsenic from drinking water. *Res. Chem. Intermed.* **2014**, *40*, 447–485.
50. Mahimairaja, S.; Bolan, N.S.; Adriano, D.; Robinson, B. Arsenic contamination and its risk management in complex environmental settings. *Adv. Aron.* **2005**, *86*, 1–82.
51. Winkel, L.; Berg, M.; Stengel, C.; Rosenberg, T. Hydrogeological survey assessing arsenic and other groundwater contaminants in the lowlands of Sumatra, Indonesia. *Appl. Geochem.* **2008**, *23*, 3019–3028.
52. Buschmann, J.; Berg, M.; Stengel, C.; Sampson, M.L. Arsenic and manganese contamination of drinking water resources in Cambodia: Coincidence of risk areas with low relief topography. *Environ. Sci. Technol.* **2007**, *41*, 2146–2152.
53. Adams, S.; Titus, R.; Pietersen, K.; Tredoux, G.; Harris, C. Hydrochemical characteristics of aquifers near Sutherland in the Western Karoo, South Africa. *J. Hydrol.* **2001**, *241*, 91–103.
54. Schettler, G.; Oberhansli, H.; Stulina, G.; Mavlonov, A.A.; Naumann, R. Hydrochemical water evolution in the Aral Sea Basin. Part I: Unconfined groundwater of the Amu Darya Delta—Interactions with surface waters. *J. Hydrol.* **2013**, *495*, 267–284.
55. Ayers, R.S.; Westcot, D.W. *Water Quality for Agriculture*; FAO: Rome, Italy, 1985; Volume 29.
56. Rasool, A.; Farooqi, A.; Masood, S.; Hussain, K. Arsenic in groundwater and its health risk assessment in drinking water of Mailsi, Punjab, Pakistan. *Hum. Ecol. Risk Assess Int. J.* **2015**, doi:10.1080/10807039.2015.1056295
57. Tuakuila, J.; Lison, D.; Mbuyi, F.; Haufroid, V.; Hoet, P. Elevated blood lead levels and sources of exposure in the population of Kinshasa, the capital of the Democratic Republic of Congo. *J. Expo. Sci. Environ.* **2013**, *23*, 81–87.
58. Taylor, M.P.; Winder, C.; Lanphear, B.P. Australia's leading public health body delays action on the revision of the public health goal for blood lead exposures. *Environ. Int.* **2014**, *70*, 113–117.

59. Public Education and Supplemental Monitoring Requirements. Available online: https://www.law.cornell.edu/cfr/text/40/141.85. (accessed on 18 April 2015).
60. PAK-EPA. *National Standards for Drinking Water Quality (NSDWG)*; Pakistan Environmental Protection Agency (PAK-EPA); Ministry of Environment: Government of Pakistan, Islamabad, Pakistan, 2008.
61. Karim, M.D.M. Arsenic in groundwater and health problems in Bangladesh. *Water Res.* **2000**, *34*, 304–310.

2

Developing Medical Geology in Uruguay

Nelly Mañay

Toxicology & Environmental Hygiene Department, Faculty of Chemistry, University of the Republic of Uruguay, Gral, Flores 2124, 11800 Montevideo, Uruguay; E-Mail: nmanay@fq.edu.uy;

Abstract: Several disciplines like Environmental Toxicology, Epidemiology, Public Health and Geology have been the basis of the development of Medical Geology in Uruguay during the last decade. The knowledge and performance in environmental and health issues have been improved by joining similar aims research teams and experts from different institutions to face environmental problems dealing with the population's exposure to metals and metalloids and their health impacts. Some of the Uruguayan Medical Geology examples are reviewed focusing on their multidisciplinary approach: Lead pollution and exposed children, selenium in critically ill patients, copper deficiency in cattle and arsenic risk assessment in ground water. Future actions are also presented.

Keywords: Uruguay; medical geology; lead; arsenic; selenium; copper

---

1. Introduction

The emerging discipline of Medical Geology has been developed in Uruguay during the last decade linking Environmental Toxicology, Epidemiology, and Human and Veterinary health with Geology and Analytical studies, which have all contributed to scientific research in this field in Uruguay. The knowledge and application of these disciplines have been improved by joining research teams and experts from different institutions with community delegates to face environmental health problems arising from metal and metalloid exposure. Medical Geology has also been a matter of discussion in ecohealth symposiums to understand the relationships among ecosystems and human health impacts providing additional sociological studies.

The toxicology research team at the Faculty of Chemistry in Uruguay has been involved in this emerging discipline since 2002, studying metal and metalloid exposure and their environmental health impacts within the Medical Geology International group (IGCP project # 454) and the International Medical Geology Association (IMGA), created in 2005 [1] . Several contributions have been presented in scientific events, which were carried out locally and regionally, strengthening the integration of the biosciences, public health and geosciences with local communities and facilitating research and training opportunities among them.

2. Objectives

We present a review of these experiences in Uruguay, focusing on the development of a multidisciplinary and transdisciplinary approach. Available data concerning lead pollution as well as other research issues with regards to metals and metalloids like selenium, copper and arsenic are reviewed. We describe the Medical Geology field in Uruguay with some examples such as environmental lead exposure in children and selenium and copper deficiency in human and cattle populations and their related factors, in addition to recent studies on distribution, mobility and exposure to arsenic from ground water. These examples are described as follows:

Lead pollution

The lead contamination in Uruguay, as in other countries in the region, is mainly due to its industrial sources (metallurgies, manufacture and recycling of batteries, foundries *etc*.). Generally, non-occupational lead exposure is caused by living in manufacturing areas or by the improper handling of lead-containing materials and solid waste, which poses an important health risk, with children being the most affected population [2]. Lead and other heavy metal exposure in Uruguayan populations has been studied at the Faculty of Chemistry for a long time with QA/QC analytical results [3]. Those scientific research publications turned out to be the only background data available for the whole country from when lead pollution first received official attention in 2001 [4-6], when the "La Teja neighborhood case" arose.

The first instance was a child from La Teja who showed blood lead levels (BLL) higher than 20 ug/dL, after which, several other cases of even higher values appeared in that neighborhood, as well as in other areas of Montevideo and throughout the whole country. The worst situation was in the slum settlements of La Teja, where the ground showed more than 3,000 ppm of lead in the soil due to scrap land fillings. This was later found in those areas because, foundries and metallurgical manufacturing industries had settled down during the last century, but most of them were no longer active due mainly to economic reasons, leaving their solid waste behind [5].

The community affected by lead contamination began a broad mobilization demanding solutions from the health and environmental authorities. As a response, the Health Ministry established an interinstitutional and multidisciplinary committee, including delegates from health, environmental, labor, educational, and social security institutions and community NGOs, among others. The University of the Republic was the main institution responsible for technical advice and support.

Lead pollution in Uruguay was then considered a Medical Geology issue, which highlighted the importance of the multidisciplinary, transdisciplinary and interinstitutional approach to provide solutions for the management of the health risks faced by thousands of affected children who were exposed to lead mainly due to the contaminated soil.

As a consequence of this approach, blood lead screening programs and lead protocols were implemented for Uruguayan children, specialized children health care centers were created and most blood lead levels determinations for health controls were confirmed at the Faculty of Chemistry. Moreover, many laws were approved, as well as several research projects which were being carried out [6].

The severity of the discovered lead pollution required official governmental actions, in order to reduce sources of lead contamination as well as to assess health impact on children who had been exposed to environmental or industrial lead pollution.

As those actions to reduce public exposure to lead, became consistent, lead studies performed by the toxicology team at the Faculty of Chemistry were reviewed to compare BLLs changes in Uruguayan populations, after the leaded gasoline was phased out in 2003 [7]. This report included comparisons of similar populations (children, exposed and unexposed adults, and lead workers) that were sampled within a 10-yr period. BLL determinations were all performed using atomic spectrometry at the Faculty of Chemistry using appropriate quality controls. The studies reviewed by the report, which were carried out in 2004, involved the sampling of children (n = 180), nonoccupationally exposed adults (n = 714), and lead workers (n = 81). A framework was established to correlate BLL with variables such as age, sex, area of residence, available environmental lead data, and possible lead exposure sources. To assess the change in risk, analytical results were statistically compared with similar screening studies results that were performed in 1994 by the same team.

Children in 1994 showed a positive relationship between BLL and traffic intensity, and 40% of their BLL exceeded 10 ug/dL, while in 2004, only 7% were above that intervention level. Results showed significantly lower BLL levels in children (5.7 ug/dL) and non occupationally exposed adults (5.5 ug/dL) than similar populations sampled in 1994 (9.9 ug/dL and 9.1 ug/dL, respectively). However, workers occupationally exposed to lead did not show significant BLL differences between 1994 and 2004, and their mean BLL values were still high (49.0 Pb ug/dL *vs.* 42.0 Pb ug/dL, respectively). In order to improve this, new laws have also been approved to address lead occupational exposure which required BLL assessment to be periodically monitored as part of the workers health certificate protocol.

It was shown that significant improvements in preventing nonoccupational lead exposure have been made and that this outcome can presumably be attributed to the phase-out of leaded gasoline and to improvements in nutrition, hygiene, and related habits for children as well as a favorable response to the official multidisciplinary actions. These changes suggest that the contribution of environmental lead to the overall exposure of children and non occupationally exposed adults in Uruguay is decreasing.

Recent studies have also demonstrated that there has been a significant change in preventing lead exposure due to the public's sensitization, along with the integration of multidisciplinary actions promoted. As a conclusion, the problem of lead contamination in Uruguay has been considered an important and unique experience in Medical Geology development [6,7].

Selenium deficiency and SIRS/MOD

A research study [8] was carried out by a multidisciplinary Medical Geology team including physicians, bioinorganic chemists and analytical toxicologists regarding Uruguayan serum selenium (Se) levels and glutathione peroxidase (GPx) activity in relation to oxidative stress such as systemic inflammatory response syndrome (SIRS) and multiple organ dysfunction (MOD).

Selenium status was evaluated in critically ill Uruguayan patients with and without SIRS in comparison with healthy subjects. Serum Se levels and GPx activity were measured in healthy subjects and patients without SIRS, with SIRS and with SIRS-MOD, who had been admitted to the Intensive Care Unit (ICU) in the Hospital de Clinicas of Montevideo. GPx activity was determined by an indirect method based on the oxidation of glutathione (GSH) to oxidized glutathione (GSSG), catalyzed by GPx, which was then coupled to the recycling of GSSG to GSH using glutathione reductase and NADPH. Se in serum was analyzed by graphite furnace atomic absorption spectrometry in our lab.

The results were expressed in mean values. As a preliminary conclusion, average Se levels in Uruguay (79 ug/L) seemed to be lower than in other populations, and these results have been confirmed by further research. SIRS is associated with Se depletion. For this reason, early Se supplementation could improve the results and prognosis in critically ill patients with SIRS [9].

Copper deficiency in cattle

With regards to bovine health and geology, serum copper levels were studied in dairy cattle in eight locations throughout the Department of Salto, in Uruguay using a geomedical approach. The overall incidence of hypocupraemia was in 30%, which was not homogeneously distributed since some farms were almost exempt from hypocupraemical individuals. One of the developed copper complexes like Cu(Phe)2 proved to be the best at improving Cu status and its efficacy was further tested in a hypocupraemic herd, showing that the treated cattle maintained the serum copper level at an adequate level for at least 100 days. At the same time, analyses of copper, molybdenum, sulphur and phosphorous levels in grass were conducted throughout the year. The results showed that the copper content in grass was under adequate levels for most of the year, and the deficiency was more critical in autumn. Although the molybdenum and sulphur levels were low enough not to expect them to interfere with copper absorption, the Mo content may have been enhancing the copper deficiency [10].

Arsenic in ground water

A thesis project and a multidisciplinary project have been carried out by environmental geologists and chemical toxicologists to look for Arsenic and other toxic metals in groundwater from the Raigon Aquifer in southwest Uruguay [11]. The groundwater quality has been the target of multiple studies in Uruguay. In particular, the Raigón Aquifer is of special interest because of its importance as a hydro-resource in the southern zone of Uruguay and for being responsible for a great part of the dairy farm water supply. Thus, little attention has been paid to the presence of toxic elements in the water. Preliminary research work done by this team has determined that arsenic levels were higher than

0.01 mg/L in water samples from this aquifer. This issue leads to the supposition that the population, as well as industrial and agricultural activities, could be consuming water with arsenic concentrations over the international maximum recommended limits of 0.01 mg/L. As it is fully described, these arsenic water levels may contribute to health problems over a long-term exposure [12]. The sampling campaign was done in fall 2007 and almost a hundred wells, with lithological profile available, were sampled with standard protocols, as representative of the aquifer.

The analysis were performed by ICP-MS and the results showed 80% samples with arsenic levels exceeding 0,01 mg/L ranging from 0,001 mg/L to an arsenic maximum concentration of 0.03 mg/L [13]. Therefore, this project is facing a typical interactive problem between geology and health (Medical Geology) and it requires a systematic evaluation of the toxicological interest, geological materials (chemical laboratory analyses) and the risks to the exposed population (human and animal ones) to characterize the water supply in connection with its toxic metal and metalloids contents. This research contributed to the assessment of exposure risks to human and animal populations, and eventually to the management and/or specific treatment of these resources to prevent long-term epidemiological problems.

In addition, since 2006, this arsenic Uruguayan working team, has been taking part in an Iberoamerican network project [14] regarding arsenic distribution, analytical methodologies development and remediation, and it is now developing feasible analytical methodologies for arsenic speciation.

Training Courses and Future actions

Medical Geology is delivered as a curricular course to undergraduate students in the Faculty of Chemistry and updating training courses on Medical Geology have been carried out in Uruguay periodically since 2005 by one or all of the leaders, Drs Centeno, Finkelman and Selinus, to professionals, postgraduate students, bio scientists and geoscientists.

Future actions have also been planned to continue developing Medical Geology in this country. Uruguay hosted the 3rd Hemispherical Conference held in Montevideo, to promote interdisciplinary discussions and contributions from the geosciences and biosciences scientific communities to share the recent advances on environmental and health problems in this part of the world [15] and a project on a expert diploma with a similar program to those offered in other Universities, will be submitted to the University of the Republic's authorities for consideration in the near future.

3. Final Considerations

In this presentation we updated the experience of Medical Geology in Uruguay, including some research studies that are being carried out. We emphasized the importance of the integration of the different University activities with the social and political actions for the management of all of these environmental health risk situations.

The main results of this new scientific approach in Uruguay are the development of feasible technologies, diagnosis tools, health impairment, and social inclusion. We conclude that Medical

Geology is a growing field with multiple applications to solve local and regional health issues in Uruguay.

References

1. International Medical Geology Association (IMGA). Available online: http://www.medicalgeology.org/ (accessed on 28 September 2009).
2. Cousillas A.; Mañay N.; Pereira L.; Alvarez C.; Coppes Z. Evaluation of Lead Exposure in Uruguayan children. *Bull. Environ. Contam. Toxicol.* **2005**, *75*, 629-636.
3. Mañay N.; Pereira L.; Cousillas Z. Lead Contamination in Uruguay. *Rev. Environ. Contam. Toxicol.* **1999**, *159*, 25-39.
4. Mañay, N. La Contaminación por Plomo y su Repercusión Sobre la Salud en Uruguay: Antecedentes y Situación Actual. *Rev. Asoc. Quím. Farm. Uruguay (2ª. Epoca)* **2001**, *31*, 3-8.
5. Mañay, N.; Alonso, C.; Dol, I. Contaminación por plomo en el barrio La Teja, Montevideo-Uruguay. In Suplemento de 2003 "Experiencia Latinoamericana". *Salud Publ. Méx.* **2003**, *45*, 268-275.
6. Mañay, N.; Cousillas, A.Z.; Alvarez, C.; Heller, T. Lead Contamination in Uruguay: The "La Teja" Neighborhood Case. *Rev. Environ. Contam. Toxicol* **2008**, *195*, 93.
7. Manay, N.; Alvarez, C.; Cousillas, A.; Pereira, L.; Baranano, R.; Heller, T. Changes in Blood Lead Levels in Uruguayan Populations. *Met. Ions Biol. Med.* **2006**, *9*, 530-534.
8. Manzanares, W.; Torre, M.H.; Biestro, A.; Pittini, G.; Mañay, N.; Fracchin, G.; Rampoldi, O. Serum Selenium and Glutathione Peroxidase activity in critically ill patients with Systemic Inflammatory Response and Multiple Organ Dysfunction Syndroems: Preliminary data. *Met. Ions Biol. Med.* **2006**, *9*, 535-539.
9. Manzanarez, W.; Biestro, A.; Torre, M.; Pittini, G.; Facchin, G.; Mañay, N. Hardi, G. Serum selenium and glutathione peroxidase-3 activity: biomarkers of systemic inflammation in the critically ill? *Intensive Care Med.* **2009**, *35*, 882-889.
10. Torre, M.; Viera, I.; Facchin, G.; Kremer, E.; Baran, E.; Porochin, T.; DiDinato, V.; Irigoyen, C.; Saldaña, S.; Bussi, J.; Onhanian, M.; Fuentes, J. Incidence of hypocupraemia in cattle in northern Uruguay and its alleviation with an injected Cu–Phenylalanine complex. *Livestock Prod. Sci.* **2005**, *95*, 49-56.
11. *Environmental Health Criteria 224: Arsenic and Arsenic Compounds. International Programme on Chemical Safety II. WHO Task Group on Environmental Health Criteria for Arsenic and Arsenic Compounds III Series*, 2nd ed.; WHO: Geneva, Switzerland, 2001; p. 114.
12. Guérèquiz, A.R.; Mañay, N.; Goso, C.; Bundschuh. J. Assesment of the environmental risk caused by the presence of arsenic in the western area of the Raigon aquifer, department of San Jose, Uruguay. Project presentation. In *Workshop of as in Ibero-América, Abstract Book*; Available online: http://www.cnea.gov.ar/xxi/ambiental/Iberoarsen/docs/libroresumenes-taller-2006.pdf (accessed on 28 September 2009).

13. Guerequiz, R.; Mañay, N.; Goso, C.; Fernandez, J.; Garcia, M. Environmental Risk Assessment of Arsenic in the Raigon Aquifer, Uruguay: Research Advancements. PA23 In *II International Congress: Arsenic in the Environment: From Nature to Humans*, Valencia, Spain, 2008; Available online: http://www.adeit.uv.es/As2008valencia/ (accessed on 28 September 2009).
14. Litter, M.; Red Temática 406RT0282 CYTED. *El Arsénico en Iberoamérica. Distribución, Metodologías Analíticas y Tecnologías de Remoción*, 2006; Available online: http://www.cnea.gov.ar/xxi/ambiental/Iberoarsen/english/participantes.asp (accessed on 28 September 2009).
15. 3rd Conference on Medical Geology, 12–16 October 2009, Montevideo: Uruguay. Available online: www.geologiamedica.com (accessed on 28 September 2009).

3

The Legacy of Uranium Development on or Near Indian Reservations and Health Implications Rekindling Public Awareness

Anita Moore-Nall

Department of Earth Sciences, Montana State University, P.O. Box 173480, Bozeman, MT 59717, USA; E-Mail: amoorenall@yahoo.com or anita.moorenall@msu.montana.edu

Academic Editors: Jose A. Centeno, Robert B. Finkelman and Olle Selinus

---

Abstract: Uranium occurrence and development has left a legacy of long-lived health effects for many Native Americans and Alaska Natives in the United States. Some Native American communities have been impacted by processing and development while others are living with naturally occurring sources of uranium. The uranium production peak spanned from approximately 1948 to the 1980s. Thousands of mines, mainly on the Colorado Plateau, were developed in the western U.S. during the uranium boom. Many of these mines were abandoned and have not been reclaimed. Native Americans in the Colorado Plateau area including the Navajo, Southern Ute, Ute Mountain, Hopi, Zuni, Laguna, Acoma, and several other Pueblo nations, with their intimate knowledge of the land, often led miners to uranium resources during this exploration boom. As a result of the mining activity many Indian Nations residing near areas of mining or milling have had and continue to have their health compromised. This short review aims to rekindle the public awareness of the plight of Native American communities living with the legacy of uranium procurement, including mining, milling, down winders, nuclear weapon development and long term nuclear waste storage.

Keywords: uranium; Native Americans; community based participatory research; abandoned mines; reservations

---

1. Introduction

Native American communities on American Indian reservations located with natural resources on or near their lands may be at a greater risk for environmentally induced ailments [1]. The impact of natural resource development has not always been fully recognized with respect to the cultural and health effects of the people and animals of these lands. Sometimes the effects are not realized until after the fact when problems associated with resource extraction or cleanup may already be impacting the health of the population [2–8]. On some reservations a lack of education and knowledge about the effects of geologic materials such as uranium and coal led to long term health problems when resources were developed [7]. In this short review the effects of uranium procurement will be addressed, though many other factors may also be contributing to poor health of the Native American populations with natural resources on or near their lands.

Technologically-enhanced, naturally-occurring radioactive material (TENORM) is produced when activities such as uranium mining or milling concentrate or expose radioactive materials that occur naturally in ores, soils, water, or other natural materials [9]. Radioactive materials can be classified under two broad headings: man-made and naturally occurring radioactive materials (NORM). Both of these materials affect many Americans but especially the Native American populations in the United States and Canada, whose designated lands host uranium deposits. Mining of uranium by underground and surface methods produces bulk waste material, including tailings and overburden. During mining the waste rock and soil have little or no practical use, they are generally stored on land near the mine site [10,11]. These materials contain NORM which may become dispersed in the environment through airborne dust and contaminated water. Continued exposure to these materials can cause severe health problems [10,12]. Abandoned conventional uranium mines often contain other hazardous contaminants, such as metals. For example, the carcinogen arsenic may be a problem at some uranium mines, contributing to increased health risks [11].

1.1. The Quest for Uranium

The origin of the Department of Energy is traced to World War II and the Manhattan Project effort to build the first atomic bomb [13]. The "Manhattan Project" was conducted mainly at the Los Alamos National Scientific Laboratory, a huge fortified compound created in 1943 [14] on the Pajarito Plateau, northwest of Santa Fe, New Mexico, on land supposedly reserved for the exclusive use and occupancy of the San Ildefonso Pueblo [15]. Uranium, the key material used in the lab's experiments and eventual fabrication of prototype nuclear weapons, was mined and milled in four centers of the nearby Navajo Reservation [6,9,16] including reservation land near Shiprock, New Mexico; Monument Valley, Utah; Church Rock, New Mexico; and Kayenta, Arizona. Hanford, a uranium enrichment/plutonium manufacturing facility, was added in 1943, near the town of Richland, on Yakima land in eastern Washington [16,17]. The Hanford area bordering the Columbia River was home to several tribes of Native Americans for centuries. Remnants, artifacts, and burial sites associated with historical Native American activity are found throughout the Site and are protected by law [16]. On 16 July 1945, the world's first atomic bomb was detonated 200 miles south of Los Alamos at Trinity Site on the Alamogordo bombing range [13,14], now the White Sands Test Range, adjoining the Mescalero Apache Reservation. It is this quest for uranium and these different aspects of the procurement plus the disposal and storage of waste that continues to contribute to poor health among many Native American populations. Many cancer clusters and other ailments are attributed to this quest.

1.2. Uranium Production on Native American Lands

The uranium production peak spanned from approximately 1948 to the early 1980s primarily to produce uranium for weapons and later for nuclear fuel [9,10]. Thousands of mines, mainly on the Colorado Plateau, were developed in the western U.S. during the uranium boom. Native Americans in the area including the Navajo, Southern Ute, Ute Mountain, Hopi, Zuni, Laguna, Acoma, and several other Pueblo nations, with their intimate knowledge of the land often led miners to uranium resources during this exploration boom [5,8]. There are about 4000 uranium mines with documented production [10]. With information provided by other federal, state, and tribal agencies, the Environmental Protection Agency (EPA) has identified 15,000 abandoned uranium mine locations with uranium occurrence in 14 western states with about 75% of those on federal and tribal lands [10]. The majority of these sites were conventional (open pit and underground) mines [10]. Between 1950 and 1989 surface and underground mines in the U.S. produced more than 225 million tons of uranium ore [8]. Figure 1 shows the abandoned uranium mines in the western United States.

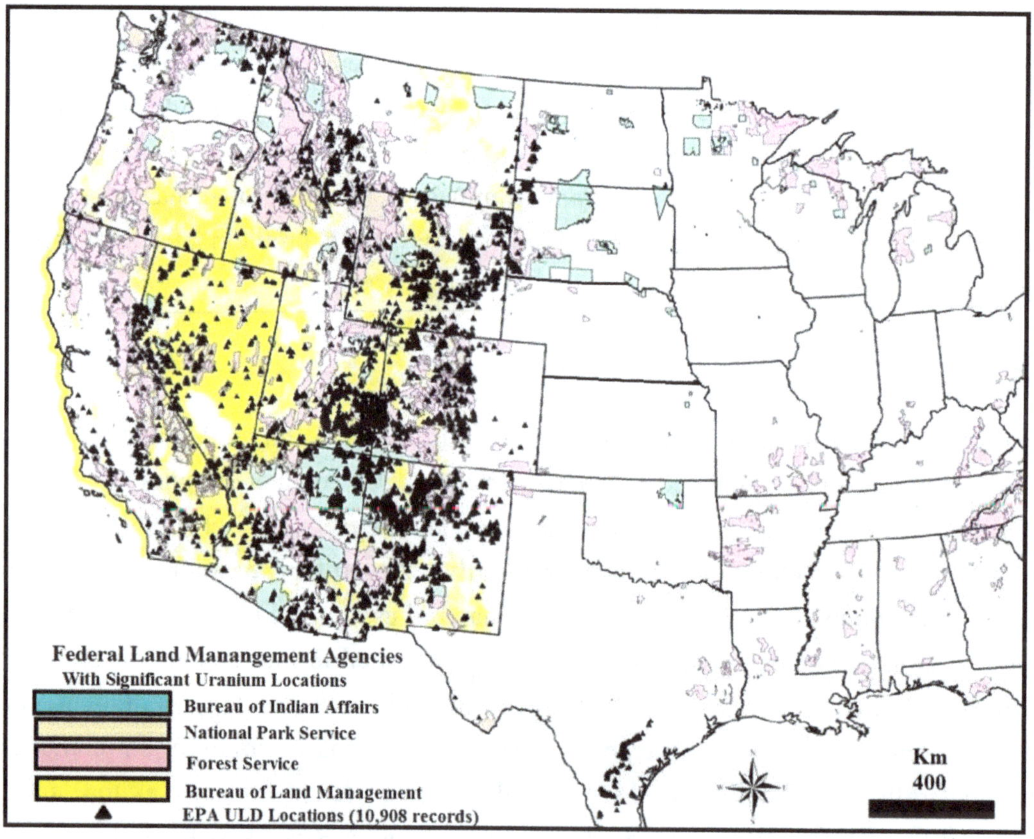

Figure 1. Uranium locations from Environmental Protection Agency (EPA) database and Federal Lands. The green federal lands are Native American reservations. About three-fourths of the uranium locations in the EPA Uranium Location Database are on Federal Lands. Figure is modified from Geographic Analysis on the Location of Uranium Mines [9].

1.2.1. The Navajo Nation

The Navajo Nation was one of the Indian nations heavily affected by this activity with more than a thousand mines and four uranium mills on the reservation lands [5,6,8]. When mining came to the reservation the Navajo men were ready to gain employment and the close work seemed ideal. What they didn't realize was that they were being exposed to radiation when they worked and brought it home with them in their clothing to their families [6]. Energy material may contain harmful chemical substances that, if mobilized into air, water, or soil, can adversely impact human health and environmental quality [18]. As a result of the mining activity much of the population of the Navajo Nation residing near the areas of mining or milling has had their health compromised. Many of the miners developed cancers; some were lung cancer from inhalation of radioactive particles, *i.e.*, exposure to radon [6]. Of the 150 Navajo uranium miners who worked at the uranium mine in Shiprock, New Mexico until 1970, 133 died of lung cancer or various forms of fibrosis by 1980 [19]. Other potential health effects include bone cancer and impaired kidney function from exposure to radionuclides in drinking water [12]. The government and the mining companies failed to inform the people of the Navajo Nation that working with uranium might be hazardous to one's health [2–8]. The Public health Service even conducted a study to document the development of illnesses as the mining progressed without consent or presenting the data to the miners involved [5,8]. Most of the 1000 unsealed tunnels, unsealed pits and radioactive waste piles still remain on the Navajo reservation today, with Navajo families living within a hundred feet of the mine sites [9,20]. Some of the homes were built with tailings material and much of the water is contaminated on the reservation [20]. Figure 2 shows a sign erected by the Navajo and U.S. EPA which is typical for many of the water sources on the reservation.

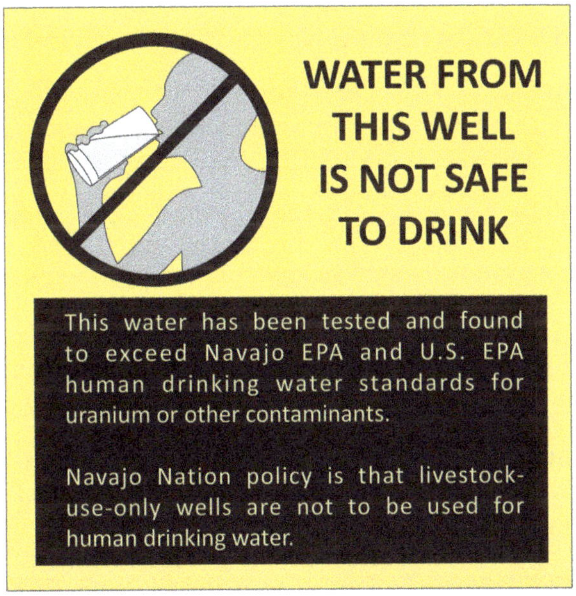

Figure 2. Sign erected by the Navajo and U.S. EPA which is typical for many of the water sources on the reservation. Figure from EPA Pacific Southwest Region 9 Addressing Uranium Contamination on the Navajo Nation [21].

1.2.2. Laguna Pueblo Tribe

The Village of Paguate (Laguna Pueblo), 40 miles west of Albuquerque, New Mexico was host to the largest open-pit uranium mine in the United States, the Jackpile Mine [22,23]. The mine was the largest producer of uranium ore in the Grants District [24]. Though the site was officially reclaimed in 1995 it is being considered for a National Priorities Listing (NPL) with the EPA after a Record of

Decision (ROD) Compliance Assessment for Jackpile-Paguate Uranium Mine was performed to determine if the post-reclamation had met the requirements of the Environmental Impact Statement and ROD. This report concluded that reclamation of the mine was still not complete. The Laguna Pueblo, representing a population of about 8000, rejected mining company offers to operate a uranium mill on tribal land. The mill was built just down the road at Bluewater, now another Superfund site [25].

1.2.3. The Eastern Shoshone and Northern Arapaho Nations

Uranium mining and processing has also left a legacy of contaminated groundwater and tailings on the Wind River Reservation, Wyoming, home to Eastern Shoshone and Northern Arapaho Indians. Increased incidences of cancers among its peoples are attributed to the old Susquehanna-Western uranium mill tailings site [26]. The site is a few miles southwest of Riverton, the ninth most-populated city in Wyoming. In some areas of the Wind River Indian Reservation groundwater contamination is so bad that the Department of Energy (DOE) estimates drinking water from contaminated aquifers could make residents up to 10 times more likely to develop cancer than the general population [26]. Uranium was not mined on the Wind River Reservation but uranium mined in the Pryor Mountains, Montana and Northern Bighorn Mountains, Wyoming was some of the ore processed there.

1.2.4. The Sioux Nations

Uranium mining in South Dakota, Wyoming, Montana, and North Dakota began in the middle of the 1950s [1]. More than 1000 open-pit uranium mines and prospects can be found in the four state region according to U.S. Forest Service maps. There were numerous uranium mines throughout the southern Black Hills National Forest as well as in Custer National Forest near the Lakota-Sioux lands in the Black Hills of South Dakota, which also had mines [1]. Most of these have not been reclaimed.

1.2.5. The Spokane Nation

The only uranium mining in Washington State was on the Spokane Indian Reservation. The mines were the Sherwood Uranium Mine and the Midnite Uranium Mine, which opened in the 1950s to produce uranium for the U.S.-Soviet nuclear arms race [27]. Just as on the Navajo reservation the mines brought needed employment to the reservation at that time and the miners were not informed of the dangers uranium mining [28]. About 33 million tons of radioactive waste rock and ore remain at the 350-acre site above the Spokane River [27]. The mines have been closed since the 1980s. The Midnite Mine site, the larger of the two uranium mines on the reservation is a superfund site [27]. Newmont Mining Co. (Greenwood Village, Colorado, USA) and its subsidiary, Dawn Mining Co. (Ford, Washington, USA) expects to begin cleanup of the Midnite Mine in 2015 [27]. "The plan is to fill in open pits left from the mine excavations with the waste rock and ore. The pits would be capped to keep radon gas from escaping. Groundwater in the pits will be collected and treated and then piped 7 miles to the Spokane River" stated a consultant from Newmont [27]. "Newmont already collects and treats water at the old mine site, but that water is currently discharged into Blue Creek, a tributary of the Spokane River. Discharging the treated wastewater directly into the Spokane River will reduce the impacts to Blue Creek, where the tribe is working to re-establish a native redband trout run" stated the Superfund director for the Spokane

Tribe [27]. "The water discharged into the Spokane River must meet the tribe's water quality standards for radionuclides, heavy metals and other pollutants, which are stricter than state and federal standards. The cleanup work is also subject to permits from the U.S. Environmental Protection Agency" [27] Members of the Spokane Tribe who worked at the mine or who live on the reservation are questioning the high rates of cancer on the reservation [28].

The Spokane Tribe teamed up with the Washington Department of Health and the Northwest Indian Health Board to track cancer rates among the tribe's 2700 members living with the legacy of the mining from the Sherwood Uranium Midnite Uranium Mines [28]. Study results are pending [28].

1.3. Nuclear Weapons Development

Pacific Northwest tribal groups on nine reservations in Washington, Idaho and Oregon were impacted by Hanford Nuclear reservation activities [29]. The Hanford Nuclear site is located on 1518 square km of shrub-steppe desert in southeastern Washington State [17] surrounded by these nine reservations (Figure 3).

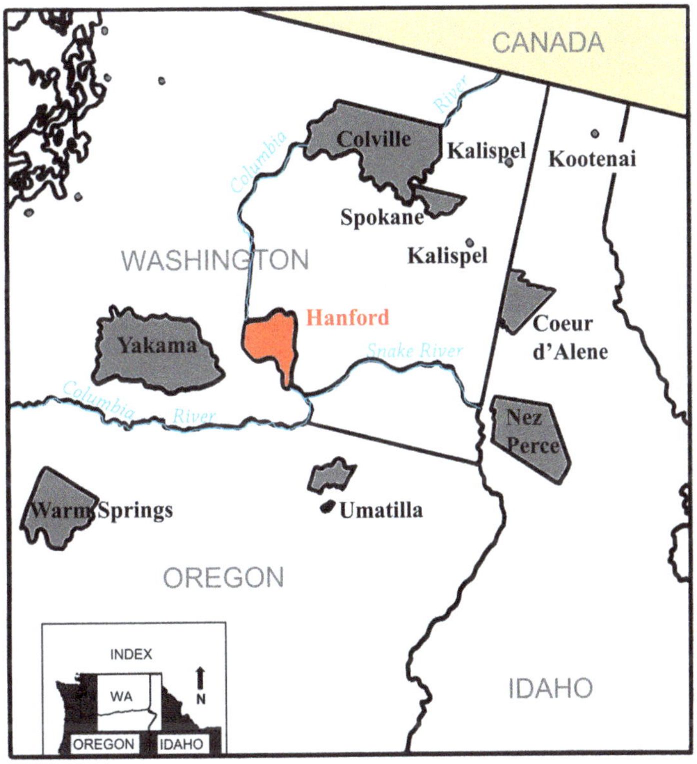

Figure 3. Hanford Nuclear Reservation, shown in red, was located in the state of Washington. Nine Native American reservations surround it. Figure modified from Edward Liebow in Hanford, Tribal Risks, and Public Health [29].

The people of these reservations traditionally used [17] and continue to use the lands and resources from the Columbia River Plateau region including land that was ceded to the government for which they retained hunting and gathering privileges [29]. Thus, they may have been exposed to more radiation and contaminants than the general public in practicing traditional lifestyles while fishing, hunting game, food gathering (berries, root plants, *etc.*) harvesting medicinal plants and traditional practices (*i.e.*, sweats), as well as social and spiritual interaction networks [29]. This region was contaminated by Hanford activities through primarily two distinct forms: airborne and river-borne releases, both normal operations and some accidental releases [29]. During the period from 1944 to 1972 Hanford released 25 million curies of radioactive contamination into the environment as a comparison the Chernobyl plant released between 35 and 49 million curies of iodine-131 (I-131) [29]. Five of the reservations, the Colville Confederated Tribes, Spokane, Kalispel, Kootenai, and Coeur D'Alene are primarily downwind of Hanford Nuclear site's 1450 square kilometer area (Figure 3) and would have been exposed to the airborne release of radioactive contamination for the most part normal by-product of chemical reactions used to separate weapons-grade plutonium from enriched uranium reactor rods, *i.e.*, I-131 with less of a contribution of the river borne releases [29]. The other four reservations, the Nez Perce, Confederated Tribes of the Umatilla, Confederated Tribes and Bands of the Warm Springs and the Yakama Nation are known to consume large quantities of fish and likely received higher doses of river borne releases which resulted from both accidental releases and normal operations that used Columbia River water to cool weapon-production reactor cores [29]. Additionally, liquid waste that had been poured onto the ground or held in ponds or trenches at the Hanford reservation evaporated or soaked into the soil on the site [30]. The waste contaminated some of the soil and is thought to have also created underground "plumes" of contaminants [30] which could also affect the tribes who consumed native food sources in the area. These nine reservations were all part of the Intertribal Council on Hanford Health Projects established in 1994 when all tribal governing bodies involved agreed on bylaws and operations plans for the council [29]. The group sought to give the tribal perspective of the information needed for estimating radiation doses from distinctive traditional lifestyles of the represented tribes and protect their sovereignty in public health research while also ensuring the scientific integrity of the research involving their people and land [29]. The final report of the federal government's Hanford Thyroid Disease Study (HTDS), a dose-based analysis epidemiological study conducted under contract by researchers at the Fred Hutchinson Cancer Research Center in Seattle from 1989 to 2002 [30], showed northwest U.S. residents with childhood radiation exposures from Washington State's Hanford nuclear site had similar risk levels for thyroid cancer and other thyroid disease regardless of their radiation dose [31]. Many people were dissatisfied with the results of the report and have lawsuits pending [30]. The study was not specific to Native American communities though "the authorizing language which provided funding for the study specifically required that thyroid disease among Native Americans be studied. However, no study focusing on thyroid disease among Native Americans was ever completed." ([29], p. 152). According to the HTDS summary report: "based on information from Native American Tribes and Nations, a study such as the HTDS in Native American populations alone was not feasible because it would have too little chance of detecting any health effects from Hanford's iodine-131" [32]. Native Americans were included in the HTDS if they were identified in the group that made up the study cohort [32]. The study used computer programs from Hanford Environmental Dose Reconstruction Project (1987–1994) and interviews with participants to estimate I-131 doses for 3440 people born between 1940 and 1946 to mothers living in seven Washington counties, took nearly 13 years to complete and cost $18 million dollars [31]. The site is an environmental cleanup project that approximately 11,000 Hanford employees are involved with today [30].

1.4. Milling and Abandoned Mills

Over ninety percent of all milling done in the U.S. occurred on or just outside the boundaries of American Indian reservations [33]. Mills logically would be located near the production or mine sites for infrastructure, thus many mills were on or near the reservations where uranium mining was operating. A disaster of huge consequence for the Navajo Nation occurred at the Church Rock uranium mill spill on 16 July 1979, in New Mexico when United Nuclear Corporation's Church Rock uranium mill tailings disposal pond breached its dam [34]. Over 1000 tons of solid radioactive mill waste and 93 million gallons of acidic, radioactive tailings solution flowed into the Puerco River, and contaminants traveled 130 km downstream onto the Navajo Nation [35]. The mill was located on privately owned land approximately 27 km north of Gallup, New Mexico, and bordered to the north and southwest by Navajo Nation Tribal Trust lands [35]. Local residents, who were mostly Navajos, used the Puerco River for irrigation and livestock and were not immediately aware of the toxic danger [34]. The Navajo Nation asked the governor of New Mexico to request disaster assistance from the U.S. government and have the site declared a disaster area, but he refused, limiting disaster relief assistance to the Navajo Nation [34]. In terms of the amount of radiation released, the accident was larger in magnitude than the Three Mile Island accident of the same year [34] but received little public attention. This was likely due to the remoteness and sparsely populated area of the Navajo Nation which was impacted by the spill. The area was inhabited by mainly Navajo people, many who only spoke their native tongue [34]. This is in contrast to the highly populated area of Middletown, Pennsylvania located three miles from the Three Mile Island Nuclear Generating Station where the TMI accident occurred. Possibly the greater significance of a nuclear power plant *versus* a tailings dam may also have influenced media coverage.

2. Indian Health Service, Census Data and Health Disparities

2.1. Indian Health Service

To evaluate health issues of Native American populations one must be aware of the unique relationship that American Indians and Alaska Natives (AI/AN) have with the federal government. The provision of health services to members of federally-recognized tribes grew out of the government-to-government relationship, established in 1787, between the federal government and Indian tribes in exchange for tribal lands. This relationship is based on Article I, Section 8 of the Constitution, and has been given form and substance by numerous treaties, laws, Supreme Court decisions, and Executive Orders [36,37]. The Indian Health Service (IHS), an agency within the Department of Health and Human Services, is responsible for providing federal health services to AI/AN. Approximately 2 million of the 3.4 million AI/AN, members of 566 federally recognized tribes across the U.S., are served by the IHS [36,37]. The organization has fulfilled the federal government's responsibility since 1955. The AI/AN health system has evolved greatly since then and now consists of IHS hospitals and health centers managed by the federal government, tribally managed services, and urban Indian health programs [38]. There are 12 Area offices, which are further divided down into 168 Service Units that provide care at the local level; most of these are rural primary care systems and are staffed by 70% native employees [36].

Tribal involvement and collaboration is an important aspect of the IHS in meeting the health needs of its service population [37]. Tribal delegation meetings are a form of tribal consultation where elected tribal officials meet with the IHS Director or senior staff to discuss health policy and program management issues related to the provision of health services to the Indian population. The IHS has an official Tribal Consultation Policy [37]. There are also programs with committees, task forces, boards and workgroups set up within the IHS system to address different aspects of policy and communication between the tribes and the federal government.

One of these programs is the Environmental Health Services (EHS) program. It includes the specialty areas of injury prevention and institutional environmental health. The IHS EHS program identifies environmental hazards and risk factors in tribal communities and proposes control measures to prevent adverse health effects. These measures include monitoring and investigating disease and injury in tribal communities; identifying environmental hazards in community facilities such as food service establishments, Head Start Centers, community water supply systems, and health care facilities; and providing training, technical assistance, and project funding to develop the capacity of tribal communities to address their environmental health issues [38]. The current IHS director is Yvette Roubideaux, M.D., M.P.H., a member of the Rosebud Sioux Tribe, South Dakota; she has served since May of 2009.

2.2. Census Data and Disparities

In the 2010 U.S. Census, 5.2 million people (about 1.7% of the U.S. population) identified themselves as AI/AN, solely or in combination with one or more racial/ethnic groups [39]. This population is concentrated in the west and south and proximate to AI/AN areas (reservations/trust lands) for most of the population [39]. AI/AN people consistently experience lower health status when compared with other Americans. The health status of AI/AN is affected by a number of environmental hazards, such as living in remote and isolated locations that expose residents to severe climatic conditions, hazardous geography, and disease-carrying insects and rodents, limited availability of housing and extensive use of sub-standard housing, unsanitary methods of sewage and waste disposal, and unsafe water supplies [40]. Lower life expectancy and the disproportionate disease burden exist possibly due to inadequate education, disproportionate poverty, discrimination in the delivery of health services, cultural differences and geographic location [40]. This population is concentrated in the west and south and proximate to AI/AN areas (reservations/trust lands) for most of the population [39]. AI/AN have the highest national poverty at 27.0%; nine states had poverty rates of about 30% or more for AI/AN: Arizona, Maine, Minnesota, Montana, Nebraska, New Mexico, North Dakota, South Dakota, and Utah [39]. There are many interwoven quality of life issues associated with life in native settings. These are broad issues deeply rooted in economic adversity, poor social conditions and a struggle to maintain a cultural identity while assimilating with U.S. society. A major cause of poverty in Native American communities is the persistent lack of opportunity; even most of the communities with natural resources on their lands are faced with high poverty. The Economic Research Service reports that Native American communities have fewer full-time employed individuals than any other high-poverty community. Mortality rates in AN populations are 60% higher than those of the U.S. white population [41,42], and mortality in AI populations are about twice that of the general U.S. population [43]. In addition, AI/AN have the lowest cancer survival rates among any racial group in the United States [44]. Native Americans in the Northern Plains region have a cancer mortality rate approximately 40% higher than that of the overall population [45].

There is sufficient evidence of disparities in health care financing, access to care, and quality of care to conclude that American Indians and Alaska Natives are disadvantaged in the health care system [33,34]. Comparing per capita personal health care expenditures on user population the IHS expenditure is $2741 while the total U.S. population expenditure is $7239 [37]. Due to the remoteness of many of the IHS facilities and funding available not all IHS facilities have the capabilities to address all the needs of the population. Contract health services (CHS) are purchased based on a priority system. The IHS is the Payor of Last Resort which requires patients to exhaust all health care resources available to them from private insurance, state health programs, and other federal programs before IHS can pay through the CHS program [40].

2.2.1. Toxic Waste Storage

When conditions exist of such extreme poverty for many Native American communities they have been approached by companies wanting to store toxic wastes on their lands. This creates hard situations for some tribes who would like the added "income" but desire to have a safe environment to live in. The Mescalero Apache, Prairie Island Mdewakanton, Minnesota Sioux, Skull valley Goshutes, Lower Brule, two Alaskan native communities, Chickasaw, Sac and Fox, Eastern Shawnee, Quassarie, Ponca. Tribes have all applied to be sites for Monitored Retrievable Storage (MRS), a temporary solution to the problem of storing vast amounts of high-level nuclear waste [46]. The safety of these sites is still under question.

2.2.2. Radiation Exposure Compensation Act

The Radiation Exposure Compensation Act passed in 1990 and amended in 2000 [46], was set up to make partial restitution to the people who contracted cancer and a number of other specified diseases as a direct result of mining, mill working or their exposure to atmospheric nuclear testing undertaken by the United States during the Cold War [6]. For miners the requirements such as whether the miner was a smoker, how long they had worked, whether the mine(s) they were employed in had radon exposure monitoring, medical proof of lung cancer or a nonmalignant respiratory disease, *etc.* made it very difficult for the people to be accepted in the program. Many miners were designated as smokers even though they may have only smoked the equivalent of a pack of cigarettes over a year, in ceremonial practices which increased the WLM (working level months—a measure of radon exposure based on Social Security work records and exposure to radon) required to 500 unless they contracted lung cancer under age 45 then it was 300 WLM [6]. The stringent, often impossible requirements made attaining this compensation hard for most of the victims involved. Many of the people are still trying to be compensated.

3. Discussion and Conclusions

The legacy of uranium procurement has left a legacy of long-lived health effects for many Native Americans and Alaska Natives in the United States. There have been a number of studies that are starting to address the health impacts of this legacy. The largest population and some of the most impacted people are the tribes living in the southwestern USA, especially the Navajo. A consortium of federal and tribal agencies reported that a five-year, $110 million project to clean up uranium contamination in the Navajo

Nation had addressed the most urgent risks there [47]. But the report also said that in the last five years the agencies have learned much more "about the scope of the problem and it is clear that additional work will be needed" [47]. The consortium included the U.S. Environmental Protection Agency, the Bureau of Indian Affairs, Nuclear Regulatory Commission, Department of Energy and Indian Health Service. The project started in 2007 to tackle the widespread uranium contamination on Navajo lands left over from the nation's atomic weapon production programs. Among their accomplishments, the agencies reported that they have cleaned up nine abandoned uranium mines, rebuilt 34 homes and replaced contaminated soil at 18 sites, many near homes. The agencies also assessed the status of 520 mines, 240 water sources and 800 homes and public structures, exceeding goals set in the five-year plan, the report said [48,49]. It added that officials shut down three contaminated wells and hauled clean water to affected areas of the Navajo Nation or started projects to pipe in water.

Another study in the Eastern Agency of the Navajo Nation in New Mexico [50], studied environmental uranium contamination in a former mining and milling area. Despite decades of inactivity in the mines and mills, environmental contamination was widespread, often in proximity to homes, areas grazed by livestock, and locations frequented by children and families. The uranium contamination in this area was predominantly in the highly soluble chemical forms that could be spread when disturbed or by the bursts of precipitation that occur in this semiarid region at certain times of the year [50].

The Navajo Birth Cohort Study will use Community Based Participatory Research (CBPR) methods [51] and is a collaborative effort to better understand the relationship between uranium exposures and early developmental delays on the Navajo Nation [52]. The five-year Study is funded by Congress at the request of the Navajo Nation and in response to concerns expressed by women about health impacts of living near abandoned uranium mines [53]. Partners in the Study include the Centers for Disease Control and Prevention/Agency for Toxic Substances and Disease Registry, Navajo Area Indian Health Service, Navajo Nation Division of Health, University of New Mexico Community Environmental Health Program, UNM Pediatrics Department Center for Development and Disability, and Southwest Research and Information Center [53]. Eligible women are between the ages of 14 and 45 who have lived on the Navajo Nation for five years, are pregnant, and will deliver at the designated hospitals in Chinle, Gallup, Shiprock, Ft. Defiance, and Tuba City [53].

This short review only provides a quick glance at the continuing legacy of long-lived health effects for many Native American populations due to uranium procurement in the United States. The reader is encouraged to explore some of these topics and become aware of the issues. Native American communities, those on and near reservations, consistently experience lower health status when compared with other Americans. To be able to set up medical geology studies as collaborations within these separate nations, it is important that traditional knowledge is incorporated into the study plans. The non-Native American exposure doses and other variables within each unique study may underestimate necessary values within a study related to Native American communities. Without weighting standard values differently in applied models, or considering different types of variables in GIS and other geospatial tools, the results of the studies may not truly represent the Native American or Alaska Native populations and the effects of the environment or toxic indicator which is studied.

Medical Geology has been shown to be an effective tool in many applications around the world. The sample size of many of the Native American and Alaska Native communities is small for large statistical studies, but increased homogeneity in the small sample sizes due to cultural and traditional values may provide good results, which can be implemented to improve health conditions of the people involved. Funding for projects will also need to be collaborative. Working with programs like the Tribal ecoAmbasadors Program, National Institute of Health, National Science Foundation, the U.S. Geological Survey, IHS and Tribal colleges may yield productive studies that can be used to help improve the overall health of these communities. The use of community-based participatory research approaches that incorporate Native American social networks can be effective in helping to achieve policy changes to address health issues.

Acknowledgments

Funding for research: Alfred P. Sloan Graduate Scholarship Programs—Minority Ph.D. Component/Sloan Indigenous Graduate Partnership; Montana State University—Dennis and Phyllis Washington Foundation Native American Graduate Fellow; HOPA Mountain Program. Note: The content is solely the responsibility of the author; it has not been formally reviewed by any of the funders.

References

1. Moore-Nall, A.L.; Lageson, D.R. Lower health status on Indian Reservations a geologic or geographic correlation associated with natural resources? In Proceedings of the 5th International Conference on Medical Geology, Arlington, VA, USA, 25–29 August 2013.
2. Brugge, D.; Benally, T.; Harrison, P.; Austin-Garrison, M.; Begay, L.F. Memories come to US in the rain and the wind: Oral histories and photographs of Navajo Uranium miners and their families. In *The Navajo Uranium Miner Oral History and Photography Project*; Tufts School of Medicine: Boston, MA, USA, 1997; pp. 1–63.
3. Brugge, D.; Benally, T. Navajo Indian voices and faces testify to the legacy of uranium mining. *Cult. Surviv. Q.* **1998**, *22*, 16–19.
4. Brugge, D.; Benally, T.; Harrison, P.; Austin-Garrison, M.; Stilwell, C.; Elsner, M.; Bomboy, K.; Johnson, H.; Fasthorse-Begay, L. The Navajo Uranium miner oral history and photography project. In *Dine Baa Hane Bi Naaltsoos: Collected Papers from the Seventh through the Tenth Navajo Studies Conferences*; Piper, J., Ed.; Navajo Nation Historic Preservation Department: Window Rock, AZ, USA, 1999; pp. 85–96.
5. Brugge, D.; Goble, R. The history of Uranium mining and the Navajo people. *Am. J. Public Health* **2002**, *92*, 1410–1419.
6. Brugge, D.; Goble, R. A documentary history of Uranium mining and the Navajo people. In *The Navajo People and Uranium Mining*; Brugge, D., Benally, T., Yazzie-Lewis, E., Eds.; UNM Press: Albuquerque, NM, USA, 2007; pp. 25–47.
7. Yazzie-Lewis, E.; Zion, J. Leetso, the powerful yellow monster a Navajo cultural interpretation of Uranium mining. In *The Navajo People and Uranium Mining*; Brugge, D., Benally, T., Yazzie-Lewis, E., Eds.; UNM Press: Albuquerque, NM, USA, 2007; pp. 1–10.

8. Johnston, B.R.; Dawson, S.E.; Madsen, G.E. Uranium mining and milling, Navajo experiences in the American southwest. In *Half-Lives & Half-Truths, Confronting the Radioactive Legacies of the Cold War*; Johnston, B.R., Ed.; School for Advanced Research Press: Santa Fe, NM, USA, 2007; pp. 97–117.
9. Technical Report on Technologically Enhanced Naturally Occurring Radioactive Materials from Uranium Mining Volume 2: Investigation of Potential Health, Geographic, and Environmental Issues of Abandoned Uranium Mines, EPA 402-R-08-005, April 2008. Available online: http://www.epa.gov/radiation/docs/tenorm/402-r-08–005-volii/402-r-08-005-v2.pdf (accessed on 20 December 2014).
10. Uranium Mining Wastes. What is the History of Uranium Mining in the U.S.? Available online: http://www.epa.gov/radiation/tenorm/uranium.html#history (accessed on 20 December 2014).
11. Abandoned Mine Lands Portal. Available online: http://www.abandonedmines.gov/wbd_um.html (accessed on 20 December 2014).
12. Brugge, D.; Buchner, V. Health effects of uranium: New research findings. *Rev. Environ. Health* **2011**, *26*, 231–249.
13. Manhattan Project. Energy.gov Office of Management. Available online: http://energy.gov/management/office-management/operational-management/history/manhattan-project (accessed on 28 December 2014).
14. Los Alamos National Laboratory. Our History. Available online: http://www.lanl.gov/about/history-innovation/index.php (accessed on 28 December 2014).
15. Churchhill, W. A breach of trust. In *Acts of Rebellion: The Ward Churchill Reader*; Routledge: London, UK, 2002; pp. 103–130.
16. Wright, Q. The law of the Nuremberg trial. *Am. J. Int. Law* **1947**, *41*, 38–42.
17. Department of Energy Hanford. Hanford Overview and History. Available online: http://www.hanford.gov/page.cfm/HanfordOverviewandHistory (accessed on 28 December 2014).
18. Orem, W.; Tatu, C.; Pavlovic, N.; Bunnell, J.; Kolker, A.; Engle, M.; Stout, B. Health Effects of Energy Resources. U.S. Department of the Interior, U.S. Geological Survey, FS 2009-3096. Available online: http://pubs.usgs.gov/fs/2009/3096/ (accessed on 30 December 2014).
19. Ali, S.H. *Mining, the Environment, and Indigenous Development Conflicts*; The University of Arizona Press: Tucson, AZ, USA, 2003; p. 254.
20. Klauk, E. Impacts of Resource Development on Native American Lands. Available online: http://serc.carleton.edu/research_education/nativelands/navajo/humanhealth.html (accessed on 10 December 2014).
21. EPA Pacific Southwest Region 9. Addressing Uranium Contamination on the Navajo Nation. Contaminated Water Sources. Available online: http://www.epa.gov/region9/superfund/navajo-nation/contaminated-water.html (accessed on 8 December 2014).
22. Dawson, S.E.; Madsen, G.E. Uranium Mine Workers, Atomic Downwinders, and the Radiation Exposure Compensation Act (RECA). In *Half-Lives & Half-Truths, Confronting the Radioactive Legacies of the Cold War*; Johnston, B.R., Ed.; School for Advanced Research Press: Sante Fe, NM, USA, 2007; pp. 117–143.
23. Eichstaedst, P. If You Poison Us: Uranium and Native Americans; Red Crane Books: Santa Fe, NM, USA, 1994; p. 194.

24. Jackpile Mine (Jackpile-Paguate), Laguna District, Cibola Co., New Mexico, USA. Available online: http://www.mindat.org/loc-33622.html (accessed on 28 December 2014).
25. Native Sun News: Laguna Pueblo Still Affected by Uranium Mine. Available online: http://www.indianz.com/News/2014/014847.asp (accessed on 28 December 2014).
26. Schilmoeller, J. Decades of Environmental Injustice: Wyoming Indian Reservation Faces High Cancer Rates. Mint Press News. Available online: http://www.mintpress.net/decades-of-environmental-injustice-wyoming-indian-reservation-faces-deteramental-rates-of-cancer/ (accessed on 13 December 2012).
27. Cleanup of Midnite Mine on Reservation to Begin by 2015. The Spokesman-Review. Available online: http://www.spokesman.com/stories/2013/nov/21/cleanup-of-midnite-mine-on-reservation-to-begin/ (accessed on 8 December 2014).
28. Spokane Tribe Members Worked Gladly in Uranium Mines. The Spokesman-Review. Available online: http://www.spokesman.com/stories/2011/jun/05/i-watch-them-die-young-and-old/ (accessed on 8 December 2014).
29. Liebow, E. Hanford, tribal risks, and public health in an era of forced federalism. In *Half-Lives & Half-Truths, Confronting the Radioactive Legacies of the Cold War*; Johnston, B.R., Ed.; School for Advanced Research Press: Santa Fe, NM, USA, 2007; pp. 145–165.
30. Department of Energy Hanford. Hanford Cleanup. Available online: http://www.hanford.gov/page.cfm/HanfordCleanup (accessed on 28 December 2014).
31. Reynolds, T. Final Report of Hanford Thyroid Disease Study Released. *J. Natl. Cancer Inst.* **2002**, *94*, 1046–1048.
32. Centers for Disease Control and Prevention, HTDS Guide—How the Study Was Conducted. Available online: http://www.cdc.gov/nceh/radiation/hanford/htdsweb/guide/conduct.htm (accessed on 16 January 2015).
33. Prados, J. *Presidents' Secret Wars: CIA and Pentagon Secret Operations since World War II*; William Morrow & Co.: New York, NY, USA, 1986; pp. 255–256.
34. Brugge, D.; de Lemos, J.L. The Sequoyah Corporation fuels release and the church rock spill: Unpublicized nuclear releases in American Indian communities. *Am. J. Public Health* **2007**, 97, 1595–1600.
35. Pasternak, J. *Yellow Dirt: A Poisoned Land and a People Betrayed*; Free Press: New York, NY, USA, 2010; p. 149.
36. Dixon, M.; Roubideaux, Y. *Promises to Keep: Public Health Policy for American Indians and Alaska Natives in the 21st Century*; American Public Health Association: Washington, DC, USA, 2001; p. 311.
37. Indian Health Service (IHS) Website. Available online: http://www.ihs.gov/index.cfm?module=ihsIntro (accessed on 11 March 2013).
38. Lillie-Blanton, M.; Roubideaux, Y. Understanding and addressing the health care needs of American Indians and Alaska natives. *Am. J. Public Health* **2005**, *95*, 759–761.
39. Census 2010 Brief: The American Indian and Alaska Native population: 2010. Available online: http://www.census.gov/prod/cen2010/briefs/c2010br-10.pdf (accessed on 11 March 2013).
40. Indian Health Service (IHS) Environmental Health Services Fact Sheet. Available online: http://www.ihs.gov/factsheets (accessed on 11 March 2013).

41. Day, G.E.; Lanier, A.P. Alaska native mortality, 1979–1998. *Public Health Rep.* **2003**, *118*, 518–530.
42. Hoover, E.; Cook, K.; Plain, R.; Sanchez, K.; Waghiyi, V.; Miller, P.; Dufault, R.; Sislin, C.; Carpenter, D.O. Indigenous peoples of North America: Environmental exposures and reproductive justice. *Environ. Health Perspect.* **2012**, *120*, 1645–1649.
43. Kunitz, S.J. Changing patterns of mortality among American Indians. *Am. J. Public Health* **2008**, *98*, 404–412.
44. Native American Health Care Disparities Briefing Executive Summary; Office of the General Counsel U.S. Commission on Civil Rights: 2004; p. 52. Available online: http://www.law.umaryland.edu/marshall/usccr/documents/nativeamerianhealthcaredis.pdf (accessed on 11 March 2013).
45. Rogers, D.; Petereit, D. Cancer disparities research partnerships in Lakota Country: Clinical trials, patient services, and community education for the Oglala, Rosebud, and Cheyenne River Sioux Tribes. *Am. J. Public Health* **2005**, *95*, 2129–2132.
46. Nuclear War: Uranium Mining and Nuclear Tests on Indigenous Lands. Available online: http://www.culturalsurvival.org/publications/cultural-survival-quarterly/united-states/nuclear-war-uranium-mining-and-nuclear-tests- (accessed on 8 December 2014).
47. RECA Radiation Exposure Compensation Act: Radiation Exposure Compensation Program—About the Program United States Department of Justice. Available online: http://usdoj.gov/civil/torts/const/reca/about.htm (accessed on 30 December 2012).
48. Agencies Cite Progress, Work Still Remaining on Navajo Uranium Cleanup. *Chronkite News*, 24 January 2013. Available online: http://cronkitenewsonline.com/2013/01/agencies-cite-progress-work-still-remaining-on-navajo-uranium-cleanup/ (accessed on 8 December 2014).
49. EPA Pacific Southwest Region 9. Addressing Uranium Contamination on the Navajo Nation. Cleanup of Abandoned Mines. Available online: http://www.epa.gov/region9/superfund/navajo-nation/abandoned-uranium.html (accessed on 8 December 2014).
50. DeLemos, J.L.; Bostick, B.C.; Quicksall, A.N.; Landis, J.D.; George, C.C.; Slagowski, N.L.; Rock, T.; Brugge, D.; Lewis, J.; Durant, J.L.; Rapid dissolution of soluble Uranyl phases in arid, mine-impacted catchments near Church Rock, NM. *Environ. Sci. Technol.* **2008**, *42*, 3951–3957.
51. CDC Navajo Uranium Impact Studies: Dr. Johnnye Lewis. Available online: https://lajicarita.wordpress.com/2012/08/31/cdc-navajo-uranium-impact-studies-dr-johnnye-lewis/ (accessed on 7 December 2014).
52. Navajo Health Research: Dr. Johnnye Lewis Continues. Available online: http://lajicarita.wordpress.com/2012/09/21/navajo-health-research-dr-johnnye-lewis-continues/ (accessed on 7 December 2014).
53. Southwest Research and Information Center. Available online: http://www.sric.org/nbcs/index.php (accessed on 7 December 2014).

4

Identifying Sources and Assessing Potential Risk of Exposure to Heavy Metals and Hazardous Materials in Mining Areas: The Case Study of Panasqueira Mine (Central Portugal) as an Example

Carla Candeias [1,*], Eduardo Ferreira da Silva [1], Paula F. Ávila [2] and João Paulo Teixeira [3]

[1] GeoBioTec—Geobiosciences, Geotechnologies e Geoengineering Research Center, Geosciences Department, University of Aveiro, Campus de Santiago, Aveiro 3810-193, Portugal; E-Mail: eafsilva@ua.pt

[2] LNEG—National Laboratory of Energy and Geology, Rua da Amieira, Apartado 1089, S. Mamede de Infesta 4466-901, Portugal; E-Mail: paula.avila@lneg.pt

[3] Environmental Health Department, National Institute of Health, Rua Alexandre Herculano, 321, Porto 4000-055, Portugal; E-Mail: jpft12@gmail.com

* Author to whom correspondence should be addressed; E-Mail: candeias@ua.pt;

External Editor: Jose A. Centeno

Abstract: The Sn-W Panasqueira mine, in activity since the mid-1890s, is one of the most important economic deposits in the world. Arsenopyrite is the main mineral present as well as rejected waste sulphide. The long history is testified by the presence of a huge amount of tailings, which release considerable quantities of heavy metal(loid)s into the environment. This work assesses soil contamination and evaluates the ecological and human health risks due to exposure to hazardous materials. The metal assemblage identified in soil (Ag-As-Bi-Cd-Cu-W-Zn; potentially toxic elements (PTEs)) reflects the influence of the tailings, due to several agents including aerial dispersion. PTEs and pH display a positive correlation confirming that heavy metal mobility is directly related to pH and, therefore, affects their availability. The estimated contamination factor classified 92.6% of soil samples as moderately to ultra-highly polluted. The spatial distribution of the potential ecological risk index classified the topsoil as being of a very high ecological risk, consistent with wind direction. Non-carcinogenic hazard of topsoil, for children (1–6 years), showed that for As the non-carcinogenic hazard represents a high health risk. The carcinogenic risks, both for children and adult alike, reveal a very high cancer risk mostly due to As ingestion.

Keywords: Panasqueira mine; potential toxic elements; modified contamination degree; non-carcinogenic hazard; carcinogenic risk; potential ecological risk factor and risk index

---

1. Introduction

Mine tailings, with considerable amounts of sulfides, left in the vicinity of environmentally sensitive locations, constitute one of the greatest threats to the surrounding environment. These materials when exposed to air and water are oxidized through chemical, electrochemical, and biological reactions, forming ferric hydroxides and sulfuric acid, leading to the generation of acid mine drainage with high contents of metals and sulfates, related to the alteration of sulfides, the equilibrium of which depends on their solubility [1–5].

Soil is prone to contamination both from hydrological and atmospheric sources. When soil is the receptor of tailings drainage, originating from metal mining and smelting, this waste disposal causes a major impact, and poses serious environmental concerns [6]. As a direct result of the mining activities, soil is generally, affected over a considerable area. The soil fine fraction is usually enriched in metals, due to the relative large surface area of fine particles that facilitate adsorption and metal binding to iron and manganese oxides and to organic matter [7,8]. Wind-blown dust originating from polluted soil is responsible for the aerial dispersion of trace metals [7]. Exposure to these hazardous elements may have different pathways, e.g., through the direct ingestion of soils and dust, ingestion of vegetables grown on contaminated soil or dust adhering to plants or dust inhalation. According to several authors [9–14] the studies dealing with the bioavailability and bioaccessibility of metal(loid) contaminants in highly-polluted soil are extremely useful to understand the possible effect on biota, and particularly on human health due to the exposure to these contaminants [12,15].

Among the purposes of environmental analysis are the determination of the geochemical background and natural concentrations of the chemical constituents in environment-background monitoring, as well as to determine the concentration of harmful pollutants in environment-pollution monitoring [16]. The sorption-desorption soil characteristics generally control the mobility and availability of heavy metals [17]. Heavy metal availability in soil depends on a number of factors, including Soil Organic Matter (SOM) and pH [18]. Soil pH plays the most important role in determining metal speciation, solubility from mineral surfaces, movement and bioavailability of metals [19–21]. Several laboratory experiments have shown that heavy metal mobility and availability have a negative correlation with pH [22]. Further, [23–25] documented that metal mobility and availability increases with the decrease of soil pH, thus enhancing the uptake of heavy metals by plants and, thereby, posing a threat to human health [26].

Exposure to increasing amounts of metal(loid)s in environmental and occupational settings is a reality worldwide, affecting a significant number of individuals. Most metal(loid)s are very toxic to living organisms and even those considered as essential can be toxic when in excess. They can disturb important biochemical processes, constituting an important threat for human health. Major health effects include development retardation, endocrine disruption, kidney damage, immunological and neurological effects, and several types of cancer [27]. The identification of potential threats to human health and natural ecosystems is useful information [16]. The quantification of all the types of risks and the determination of the total risk of metal(loid)s to the exposed population through oral intake, inhalation and dermal contact [28] is also very important. Risk assessment is typically a multistep process of identifying, defining, and characterizing potentially adverse consequences of exposure to hazardous materials [28]. According to the Toxic Substances Portal [29], Ag, As, Cd, Cu, W and Zn are known to be toxic to humans, while arsenic and cadmium are classified as human carcinogens. Some studies also consider that Bi causes acute toxicity, and large doses can be fatal [30,31]. However, as Bi is considered to be one of the less toxic heavy metals, it is not included in this analysis.

In a previous paper from the same authors [32], several variables (Ag, As, Bi, Cd, Cu, W and Zn) showed moderate to strong correlation in the Panasqueira topsoil. This indicates an anthropogenic origin, especially linked to aerial transportation and deposition and/or to a geogenic origin. The main goals of the present study are: (a) establishment of the relationship between Potentially Toxic Elements (PTEs) with depth and soil pH; (b) assessment of soil contamination using a contamination factor for each pollutant; and (c) determination and evaluation of the ecological and human health risks due to exposure to hazardous materials.

2. Materials and Methods

2.1. Study Area

The active Panasqueira mine, exploited since the last decade of the 19th century, is located in Central Portugal (UTM (Universal Transverse Mercator) 29N, P 4445620.79, M 606697.31; Figure 1). It is considered to have the largest Sn-W deposit of Western Europe [33]. The geology has been extensively studied by many researchers [34–44]. Briefly, the Panasqueira deposit is a classic example of postmagmatic hydrothermal ore deposit, which is associated with Hercynian plutonism [36,41]. The paragenesis is complex with four stages of mineral formation identified: 1st stage, the oxide silicate phase (quartz, wolframite; cassiterite); 2nd phase, the main sulphide phase (pyrite, arsenopyrite, pyrrhotite, sphalerite, chalcopyrite); 3rd stage, the pyrrhotite alteration phase (marcasite, siderite, galena, Pb-Bi-Ag sulphosalts); and 4th stage, the late carbonate phase (dolomite, calcite) [38–49]. The Panasqueira deposit contains significant amounts of wolframite, arsenopyrite, chalcopyrite and cassiterite [34].

The long history of exploitation is testified by the presence of a huge amount of tailings and other debris (Figure 1b). The piles (Rio ~1.2 million m^3; Barroca Grande ~7.0 million m^3) and the mud dams (Rio ~0.7 million m^3; Barroca Grande ~1.2 million m^3) are exposed to atmospheric conditions, and are being altered by chemical, physical and geotechnical activities. On the top of the Rio tailings, an arsenopyrite stockpile (~9400 m^3) was deposited and remained exposed until 2006 [41].

Topography ranges in altitude from 350 to 1080 m [47], with deep valleys of about 9%–25% inclination, constraining the soil into a very thin layer. Climate is severe, with dry and hot summers and very cold, rainy and windy winters. The annual precipitation ranges between 1200 and 1400 mm with frequent snow falls, particularly above 700 m altitude. The mean annual temperature is 12 °C, ranging from 0 °C during the winter to 30 °C in the summer. The streams are generally dry in the summer and flooded in the winter. The prevailing wind in the area is NW-SE, with mean wind speeds of 4.22 m/s (h = 10 m), 5.55 m/s (h = 40 m) and 6.21 m/s (h = 80 m) (Figure 1c) [48–50]. The small villages around the mine have a historical dependence on soil and water use drinking water, agriculture, cattle rearing, fishing and forestry.

Figure 1. (**a**) Synthetic map of Portugal showing the location of Panasqueira mining area; (**b**) details of the study area, main geological units and soil samples grid - geological map adapted from [34,41,45]; (**c**) wind rose of the prevailing winds on the top of the mine (Barroca Grande tailing); and (**d**) on the top of a mountain 800 m north of the mine [46].

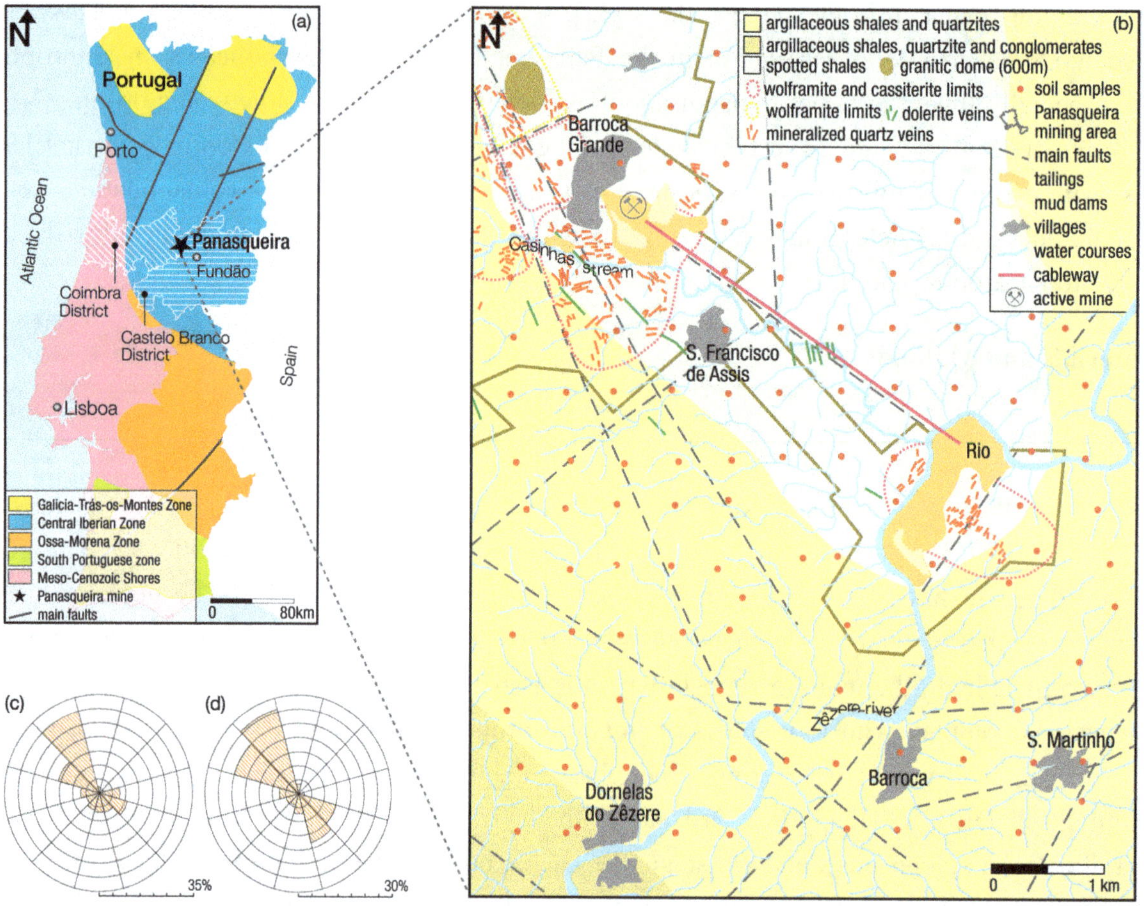

2.2. Field Sampling and Sample Preparation

Soil samples were collected according to a predefined grid (spaced ~400 m—Figure 1b). Two types of soil samples were collected at each sampling site: 122 topsoil (0–15 cm) samples and 116 subsoil samples collected below 15 cm depth. The difference in the total number of samples of each soil type is due to the presence at six sites of incipient and thin lithic soil derived from a substrate of metasediments. Topsoil samples were collected for the characterization of superficial contamination derived from the tailings, and subsoil samples to assess the extent of contamination at depth and simultaneously to identify geogenic markers. Approximately 50% of all samples were collected in duplicate. To establish the local geochemical background, 47 unaffected soil samples (Bk) were also collected outside the contaminated area (Casegas area located NE, out of the influence of the Barroca Grande prevailing winds). The coordinates of each sample were determined by GPS and georeferenced with UTM (Universal Transverse Mercator) coordinates. All soil samples were collected after clearing the soil surface of superficial debris and vegetation, and placed in polyethylene bags. Samples were dried in a thermostatically controlled oven at 40 °C, disaggregated in a porcelain mortar, sieved (<2 mm), homogenized, split into aliquots and the analytical aliquot pulverized to <170 μm in a pre-cleaned mechanical agate mill for chemical analysis.

2.3. Chemical Analysis

Soil samples were submitted for multi-element analysis at the ACME Analytical Laboratories, which is an ISO 9002 Accredited Lab (Vancouver, Canada). A sample weight of 0.5 g was leached in hot (95 °C) aqua regia (HCl-HNO_3-H_2O), and concentrations were determined by Inductively Coupled Plasma Mass Spectrometry (ICP-MS) for Ag, As, Bi, Cd, Cu, W and Zn (detection limits of Ag, Bi, Cd, Cu, W < 0.1 $mg \cdot kg^{-1}$; As < 0.5 $mg \cdot kg^{-1}$; Zn < 1 $mg \cdot kg^{-1}$).

Accuracy and analytical precision were determined using analytical results of certified reference materials (standards C3 and G-2) and duplicate samples in each analytical batch. The results were within the 95% confidence limits of the recommended values given for the certified materials. The Relative Standard Deviation (RSD) was between 5% and 10%.

Soil pH: numerous studies have verified that soil pH has a great effect on metal bioavailability [16,51,52]. The pH gives an indication of the acidity and alkalinity of soil. Many chemical reactions are pH dependent, and knowledge of the pH enables the prediction of the extent and speed of chemical reactions [53]. The procedure adopted for the determination of pH was modified from [54]. A suspension of soil was made up in five times its volume of a 0.01 mol/L solution of calcium chloride ($CaCl_2$) in water. The pH was measured using a calibrated pH-meter.

SOM: plays an important role in determining the fate of inorganic, as well as organic compounds in natural soil [55–58]. SOM can be roughly determined by measuring weight loss before and after ashing at 430 °C. Results are typically accurate to 1%–2% for soil with over 10% organic matter [53]. The procedure adopted was modified from [53]. Approximately 5 g of each sieved sample (<2 mm) was placed in a crucible and dried at 105 °C for 24 h. After cooling in a glass desiccator its weight was determined in a mass balance (resolution 0.001 g). The difference in weight gives the water content of each soil sample. The crucibles were then placed in a muffle furnace at 430 °C for 20 h. After cooling in a glass desiccator, the weight was measured on the same mass balance. The difference from the dry state gives the soil organic content (%).

2.4. Data Treatment of Data

Pearson's product-moment linear correlation coefficient matrix (*r*) was estimated in order to determine the extent of the relationship between the PTEs, pH and SOM [53]. The normality of statistical distribution of all data was verified by the Kolmogorov-Smirnov test ($\alpha = 0.05$) and Q-Q plots. The non-normal data were subjected to a non-parametric test or converted logarithmically to ensure the validity of the results. The statistical analysis was performed using Six Sigma Statistica® (Stat Software Inc, Tulsa, OK, USA) and IBM® SPSS® Statistics software (IBM, New York, NY, USA).

Analysis of Variance (ANOVA) was carried out in order to assess the relationship between the Potentially Toxic Elements and the independent variables (depth, pH and SOM), by a two-way ANOVA test, according to the following expression:

$$Z_{ijk} = \mu + \alpha_i + \beta_j + \gamma_{ij} + \varepsilon_{ijk} \quad (1)$$

where, Z = the kth observation of the PTE taken at jth depth (j = 1 or 2) and ith soil property (i = 1 or 2), μ = the overall mean estimated, α = the depth effect, β = the soil property (pH or SOM), γ = the interaction between depth and the soil property, and ε = the residual error [59–61].

Log_{10} transformation was applied to PTEs in order to convert the data to a normal or near-normal distribution and homogeneity of variances (Levene's test, $p < 0.05$). For the two-way analysis of variance, samples were classified according to pH values (very acid (3.0, 4.0), acid (4.0, 6.0) and neutral (6.0, 7.0)) and SOM ((3.6, 10.0) and (10.0, 39.0) in %). It should be noted that the SOM classes established, were only defined for statistical purposes. In the cases where there were only two samples with neutral pH, this particular class was not considered further.

Contamination Factor and Modified Degree of Contamination was estimated using the method proposed by [62] in sediment pollution studies, but is also applied to soil studies [63,64]. It is based on the calculation, for each pollutant, of a contamination factor (CF_i) which is the ratio obtained by dividing the mean concentration of each metal in soil (C_i) by its corresponding baseline or background value (estimated from samples collected outside the area influenced by the mining activities) according to [65], and as explained in [6], *i.e.*, the background value, C_b (mg kg^{-1}), for the studied elements is as follows: Ag = 0.05; As = 22; Bi = 0.3; Cd = 0.01; Cu = 28; W = 0.35; Zn = 58) [64] (Table 1):

$$CF_i = C_i / C_b \quad (2)$$

Table 1. Classification and description of the Contamination factor (*CF*) [62] and the Modified contamination degree (*mCd*) [66].

CF Value	Level of the Contamination Factor	mC_d Value	Modified Contamination Degree Gradations
$0 \leq CF < 1$	Low	$0 \leq mC_d < 1.5$	None to very low
		$1.5 \leq mC_d < 2$	Low
$1 \leq CF < 3$	Moderate	$2 \leq mC_d < 4$	Moderate
$3 \leq CF < 6$	High	$4 \leq mC_d < 8$	High
$6 \leq CF$	Very high	$8 \leq mC_d < 16$	Very high
		$16 \leq mC_d < 32$	Extremely high
		$32 \leq mC_d$	Ultra high

In [66] is presented a modified and generalized form of the [62] equation for the calculation of the overall degree of contamination (mC_d) for each sample as below:

$$mC_d = \left(\sum_{i=1}^{7} CF_i \right) / 7 \quad (3)$$

where CF_i is the contamination factor computed for each of the seven pollutants (Ag, As, Bi, Cd, Cu, W, Zn) considered in this study. In [66] is defined seven mC_d degrees as shown in Table 1.

Potential ecological risk factor and risk index (*PERI*): is defined as the sum of the risk factors, which quantitatively defines the potential ecological risk of a contaminant in a sample, *i.e.*:

$$PERI_i = \sum_{i=1}^{7} EF_i = \sum_{i=1}^{7} CF_i \cdot TF \quad (4)$$

where $PERI_i$ is the Potential Ecological Risk Index for each sample (*i*); EF_i is the monomial potential ecological risk factor; CF_i is the single contamination factor (Equation (2)); and *TF* is the heavy metal toxic-response factor for each element. Soil toxic-response factors were computed for the seven selected elements according to the toxic factor requirements proposed by [62]. For this estimation there were used reference guide values of igneous rock types, soil, freshwater and land plants proposed by [67], and the land animals reference values proposed by [68]. The TF values obtained were: Zn = 1 < Cu = 2 < As = 5 < W = 15 < Bi = 20 < Cd = 30 < Ag = 35. In [62] are defined five *EF* classes and four *PERI* degrees, as shown in Table 2.

Table 2. Monomial potential ecological risk factor (*EF*) and Potential ecological risk index (*PERI*) classification levels [62].

EF	Ecological Potential Risk for Single Substance	*PERI*	Ecological Risk
$0 \le EF < 40$	Low	$PERI < 150$	Low
$40 \le EF < 80$	Moderate	$150 \le PERI < 300$	Moderate
$80 \le EF < 160$	Considerable	$300 \le PERI < 600$	Considerable
$160 \le EF < 320$	High	$600 \le PERI$	Very high
$320 \le EF$	Very high		

Human health risk assessment calculations were based on the assumption that residents, both children and adults, are directly exposed to soil through three main pathways (a) ingestion; (b) dermal absorption and (c) inhalation of soil particles present in the air [69–72]. Ingestion of soil (i) occurs by eating soil particles and/or licking contact surfaces (e.g., hands). It is assumed that children present a higher ingestion rate, due to hand-to-mouth intake. Dermal absorption (ii) occurs through exposed skin, while soil is inhaled (iii) both by mouth and nose during breathing. Particles <10 µm (PM_{10}) are the more relevant in this process, although larger fractions of inhaled soil are, probably, decomposed in the gastrointestinal track. It is assumed that all contaminants are absorbed, both by the gastrointestinal tract or the lung [72]. Equations (5)–(7) were used to estimate the chronic daily intake of each exposure route considered [28,69,70,73], supplemented by specific quantitative information (Table 3):

$$CDI_{\text{ing}} = C_{\text{soil}} \times \frac{\text{Ing}R \times EF \times ED}{BW \times AT} \times 10^{-6} \quad (5)$$

$$CDI_{\text{drm}} = C_{\text{soil}} \times \frac{SA \times SAF \times DA \times EF \times ED}{BW \times AT} \times 10^{-6} \quad (6)$$

$$CDI_{\text{inh}} = C_{\text{soil}} \times \frac{\text{Inh}R \times EF \times ED}{PEF \times BW \times AT} \quad (7)$$

Table 3. Variables for estimation of soil residential risk in the Panasqueira mining area.

Parameters	Meaning	Values		Reference
		Child	Adult	
ABS_{gi}	fraction of contaminant absorbed in gastrointestinal tract	Ag 0.04; As 1.00; Cd 0.025; Cu 1.00; W 1.00; Zn 1.00		[28]
ABS_{drm}	fraction of contaminant absorbed dermally from soil	As 0.03; Cd 0.001		[28]
AT_c (d)	averaging time for carcinogenic effects	$LT \times 365$		[73]
AT_{nc} (d)	averaging time for non-carcinogenic effects	$ED \times 365$		[73]
BW (kg)	average body weight	15	70	[69,72]
C_{soil} ($mg \cdot kg^{-1}$)	concentration of the element in soil	-		
DA	dermal absorption factor	0.03 for As; 0.001 for other		[28]
CDI_{ing} ($mg \cdot kg^{-1} \cdot d^{-1}$)	chronic daily intake dose through ingestion	-		Equation (5)
CDI_{drm} ($mg \cdot kg^{-1} \cdot d^{-1}$)	chronic daily intake through dermal contact	-		Equation (6)
CDI_{inh} ($mg \cdot m^{-3}$) (nc), ($\mu g \cdot m^{-3}$) (c)	chronic daily intake through inhalation	-		Equation (7)
CSF_{ing} ($(mg \cdot kg^{-1} \cdot d^{-1})^{-1}$)	chronic oral slope factor	As 1.50		[28]
CSF_{drm}	chronic dermal slope factor	CSF_{ing}/ABS_{gi}		[28]
ED (yr)	exposure duration	6	24	[73]
EF ($d \cdot yr^{-1}$)	exposure frequency	350 residents		[73]
ET ($h \cdot d^{-1}$)	exposure time	24 residents		[73]
Ing$R$ ($mg \cdot d^{-1}$)	soil ingestion rate	200	100	[73]
Inh$R$ ($m^3 \cdot d^{-1}$)	inhalation rate	7.6	20	[72]
IUR ($(\mu g \cdot m^{-3})^{-1}$)	chronic inhalation slope factor	As 4.3×10^{-3}; Cd 1.8×10^{-3}		[74]
LT (yr)	lifetime expected at birth	78 national		[75]
PEF ($m^3 \cdot kg^{-1}$)	particle emission factor	1.36×10^9		[73]
SA (cm^2)	exposed skin area	2800	5700	[73]
SAF ($mg \cdot cm^{-2}$)	skin adherence factor	0.2	0.07	[73]
RfD_{ing} ($mg \cdot kg^{-1} \cdot d^{-1}$)	chronic oral reference dose	Ag 5×10^{-3}; As 3×10^{-4}; Cd 1×10^{-3}; Cu 4×10^{-2}; Zn 0.3		[74]
RfD_{drm}	chronic dermal reference dose	$RfD_{ing} \times ABS_{gi}$		[28]
RfD_{inh} ($mg \cdot m^{-3}$)	chronic inhalation reference dose	As 1.5×10^{-5}; Cd 1×10^{-5}		[28]

The carcinogenic and non-carcinogenic side effects for each PTE were computed individually, as toxicity calculation uses different computational methods [76]. For each element and pathway, the non-cancer toxic risk was estimated by computing the Hazard Quotient (HQ, also known as non-cancer risk-Equation (8)) for systemic toxicity [73]. If HQ exceeds unity, it indicates that non-carcinogenic effects might occur. To estimate the overall developing hazard of non-carcinogenic effects, it is assumed that toxic risks have additive effects. Therefore, it is possible to calculate the cumulative non-carcinogenic hazard index (HI), which corresponds to the sum of HQ for each pathway (Equation (9)) [69,77]. Values of $HI < 1$ indicate that there is no significant risk of non-carcinogenic effects. While, values of HI > 1 imply that there is a probability of occurrence of non-carcinogenic effects, and are enhanced with increasing HI values [73]. The toxicity levels for each element were taken from The Risk Assessment

Information System (RAIS) [28]. The probability of an individual developing any type of cancer over a lifetime, as a result of exposure to the carcinogenic hazards, was computed for each pathway according to Equation (10) [78]. The carcinogenic risk was estimated by the sum of total cancer risk (Equation (11)). A cancer risk below 1×10^{-6} is considered insignificant. The result of 1×10^{-6} is classified as the carcinogenic target risk. If the cancer risk is above 1×10^{-4} it is qualified as unacceptable [69,79,80]:

$$HQ = \frac{CDI_{\text{pathway}}}{R_f D} \tag{8}$$

$$HI = \sum HQ = HQ_{\text{ing}} + HQ_{\text{drm}} + HQ_{\text{ihn}} \tag{9}$$

$$\text{Risk}_{\text{pathway}} = CDI_{\text{pathway}} \times CSF_{\text{pathway}} \tag{10}$$

$$\begin{aligned}\text{Risk} &= \sum \text{Risk}_{\text{pathway}} = \text{Risk}_{\text{ing}} + \text{Risk}_{\text{drm}} + \text{Risk}_{\text{ihn}} \\ &= CDI_{\text{ing}} \times CFS_{\text{ing}} + CDI_{\text{inh}} \times IUR + \frac{CDI_{\text{drm}} \times CSF_{\text{ing}}}{ABS_{\text{gi}}}\end{aligned} \tag{11}$$

Reference toxicity values were estimated as given in RAIS [28].

Spatial Estimation of extrapolated concentration values of chemical elements and contamination factors for the plotting of maps was based on geostatistics by extracting the necessary parameters for Ordinary Kriging from the variograms of each variable. Variograms were constructed and modelled with Surfer® (v. 8, Golden Software Inc, Golden, CO, USA), and the kriged estimations by Ordinary Kriging were also performed with Surfer®.

3. Results and Discussion

3.1. Distribution of Ag, As, Bi, Cd, Cu, W and Zn in Soil Samples

Previous studies carried out in the Panasqueira area [6,43,44], allowed, through the topsoil concentrations, the characterization of the anthropogenic soil contamination due to the presence of tailings and open air impoundments.

Descriptive statistical parameters (median and range) for pH, SOM, Ag, As, Bi, Cd, Cu, W and Zn are summarized in Table 4. The individual element values are compared with the corresponding local geochemical background levels, and also with reference values from the literature.

All samples, both topsoil and subsoil, have a pH lower than 7. In particular, topsoil pH values range from 3.2 to 6.6; 35.9% of topsoil samples have pH values between 3.0 and 4.0; 59.2% are between 4.0 and 5.0; 4.2% from 5.0 to 6.0, and 1.7% from 6.0 to 7.0, *i.e.*, generally very acid to acid according to the United States Department of Agriculture classification [81]. As shown in Figure 2 (pH (a)), it is possible to identify that the areas with higher values are located around the villages Barroca Grande, S. Francisco de Assis, Rio, Barroca, Dornelas do Zêzere and S. Martinho. Around Rio and Barroca Grande tailings, the soil pH is above the 75th percentile (<4.1). The subsoil pH ranges from 3.6 to 6.2: 23.0% of the subsoil samples have pH values between 3.0 and 4.0; 73.5% are between 4.0 and 5.0; 2.7% from 5.0 to 6.0, and 0.9% from 6.0 to 7.0, *i.e.*, also generally very acid to acid. The highest pH value found in subsoil samples was located in Rio village (Figure 2 pH (b)) on the north section of the Rio tailings. In the surroundings of S. Francisco de Assis, Barroca Grande and Dornelas do Zêzere villages, it is possible to identify some agricultural soil with pH > 4.6. Possibly these slightly higher pH values are due to land agricultural beneficiation techniques. Nevertheless, the soil of the present study area is overall classified as very acid to acid.

Figure 2. Spatial distribution of pH and soil organic matter (SOM, %) and Ag (mg kg^{-1}) for topsoil (**a**) and subsoil (**b**). Percentile class limits at P5, P10, P25, P50, P75, P90, P95 and P97.5. In blue are represented the main water courses, in grey the villages and in white the main tailings and dams. The green dashed lines represent the Ag background levels.

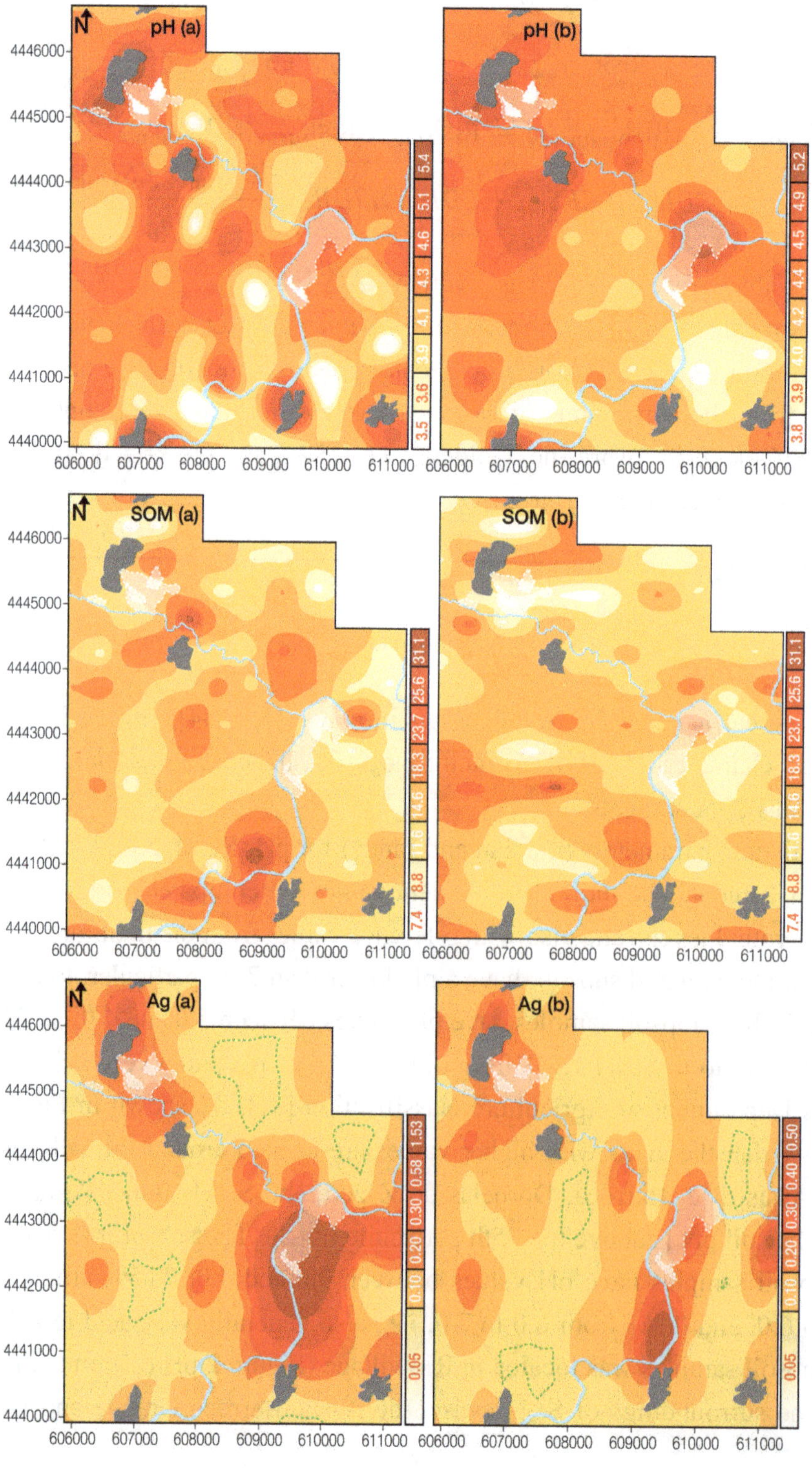

Table 4. Median, minimum and maximum concentrations values of topsoil and subsoil samples from Panasqueira mine and surrounding environment compared with international data. Casegas area, considered as representative of geochemical background (Bk).

Units		pH	SOM %	Ag $mg \cdot kg^{-1}$	As $mg \cdot kg^{-1}$	Bi $mg \cdot kg^{-1}$	Cd $mg \cdot kg^{-1}$	Cu $mg \cdot kg^{-1}$	W $mg \cdot kg^{-1}$	Zn $mg \cdot kg^{-1}$
Topsoil (n = 122)	**Median**	4.1	14.6	0.1	65	0.9	0.2	35	6	70
	Min–Max	3.2–6.6	5.7–39.0	0.05–1.7	17–1503	0.3–65	0.1–3	10–292	0.2–200	22–199
	Sk	1.59	1.2	4.72	6.98	9.21	3.77	4.80	5.40	1.38
Subsoil (n = 116)	**Median**	4.2	10.2	0.1	52	0.6	0.1	33	3	70
	Min–Max	3.6–6.2	3.6–19.5	0.1–0.6	8–350	0.2–15	0.1–1.5	12–146	0.1–29	16–192
	Sk	2.09	0.23	1.98	2.05	5.51	3.65	2.86	2.51	1.08
Geochemical background	**Topsoil**	4.2	14.5	0.1	63	0.8	0.20	34	4.4	68
	Subsoil	4.3	10.0	0.1	49	0.6	0.10	31	2.5	68
	Bk	3.98	10.5	0.05	22	0.3	0.01	28	0.4	58
Data from literature		6.0–8.0 [a]	1–20 [b]	0.07 [c]	11 [d]	0.3 [c]	0.1 [d]	16 [d]	1 [d]	55 [d]

Notes: SOM, soil organic matter; Sk, Skewness; Bk, background values, calculated according the [65] paradigm and confirmed by the [82] methods; [a] Ontario reference values [83]; [b] Normal Ranges in Soils [16,84,85]; [c] Mean World Soil [67,86]; [d] Median values for Portuguese Soil [87].

The topsoil SOM values range from 5.7% to 39.0% (see Table 4 and Figure 2 SOM (a)), while the subsoil SOM values vary from 3.6% to 19.5% (see Table 4 and Figure 2 SOM (b)). Comparing the topsoil and subsoil pH and SOM maps (Figure 2 and Table 4) is possible to observe that areas with the highest SOM values are related to areas with the lowest pH values.

To evaluate the presence of possible local anomalies the Ag (Figure 2), As, Bi, Cd (Figure 3), Cu, W, Zn (Figure 4) median and maximum values, observed in topsoil, were compared with the corresponding results in subsoil samples. Although the results tabulated in Table 4 show that Ag, As, Bi, Cu, W, and Zn present highest median and maximum values for topsoil when compared with subsoil, the paired samples t-test indicates that there are significant differences between soil samples at both depths for the elements As, Bi and W. Additionally, the results clearly show that there are higher contents in soil samples at both depths, when compared with the local geochemical background. The behavior of the topsoil element concentrations may reflect the influence of the Barroca Grande and Rio tailings and open air impoundments, possibly caused by aerial transport and deposition.

Topsoil samples, as shown in Table 5, have many strong to very strong correlation coefficients, *i.e.*, As/Ag, As/Bi, As, Cd, As/Cu, As/W, Ag/Bi, Ag/Cu, As/W, Bi/Cd, Bi/Cu, Bi/W, Cd/Cu, Cd/W, Cd/Zn, Cu/W. The strongest correlations are between Ag/Cu (0.94), As/Ag (0.90) and Bi/W (0.90). There is also a positive intermediate correlation (r = 0.31 to 0.70) between PTEs and pH. Several authors claim that heavy metal mobility holds a positive correlation with pH [18,88,89]. It is well known that pH affects heavy metal availability, since it is the major factor in controlling the ability of soil to retain heavy metals in an exchangeable form [21]. With low SOM the pH values may become relatively more important for the partitioning of metals. Most elements exhibit a weak negative correlation with SOM. For subsoil samples the PTEs correlation also presents some strong correlation coefficients (Table 5), but they are overall lower than in topsoil. The stronger correlations are between As/Bi (r = 0.75) and

Bi/Cu (r = 0.69). At this depth, pH is also the most significant soil property, presenting weak to intermediate positive correlations with the PTEs, except W.

Figure 3. Spatial distribution of As, Bi, Cd (mg·kg^{-1}) values for topsoil (**a**) and subsoil (**b**). Percentile class limits at P5, P10, P25, P50, P75, P90, P95 and P97.5. The green dashed lines represent the elements background levels. In blue are represented the main water courses, in grey the villages and in white the main tailings and dams.

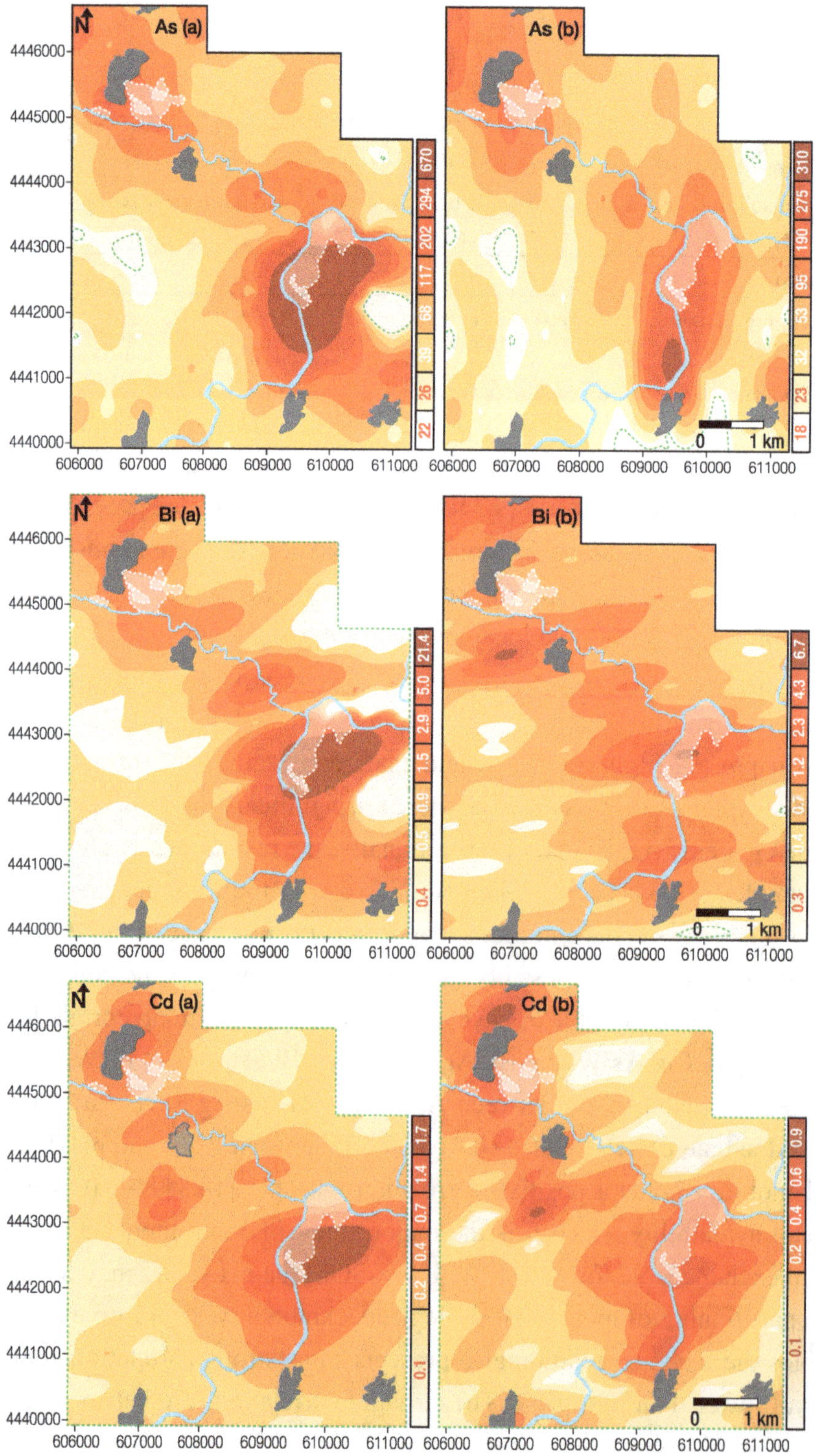

Figure 4. Spatial distribution of Cu, W, Zn (mg·kg^{-1}) values for topsoil (**a**) and subsoil (**b**). Percentile class limits at P5, P10, P25, P50, P75, P90, P95 and P97.5. The green dashed lines represent the elements background levels. In blue are represented the main water courses, in grey the villages and in white the main tailings and dams.

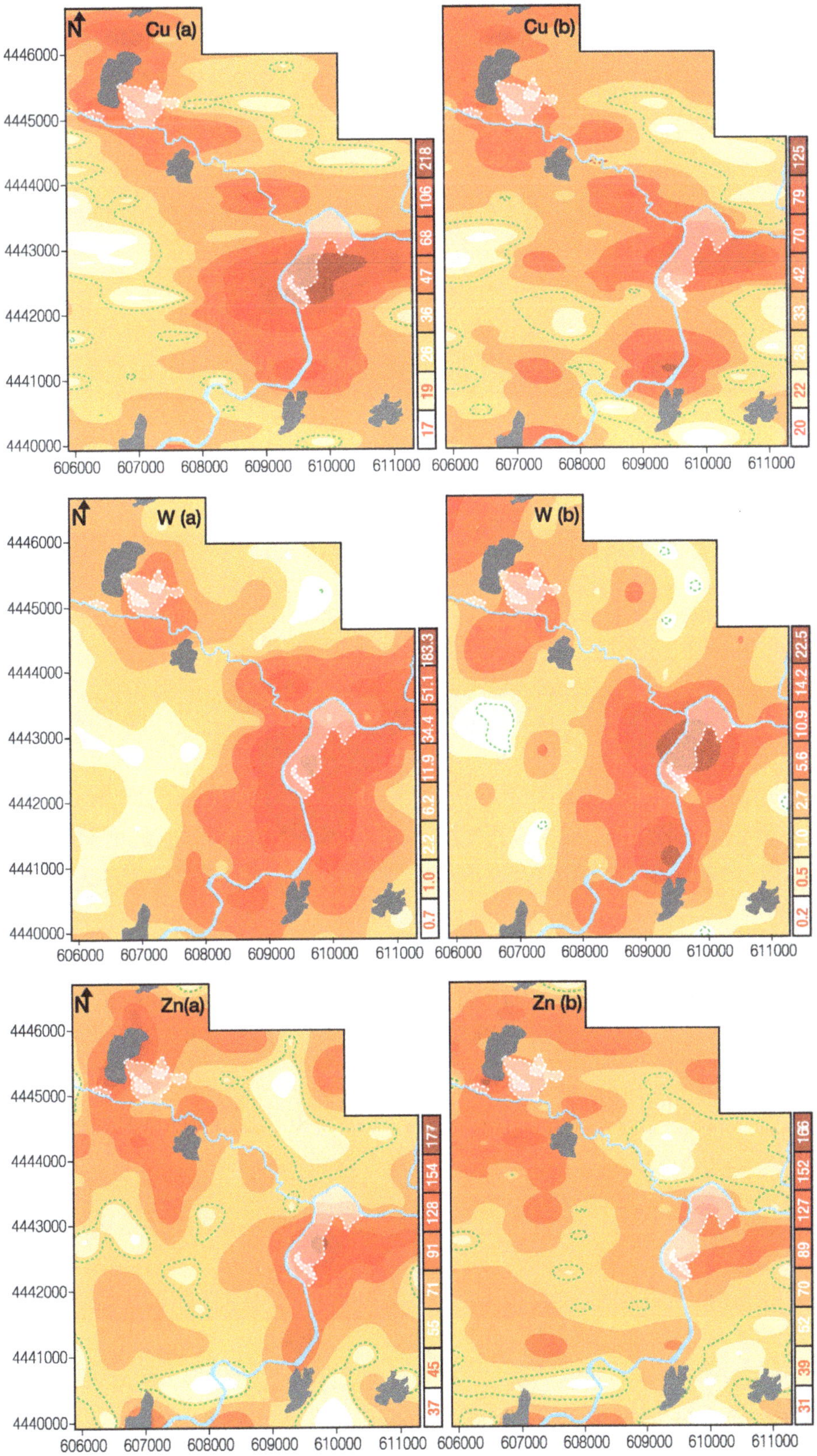

Table 5. Pearson's linear product-moment correlation coefficients for Ag, As, Bi, Cd, Cu, W, Zn, pH and SOM in topsoil (n = 122) and subsoil (n = 116) samples.

Var		Ag	As	Bi	Cd	Cu	W	Zn	pH	SOM
	Ag	1.00	**0.90** **	**0.84** **	**0.79** **	**0.94** **	**0.83** **	0.51 **	**0.70** **	−0.1
	As		1.00	**0.84** **	**0.77** **	**0.89** **	**0.81** **	0.44 **	0.37 **	−0.09
	Bi			1.00	**0.82** **	**0.87** **	**0.90** **	0.44 **	0.54 **	−0.14
	Cd				1.00	**0.86** **	**0.79** **	**0.68** **	0.42 **	−0.07
Topsoil	**Cu**					1.00	**0.80** **	**0.60** **	**0.61** **	−0.14
	W						1.00	0.38 **	0.46 **	0.01
	Zn							1.00	0.31 **	−0.15
	pH								1.00	−0.40 **
	SOM									1.00
	Ag	1.00	0.43 **	0.34 **	0.45 **	0.42 **	0.36 **	0.43 **	0.30 **	0.15
	As		1.00	**0.75** **	0.43 **	**0.59** **	0.49 **	0.30 **	0.09	−0.01
	Bi			1.00	0.50 **	**0.69** **	**0.56** **	0.35 **	0.04	−0.01
	Cd				1.00	**0.53** **	0.43 **	**0.57** **	0.17	−0.09
Subsoil	**Cu**					1.00	0.44 **	**0.56** **	0.11	−0.17
	W						1.00	0.14	−0.21 *	0.16
	Zn							1.00	0.45 **	−0.23 *
	pH								1.00	−0.35 *
	SOM									1.00

Notes: ** Correlation is significant at the 0.01 level (2-tailed); * Correlation is significant at the 0.05 level (2-tailed).

In order to identify the most important factor controlling the different PTEs spatial differences concentrations, a two-way ANOVA was performed [90]. In this study, two models were selected to group the variables, (a) depth-SOM and (b) depth-pH. The results of the test between dependent (PTEs) and independent (depth and SOM) variables (Table 6) showed that soil depth accounts for significant variations between the group means: Bi ($p = 0.035$), Cd ($p = 0.015$) and W ($p = 0.009$). The independent variable SOM shows significant variations in the concentration of As ($p = 0.021$), Bi ($p = 0.068$), W ($p = 0.013$) and Zn ($p = 0.021$). There is no significant interaction between depth and SOM. While the independent variable pH (Table 7) shows that there are significant variations with depth for most PTEs (Ag $p = 0.071$; As $p = 0.027$; Bi $p = 0.001$; Cd $p < 0.000$; W $p < 0.000$), except for Cu ($p = 0.371$). pH presents a significant variation for Ag ($p = 0.031$), W ($p = 0.001$) and Zn ($p < 0.001$). The interaction between pH*depth shows no significant variations ($p > 0.050$), except on the concentration of Cu ($p = 0.038$).

3.2. Quantitative Assessment of Soil Contamination

In this study, a simplified approach to assess soil contamination based on comparing the measured concentrations in the Panasqueira soil with the geochemical background values for Casegas was adopted. Table 8 shows the results of contamination factors (*CF*) and the modified degree of contamination (mC_d) for the selected elements in topsoil and subsoil, and also in Casegas soil.

Table 6. Two-way ANOVA results between the dependent (PTEs) and independent (depth, SOM) variables. PTEs were subjected to log-normal transformation (As, As, Cd, Cu, W and Zn with α = 0.050; Bi with α = 0.075).

Source of Variation	Dependent Variables	*df*	Mean Square	*F*	*p*-Value
Depth	Ag	1	0.223	1.624	0.204
	As	1	0.127	1.652	0.200
	Bi	1	0.333	4.484	**0.035**
	Cd	1	0.926	5.951	**0.015**
	Cu	1	0.012	0.483	0.488
	W	1	1.486	6.928	**0.009**
	Zn	1	0.062	1.933	0.166
SOM	Ag	1	0.010	0.076	0.783
	As	1	0.417	5.422	**0.021**
	Bi	1	0.251	3.371	0.068
	Cd	1	0.160	1.029	0.311
	Cu	1	0.007	0.275	0.601
	W	1	1.763	8.219	**0.005**
	Zn	1	0.173	5.372	**0.021**
Depth*SOM	Ag	1	0.051	0.373	0.542
	As	1	0.007	0.093	0.760
	Bi	1	0.001	0.008	0.928
	Cd	1	0.001	0.006	0.940
	Cu	1	0.037	1.52	0.219
	W	1	0.095	0.44	0.506
	Zn	1	0.002	0.06	0.811
Error	Ag	238	0.137	-	-
	As	215	0.077	-	-
	Bi	225	0.074	-	-
	Cd	233	0.156	-	-
	Cu	218	0.024	-	-
	W	215	0.215	-	-
	Zn	235	0.032	-	-

According the topsoil median values of the contamination factor, Bi, Cd and W present an extremely high degree of contamination, while Ag and As a high contamination factor. The results demonstrated that mC_d values vary from the minimum 1.2 in both topsoil and subsoil to the maximum of 150 in topsoil, with median values varying from 4 in subsoil to 6 in topsoil. The cumulative frequency distribution indicates that only 7.4% of the soil samples were classified as no to low degree of pollution, with mC_d values < 2.0, and the remaining soil samples (92.6%) registered moderate to ultra-high degree of pollution, with mC_d values equal or greater than 2.0 (27.9% between $2 \leq mC_d < 4$; 27.1% between $4 \leq mC_d < 8$; 19.7% between $8 \leq mC_d < 16$; 15.6% between $16 \leq mC_d < 32$ and 2.5% between $32 \leq mC_d$). The enrichment is more pronounced in topsoil (subsoil mC_d values ranged 1.2–26.4).

Table 7. Two-way ANOVA results between the dependent (PTEs) and independent (depth, pH) variables. PTEs were subjected to log-normal transformation (As, Bi, Cd, Cu, W, Zn with $\alpha = 0.050$; Ag with $\alpha = 0.075$).

Source of Variation	Dependent Variables	*df*	Mean Square	*F*	*p*-Value
Depth	**Ag**	1	0.353	3.296	**0.071**
	As	1	0.512	4.930	**0.027**
	Bi	1	0.832	10.605	**0.001**
	Cd	1	1.810	13.449	**0.000**
	Cu	1	0.019	0.805	0.371
	W	1	3.055	14.560	**0.000**
	Zn	1	0.007	0.266	0.607
pH	**Ag**	1	0.506	4.726	**0.031**
	As	1	0.031	0.301	0.584
	Bi	1	0.017	0.222	0.638
	Cd	1	0.020	0.146	0.703
	Cu	1	0.000	0.001	0.971
	W	1	2.315	11.033	**0.001**
	Zn	2	0.605	21.777	**0.000**
Depth*pH	**Ag**	1	0.116	1.085	0.299
	As	1	0.053	0.510	0.476
	Bi	1	0.082	1.040	0.309
	Cd	1	0.179	1.332	0.250
	Cu	1	0.104	4.351	**0.038**
	W	1	0.321	1.532	0.217
	Zn	2	0.077	2.769	0.065
Error	**Ag**	233	0.107	-	-
	As	230	0.104	-	-
	Bi	225	0.078	-	-
	Cd	226	0.135	-	-
	Cu	217	0.024	-	-
	W	213	0.210	-	-
	Zn	233	0.028	-	-

Table 8. Contamination Factors (*CF*) and Modified Degree of Contamination (mC_d) using geochemical background values. Casegas area is considered as representative of geochemical background.

Var		Ag_{CF}	As_{CF}	Bi_{CF}	Cd_{CF}	Cu_{CF}	W_{CF}	Zn_{CF}	mC_d
Bk	Min	1.0	0.4	0.7	1.0	0.6	0.1	0.3	0.7
	Med	1.0	1.0	1.0	1.0	1.0	1.1	1.0	1.4
	Max	8	5	9	30	6	26	2	13
Topsoil	Min	1.0	0.8	1.0	5.0	0.4	0.6	0.4	1.2
	Med	2	3	3	20	1.2	17	1.2	6
	Max	34	68	215	300	10	571	3	150
Subsoil	Min	1.0	0.4	0.7	5.0	0.4	0.1	0.3	1.2
	Med	2	2	2	10	1.1	8	1.2	4
	Max	12	16	51	150	5	84	3	26

Casegas is considered as an uncontaminated site, since it is outside the mine area and the influence of airborne polluted dust. The maximum mC_d value of 13.1, represents a very high contamination degree, which is mostly due to the Cd and W contamination factors. In this case, however, the high mC_d value is most likely due to geogenic sources, as this is a naturally enriched and mineralized zone.

The calculated mC_d values make possible the assessment of the spatial distribution of the modified degree of contamination. The first step is the determination of the spatial structure of the new variables, and the experimental variograms were used to model the data using exponential models, the extracted parameters are for topsoil: main direction = 90°; Nugget effect (C_0) = 30; Sill-Nugget effect (C_1) = 330; range of influence (length) = 1200 m; anisotropy ratio = 1.81; and for subsoil: main direction = 90°; C_0 = 0; C_1 = 19; length = 900 m; anisotropy ratio = 2.90. Estimation of the spatial distribution was then achieved by Ordinary Kriging and the respective map plotted. In Figure 5 it is possible to observe the mC_d spatial distribution revealing areas with very high values.

Figure 5 shows that soil samples collected near the Barroca Grande tailings (A), Rio tailings (C) and the mud impoundments stand out clearly, because the soil is enriched in Ag, As, Bi, Cd, Cu, W and Zn; all soil samples from both depths taken from Barroca Grande exceed the As, Bi, Cd and W baseline values for Portugal, while at Rio only Zn in some samples (25%) has concentrations that are lower than the guide value. According to [42], the Barroca Grande tailings and open impoundments have high As, Cd, Cu, Pb, W, and Zn concentrations (mean content in the more coarse tailings material As = 7142 $mg{\cdot}kg^{-1}$; Cd = 56 $mg{\cdot}kg^{-1}$; Cu = 2501 $mg{\cdot}kg^{-1}$; Pb = 172 $mg{\cdot}kg^{-1}$; Sn = 679 $mg{\cdot}kg^{-1}$; W = 5400 $mg{\cdot}kg^{-1}$ and Zn = 1689 $mg{\cdot}kg^{-1}$ and mean content in the impoundment material (rejected from the mill operations) As = 44,252 $mg{\cdot}kg^{-1}$; Cd = 491 $mg{\cdot}kg^{-1}$; Cu = 4029 $mg{\cdot}kg^{-1}$; Pb = 166 $mg{\cdot}kg^{-1}$; Sn = 454 $mg{\cdot}kg^{-1}$; W = 3380 $mg{\cdot}kg^{-1}$ and Zn = 3738 $mg{\cdot}kg^{-1}$). The mineralogy of these tailings consists of mainly quartz, muscovite, kaolinite, illite-montmorillonite, montmorillonite-vermiculite, and chlorite, and also arsenopyrite, wolframite, and natrojarosite.

Figure 5. Spatial distribution of the modified degree of Contamination (mC_d) for topsoil (**a**) and subsoil (**b**). Values were estimated on the basis of the concentration factors of Ag, As, Bi, Cd, Cu, W and Zn (A, Barroca Grande; B, S. Francisco de Assis; C, Rio).

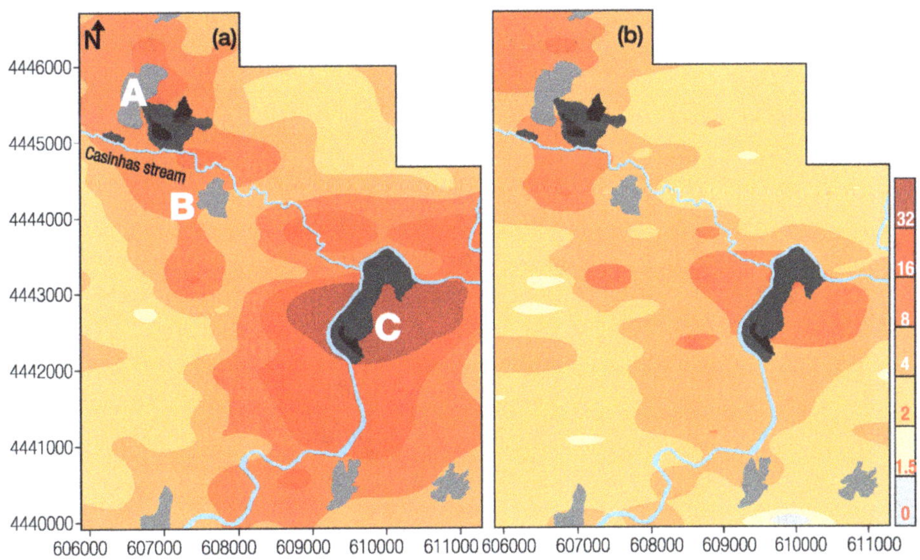

The dams at Barroca Grande may pose a significant potential threat, due to the fine-grained nature of the materials, and their location with respect to the Casinhas stream that cross S. Francisco de Assis village. The X-Ray Diffraction (XRD) analysis of the impoundment material revealed the presence of scorodite, arsenopyrite, quartz, sphalerite, hematite, and muscovite. These tailings and impoundment material are metal-enriched at such a level, likely to be toxic to the ecosystem [42]. The concentrations exceed the values defined for the 90th percentile of the South Portuguese Zone (As 157 $mg \cdot kg^{-1}$; Cu 108 $mg \cdot kg^{-1}$; Ni 62 $mg \cdot kg^{-1}$; Pb 117 $mg \cdot kg^{-1}$; Zn 134 $mg \cdot kg^{-1}$), which is indicative of enrichment in trace metals. This Ag-As-Bi-Cd-Cu-W-Zn association is quite logical and is linked to the Panasqueira ore-paragenetic association. The highest mC_d values identified near Barroca Grande (A), São Francisco de Assis (B) and Rio (C) confirms that mechanical and chemical dispersion from Barroca Grande and Rio tailings and mud impoundments occurs. Most of the samples (90% or higher of total samples) collected from Barroca Grande (A), São Francisco de Assis (B) and Rio (C) villages, exhibit mC_d values >8.0, clearly indicting a very high degree of contamination.

The Panasqueira tailings impoundments have been and are affected by surface water flows (from heavy rainfall events) that have eroded the tailings from their original location and transported the materials downstream to residential areas (namely to S. Francisco de Assis). However, the superficial flat of the tailings have dried and are susceptible to wind erosion. The relative rates of water and wind erosion and transport, in Barroca Grande, São Francisco de Assis and Rio, suggest that wind processes have similar, and in many cases greater, impact on loss and local redistribution of soil in ecosystems than an eventual erosional soil enrichment.

3.3. Potential Ecological Risk Factor and Risk Index

The topsoil and subsoil samples results for individual element potential pollution factor (*EF*) and potential ecological risk (*PERI*) are presented in Table 9. For both soil sample depths, As, Cu and Zn show a low potential ecological risk, with median values <40 (see Table 2). Tungsten also exhibits a low risk in subsoil, but a high risk in topsoil, while Bi and Ag show a moderate risk at both depths. Cadmium presents a very high ecological risk in topsoil and a high risk on subsoil. Using the median values, the topsoil risk factor is ranked as: Cd > W > Ag > Bi > As >> Cu > Zn, while for subsoil the ranking is: Cd > Ag > Bi > As > Cu = W > Zn. These results suggest a very high environmental risk, especially for Cd.

In order to estimate the global potential ecological risk in the study area, the PERI was computed. The median values classify soil samples at both depths with a very high risk (Table 9). The cumulative analysis shows that the soil samples at both depths do not display a low risk index (<150), and only 7.4% of topsoil present a moderate risk index. *PERI* classified 92.6% of topsoil samples as high to very high ecological risk. The same occurs for 61.2% of subsoil samples, which should be considered as an extensive hazard. Figure 6 displays the *PERI* spatial distribution. Topsoil has a wide area classified with a very high ecological risk, which is consistent with the wind direction, the water courses and the actual and previous exploration and beneficiation locations (Figure 6a). Subsoil also presents a very high risk index in the same topsoil areas, but with smaller area expression. These results are consistent with those mapped by the individual elements, Ag, As, Bi, Cd, Cu, W and Zn (Figures 2–4), and the modified degree of contamination (mC_d; Figure 5), with the same affected areas.

Table 9. Statistical results of the single element potential pollution factor (*EF*) and potential ecological risk (*PERI*) for topsoil and subsoil samples.

Var		Ag_{EF}	As_{EF}	Bi_{EF}	Cd_{EF}	Cu_{EF}	W_{EF}	Zn_{EF}	*PERI*
Topsoil	Min	120	4	20	150	1	9	0	224
	Mean	120	23	127	893	3	573	1	1,740
	Med	70	15	60	600	2	255	1	1,020
	Max	1,190	338	4,300	9,000	21	8,571	3	23,353
Subsoil	Min	30	4	10	125	2	2	0	173
	Mean	76	33	56	418	7	8	1	600
	Med	60	23	30	250	6	6	1	350
	Max	360	158	770	3,750	26	203	3	4,369

Figure 6. Spatial distribution of Potential Ecological Risk Index (*PERI*) for topsoil (**a**) and subsoil (**b**) in the study area.

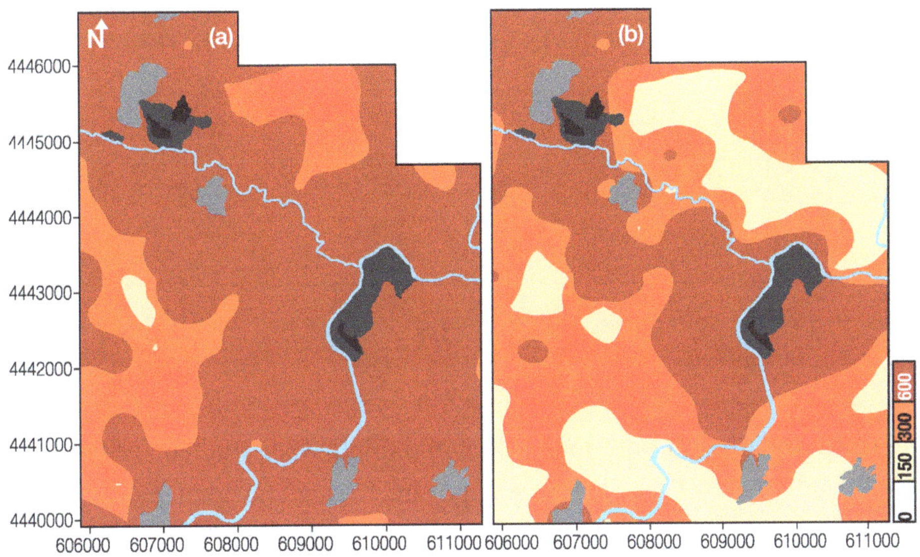

3.4. Human Health Risk Assessment

Both non-carcinogenic hazard (*HQ*) and carcinogenic risk ($Risk_{pathway}$) of topsoil in the Panasqueira mine and surrounding area, through the different pathways (ingestion, dermal and inhalation), were estimated according to the human health risk assessment model [28]. The cumulative hazard index (*HI*) and total risk ($Risk_{total}$) were also characterized for multi-pathway routes in resident population.

The non-carcinogenic effects considered the most conservative exposure condition—children (1–6 years old). The potentially toxic elements defined in this study (Ag, Cd, Cu, W and Zn), apart from As, do not present a non-carcinogenic hazard for children in the Panasqueira area (maximum $HI_{child\text{-}Ag,Cd,Cu,W,Zn} \leq 0.37$). The As non-carcinogenic hazard median values, estimated for the different exposure routes were $HQ_{ing\text{-}As}$ (2.75) >> $HQ_{drm\text{-}As}$ (0.23) >> $HQ_{inh\text{-}As}$ (0.00). $HI_{child\text{-}As}$ values ranged between 0.78 and 69.50, with a median value of 2.98 ≈ $HQ_{ing\text{-}As}$ (2.70), due to the ingestion hazard quotient ranging between 0.72 and 64.10. These results (<1—safe level) indicate that there is a cause for concern for the non-cancer health effects for children living in the Panasqueira study area, mainly due to As oral ingestion, with $HQ_{ing\text{-}As}$ showing median values above one (Figure 7).

Figure 7. Comparative boxplot distribution of the Non-carcinogenic Hazard Quotient for children of As for Ingestion (HQ_{ingAs}), Inhalation (HQ_{ihnAs}), Dermal contact (HQ_{drmAs}) routes, the Cumulative Hazard Index (HI_{As}) and the sum of the Non-carcinogenic Hazard Quotient of the other defined PTEs (Ag, Cd, Cu, W and Zn) for Ingestion ($HQ_{ingPTE(-As)}$), Inhalation ($HQ_{ihnPTE(-As)}$), Dermal contact ($HQ_{drmPTE(-As)}$) routes and the Cumulative Hazard Index ($HI_{PTE(-As)}$) for topsoil samples (tailing samples were removed) in the Panasqueira area. The extremes and outliers were removed.

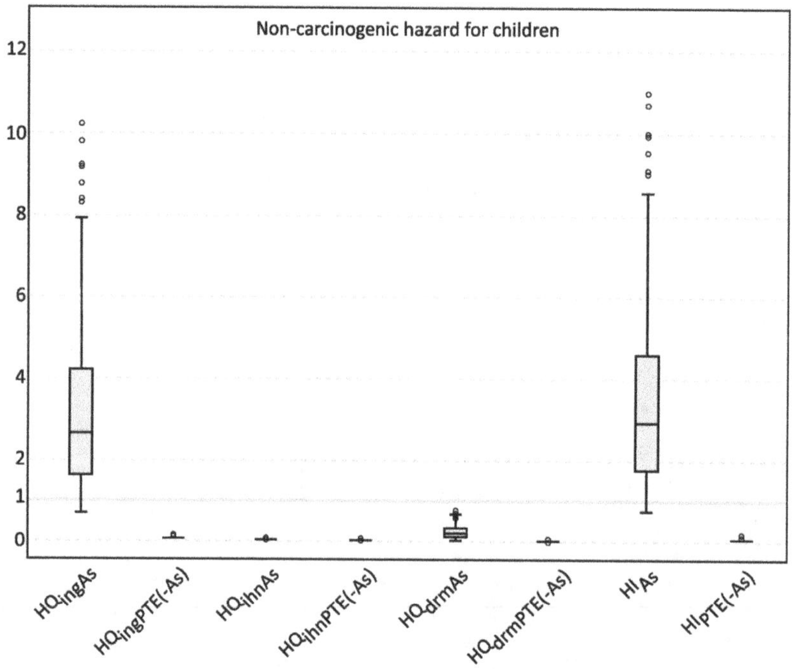

The carcinogenic risks adjusted both to children and adult were studied for the identified PTEs in this study. The median values of the different exposure routes and total risk were estimated. Their mean distribution were $Risk_{total}$ (2.62×10^{4}) ≈ $Risk_{As}$ (2.62×10^{-4}) ≈ $Risk_{ing}$ (2.39×10^{-4}) ≈ $Risk_{ingAs}$ (2.39×10^{-4}) >> $Risk_{drm}$ (2.26×10^{-5}) ≈ $Risk_{drmAs}$ (2.26×10^{-5}) >> $Risk_{inh}$ (1.32×10^{-7}) ≈ $Risk_{inhAs}$ (1.32×10^{-7}) (Figure 8). The high significance of As to cumulative carcinogenic elements risk is due to the very low risk displayed by the other elements. Furthermore, the representation of the exposure routes are distributed as: (a) $Risk_{ing}$ ≈ $Risk_{ingAs}$ ranged 3.97×10^{-5}–3.53×10^{-3}, with a median value of 1.52×10^{-4}; (b) $Risk_{drm}$ ≈ $Risk_{drmAs}$ ranged 3.76×10^{-6}–3.34×10^{-4}, with median value of 1.44×10^{-5}; and (c) $Risk_{inh}$ ≈ $Risk_{inhAs}$ ranged 2.21×10^{-8}–1.96×10^{-6}, with median value of 8.38×10^{-8}. The cumulative pathway $Risk_{total}$ ≈ $Risk_{As}$ ranged 4.35×10^{-5}–3.87×10^{-3}, with a median $Risk_{total}$ of 1.66×10^{-4} mostly due to $Risk_{ingAs}$. Intake of As may cause cancer in several human organs through ingestion, and lung and skin cancer through inhalation [28]. Moreover, the $Risk_{ing}$ represents 91.29% of cumulative risk from exposure routes, while $Risk_{drm}$ (8.69%) and $Risk_{inh}$ (0.05%) have less significance. Similar results were obtained in other studies [77,91–94]. The cumulative median $Risk_{drm}$ is > 1×10^{-6} for all samples, of which 69.67% > 1×10^{-5}, and the cumulative exposure route median $Risk_{ing}$ is > 1×10^{-5} for all samples, being 72.13% > 1×10^{-4}. These results show that there is a very high As ingestion cancer risk. The samples with higher hazard are located in and around the villages of the study area, being the more representative results found nearby the large tailing piles and open air impoundments (Figure 9). Although the median $Risk_{drm}$ value is lower and between 1×10^{-6} and 1×10^{-4}, and is considered as acceptable, it cannot, however, be negligible in the Panasqueira mining area, once all samples exceed the target value (1×10^{-6}). While the sum of exposure pathways is $Risk_{Cd} = 1.09 \times 10^{-10}$ ($<1 \times 10^{-6}$), it should be noted that it is the cumulative toxic metal and kidney index that is the main target for Cd toxicity [26,95].

Figure 8. Comparative boxplot distribution of the Carcinogenic Risk adjusted to both children and adult for total PTEs (Ag, As, Cd, Cu, W and Zn) for Ingestion ($Risk_{ing}$), Inhalation ($Risk_{inh}$), Dermal contact ($Risk_{drm}$) routes, the Cumulative Risk ($Risk_{total}$) and the Carcinogenic Risk of As for Ingestion ($Risk_{ingAs}$), Inhalation ($Risk_{inhAs}$), Dermal ($Risk_{drmAs}$) routes and the Cumulative Risk ($Risk_{As}$) for topsoil samples (tailing samples were removed) of the Panasqueira area. The extremes and outliers were removed.

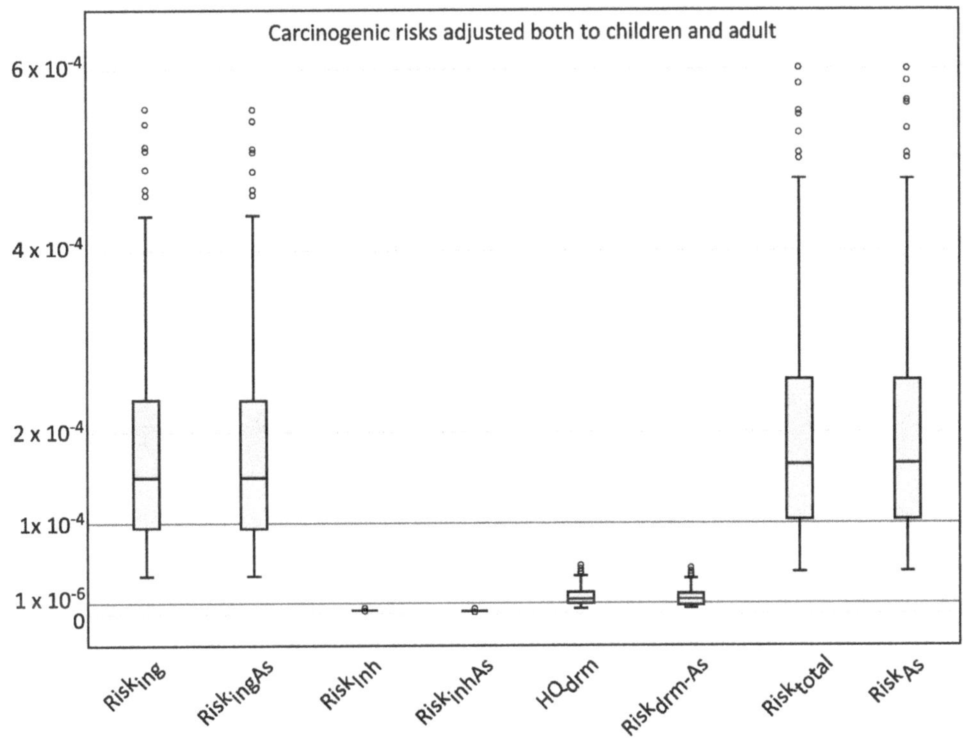

As the risk analyses showed that ingestion is the most important pathway, further studies should be carried out in order to estimate the metal bioaccessibility in human receptors, such as a simplified *in vitro* physiologically based extraction test (PBET), allowing the estimation of the percentage of the bioaccessible orally ingested fraction of each metal from soil samples [77,80,96]. Additional investigations must be made on different sample media, such as vegetables, rhizosphere, irrigation and drinking water and street dust in the local villages under influence of mining activities (such as S. Francisco de Assis and Barroca) and also in non-exposed villages considered as reference areas (such as Casegas and Unhais-o-Velho). These studies will provide the necessary data and information for the determination of the influence of the Panasqueira mine activities, through more than 110 years, on the surrounding population, and should be complemented by biological studies [97].

Figure 9. Spatial distribution of the Carcinogenic risk adjusted for both children and adult considering (**a**) ingestion; (**b**) dermal contact; (**c**) inhalation routes; and (**d**) the cumulative Risk.

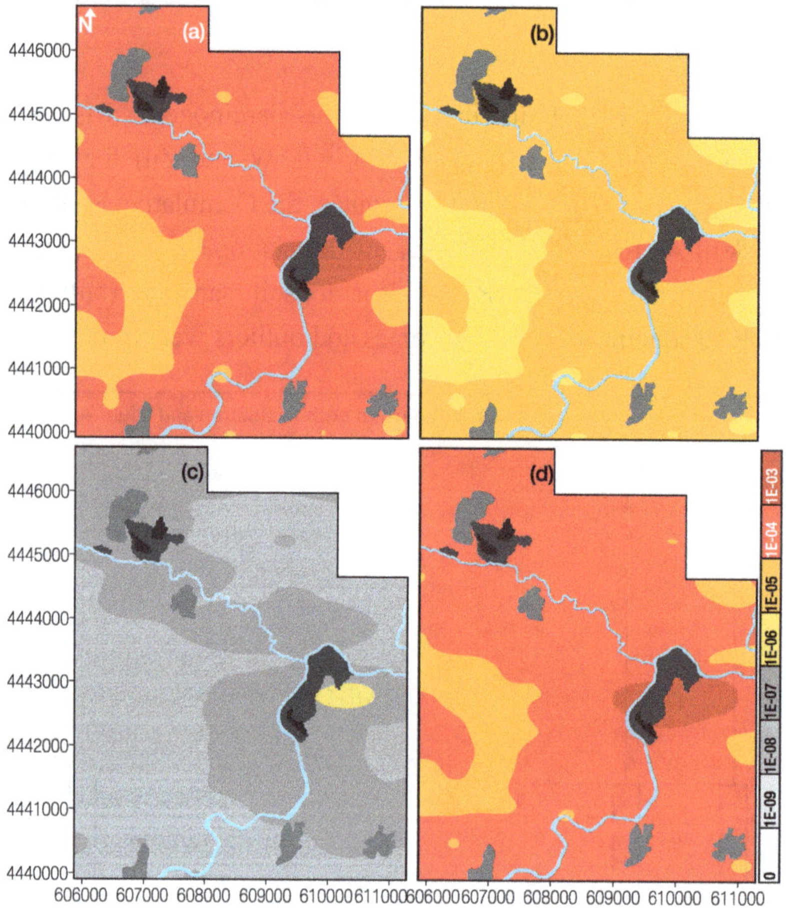

4. Conclusions

The mining and beneficiation process generates huge quantities of waste materials from the ore extraction and milling operations, which accumulate in tailings and open impoundments and are largely responsible for the high levels of metals(loid)s released into the surrounding environment. At the Panasqueira mine, the mining activities have produced sulphide-rich mine wastes that are responsible for the high levels of metals at Barroca Grande and Rio tailings. The oxidation of these sulphides may give rise to the mobilization and migration of trace metals from the mining wastes into the soil. Heavy metal soil contamination is an outstanding example of environmental risk. Metal(loid)s, such as As, Cd or Pb, for example, are toxic for humans, as well as for animals, and can even lead to death if ingested in large doses, or over large periods of time. Exposure to hazardous elements may have different pathways, such as ingestion, dermal absorption and inhalation of soil particles present in the air.

Collection of surface soil permits the characterization of anthropogenic contamination, caused by the presence of tailings and open air impoundments. Such soil, classified globally as very acid to acid, occurs in areas with very low soil pH values, which are related to areas with the highest SOM values. The metal assemblage identified in these soil types (Ag, As, Bi, Cd, Cu, W and Zn) show highest values in topsoil samples (0–15 cm), when compared with the values of the corresponding subsoil samples below 15 cm depth. Soil samples from both depths have higher contents when compared to the estimated local geochemical background. These results show the influence of the metal-rich mine wastes, stored in Barroca Grande and Rio tailings and in the open impoundments, as the main source of pollution of the surrounding environment, possibly due to aerial transport and deposition.

Very strong correlations were estimated between the PTEs and between PTEs and pH. The strongest correlations were Ag/Cu, As/Ag and Bi/W. The PTEs and pH positive correlation, confirm the findings of other studies that heavy metal mobility holds a positive correlation with pH, affecting their availability.

The ANOVA results, showed significant variations with depth, and the majority of the PTEs (Ag, As, Bi, Cd and W) and pH exhibit a significant variation for Ag, W and Zn.

According to the calculated contamination factor (*CF*) and the modified degree of contamination (mC_d), 7.4% of the soil samples were classified as having no to low degree of pollution with $mC_d < 2.0$ and 92.6% registered moderate to ultra-high degree of pollution with $mC_d \geq 2.0$. The spatial distribution of the mC_d reveals areas with a very high degree of contamination. The highest mC_d values were identified near Barroca Grande, São Francisco de Assis and Rio, and confirm the mechanical and chemical dispersion from tailings.

The risk factor estimated for individual element potential pollution factor and potential ecological risk, revealed at both soil sample depths that As, Cu and Zn have a low potential ecological risk, W low risk in subsoil, but a very high risk in topsoil samples; Ag moderate to considerable ecological risk and Cd is the worst element, exhibiting a very high environmental risk. The estimated potential ecological risk (*PERI*) classifies samples from both depths with a very high risk. In the *PERI* spatial distribution, topsoil has a wide area classified with a very high ecological risk, consistent with wind direction, water courses and current and previous exploration and beneficiation locations.

The non-carcinogenic hazard effects, determined for children (1–6 years old), indicated that the PTEs (Ag, Cd, Cu, W and Zn) do not present a non-carcinogenic hazard for children, while the As value is high, representing a risk for the non-cancer health effects for children in the Panasqueira area. The carcinogenic risk for both children and adults, revealed a very high cancer risk due to As ingestion, which may cause cancer to several human organs cancer through ingestion, and lung and skin cancer through inhalation.

Further studies should be carried out in order to estimate the metal bioaccessibility in human receptors.

Acknowledgments

This research is financially supported by FCT—Fundação para a Ciência e a Tecnologia (grants SFRH/BD/63349/2009).

Author Contributions

The original idea of the study was designed on a brainstorm meeting by all authors. E. Ferreira da Silva and J. P. Teixeira were responsible for recruitment and follow-up of study participants. All authors participated on the field work. C. Candeias and P. F. Ávila were responsible for data cleaning and analyses. C. Candeias drafted the manuscript with collaboration of all authors and it was revised by all. All authors read and approved the final manuscript.

References

1. Cohen, R.R.H.; Gorman, J. Mining-related nonpoint-source pollution. *Water Environ. Technol.* **1991**, *3*, 55–59.
2. Merson, J. Mining with microbes. *N. Sci.* **1992**, *133*, 9–17.
3. Evangelou, V.P.B.; Zhang, Y.L. A review: Pyrite oxidation mechanisms and acid mine drainage prevention. *Crit. Rev. Environ. Sci. Technol.* **1995**, *25*, 141–199.
4. Larocque, A.C.L.; Rasmussen, P.E. An overview of trace metals in the environment, from mobilization to remediation. *Environ. Geol.* **1998**, *33*, 85–91.
5. Soucek, D.J.; Cherry, D.S.; Currie, R.J. Laboratory to field validation in an integrative assessment of an acid mine drainage-impacted watershed. *Environ. Toxicol. Chem.* **2000**, *19*, 1036–1043.
6. Candeias, C. Modelling the Impact of Panasqueira Mine in the Ecosystems and Human Health: A Multidisciplinar Approach. Ph.D. Thesis, Aveiro University/Porto University, Aveiro, Portugal, 2013.
7. Rasmussen, P.E. Long-range atmospheric transport of trace metals: The need for geosciences perspectives. *Environ. Geol.* **1998**, *33*, 96–108.
8. Yukselen, M.A.; Alpaslan, B. Leaching of metals from soil contaminated by mining activities. *J. Hazard Mater.* **2001**, *87*, 289–300.
9. Chen, X.; Wright, J.V.; Conca, J.L.; Peurrung, L.M. Evaluation of heavy metal remediation using mineral apatite. *Water Air Soil Pollut.* **1997**, *98*, 57–78.
10. Bosso, S.T.; Enzweiler, J. Bioaccessible lead in soils, slag, and mine wastes from an abandoned mining district in Brazil. *Environ. Geochem. Health* **2008**, *30*, 219–229.
11. Douay, F.; Pruvot, C.; Roussel, H.; Ciesielski, H.; Fourrier, H.; Proix, N.; Waterlot, C. Contamination of urban soils in an area of Northern France polluted by dust emissions of two smelters. *Water Air Soil Pollut.* **2008**, *188*, 247–260.
12. Roussel, H.; Waterlot, C.; Pelfrêne, A.; Pruvot, C.; Mazzuca, M.; Douay, F. Cd, Pb and Zn Oral Bioaccessibility of urban soils contaminated in the past by atmospheric emissions from two lead and zinc smelters. *Arch. Environ. Contam. Toxicol.* **2010**, *58*, 945–954.
13. Juhasz, A.L.; Weber, J.; Smith, E. Impact of soil particle size and bioaccessibility on children and adult lead. *J. Hazard Mater.* **2011**, *186*, 1870–1879.
14. Ettler, V.; Kribek, B.; Majer, V.; Knesl, I.; Mihaljevic, I. Differences in the bioaccessibility of metals/metalloids in soils from mining smelting areas (Copperbelt, Zambia). *J. Geochem. Explor.* **2012**, *113*, 68–75.
15. Banza, C.L.N.; Nawrot, T.S.; Haufroid, V.; Decre, S.; de Putter, T.; Smolders, E.; Kabyla, B.I.; Luboya, O.N.; Ilunga, A.N.; Mutombo, A.M.; *et al.* High human exposure to cobalt and other metals in Katanga, a mining area of the Democratic Republic of Congo. *Environ. Res.* **2009**, *109*, 745–752.

16. Radojevic, M.; Bashki, V.N. *Practical Environmental Analysis*; The Royal Society of Chemistry: Cambridge, UK, 2006.
17. Krishnamurti, G.S.R.; Huang, P.M.; Kozak, L.M. Sorption and desorption kinetics of cadmium from soils: Influence of phosphate. *Soil Sci.* **1999**, *164*, 888–898.
18. Antoniadis, V.; Robinson, J.S.; Alloway, B.J. Effects of short-term pH fluctuations on cadmium, nickel, lead, and zinc availability to ryegrass in a sewage sludge-amended field. *Chemosphere* **2008**, *71*, 759–764.
19. Mühlbachová, G.; Simon, T.; Pechová, M. The availability of Cd, Pb and Zn and their relationships with soil pH and microbial biomass in soils amended by natural clinoptilolite. *Plant Soil Environ.* **2005**, *51*, 26–33.
20. Zhao, K.L.; Liu, X.M.; Xu, J.M.; Selim, H.M. Heavy metal contaminations in a soil-rice system: Identification of spatial dependence in relation to soil properties of paddy fields. *J. Hazard Mater.* **2010**, *181*, 778–787.
21. Zeng, F.; Ali, S.; Zhang, H.; Ouyang, Y.; Qiu, B.; Wu, F.; Zhang, G. The influence of pH and organic matter content in paddy soil on heavy metal availability and their uptake by rice plants. *Environ. Pollut.* **2011**, *159*, 84–91.
22. Sukreeyapongse, O.; Holme, P.E.; Strobel, B.W.; Panichsakpatana, S.; Magid, J.; Hansen, H.C.B. pH-dependent release of cadmium, copper, and lead from natural and sludge-amended soils. *J. Environ. Qual.* **2002**, *31*, 1901–1909.
23. Oliver, D.P.; Tiller, K.G.; Connyers, M.K.; Sattery, W.J.; Alston, A.M.; Merry, R.H. Effectiveness of liming to minimise uptake of cadmium by wheat and barley grain grown in the field. *Aust. J. Agric. Res.* **1996**, *47*, 1181–1193.
24. Braillier, S.; Harrison, R.B.; Hennry, C.L.; Dogsen, X. Liming effects on availability of Cd, Cu, Ni and Zn in a soil amended with sewage sludge 16 years previously. *Water Air Soil Pollut.* **2006**, *86*, 195–206.
25. Du Laing, G.; Vanthuyne, D.R.J.; Vandecasteele, B.; Tack, F.M.G.; Verloo, M.G. Influence of hydrological regime on pore water metal concentrations in a contaminated sediment-derived soil. *Environ. Pollut.* **2007**, *147*, 615–625.
26. Zheng, N.; Liu, J.; Wang, Q.; Liang, Z. Health risk assessment of heavy metal exposure to street dust in the zinc smelting district, Northeast of China. *Sci. Total Environ.* **2010**, *408*, 726–733.
27. Mudgal, V.; Madaan, N.; Mudgal, A.; Singh, R.B.; Mishra, S. Effect of toxic metals on human health. *Open Nutraceuticals J.* **2010**, *3*, 94–99.
28. U.S. Department of Energy. *The Risk Assessment Information System (RAIS)*; U.S. Department of Energy's Oak Ridge Operations Office (ORO): Oak Ridge, TN, USA, 2013.
29. Agency for Toxic Substances and Disease Registry. Available online: http://www.atsdr.cdc.gov/ (accessed on 23 September 2014).
30. World Health Organization (WHO). Monographs-Analytical and Toxicological Data. In *Basic Analytical Toxicology*; World Health Organization: Geneva, Switzerland, 2013.
31. *National Drug Formulary of Ethiopia*; Drug Administration and Control Authority of Ethiopia (DACAE): Addis Ababa, Ethiopia, 2007.

32. Candeias, C.; Ferreira da Silva, E.; Ávila, P.F.; Salgueiro, A.R.; Teixeira, J.P. Integrated approach to assess the environmental impact of mining activities: Multivariate statistical analysis to estimate the spatial distribution of soil contamination in the Panasqueira mining area (Central Portugal). *Environ. Monit. Assess.* **2014**, in press.
33. Smith, M. Panasqueira the tungsten giant at 100+. *Oper. Focus. Int. Min.* **2006**, *33*, 10–14.
34. Thadeu, D. Geologia do couto mineiro da Panasqueira. *Comunicações dos Serviços Geológicos de Portugal* **1951**, *32*, 5–64. (In Portuguese)
35. Bloot, C.; de Wolf, L.C.M. Geological features of the Panasqueira tin-tungsten ore occurrence (Portugal). *Bol. Soc. Geol. Port.* **1953**, *11*, 1–58.
36. Kelly, W.C.; Rye, R.O. Geologic, fluid inclusion and stable isotope studies of the tin-tungsten deposits of Panasqueira, Portugal. *Econ. Geol.* **1979**, *74*, 1721–1822.
37. Polya, D.A. Chemistry of the main stage ore-forming fluids of the Panasqueira W-Cu(Ag)-Sn deposit, Portugal: Implications for models of ore genesis. *Econ. Geol.* **1989**, *84*, 1134–1152.
38. Noronha, F.; Dória, A.; Dubessy, J.; Charoy, B. Characterisation and timing of the different types of fluids present in the barren and ore-veins of the W-Sn deposit of Panasqueira, Central Portugal. *Miner. Deposita* **1992**, *27*, 72–79.
39. Correia, A.; Naique, R.A. Minas Panasqueira, 100 Years of Mining History. In Proceedings of the International Tungsten Industrial Association (ITIA) Conference, Salzburg, Austria, 20–22 October 1998.
40. Corrêa de Sá, A.; Naique, R.A.; Nobre, E. Minas da Panasqueira: 100 anos de História. *Bol. Minas* **1999**, *36*, 3–22. (In Portuguese)
41. *e-Ecorisk, A Regional Enterprise Network Decision-Support System for Environmental Risk and Disaster Management of Large-Scale Industrial Soils, Contract n.° EGV1-CT-2002-00068*; WP3–Case Study Site Characterization, Project Management Report for the Reporting Period, Deliverable 3.1; Joanneum Research Forschungsgeselfschaft—GMBH: Frohnleiten, Austria, 2007; not published.
42. Ávila, P.; Ferreira da Silva, E.; Salgueiro, A.; Farinha, J.A. Geochemistry and Mineralogy of Mill Tailings Impoundments from the Panasqueira Mine (Portugal): Implications for the Surrounding Environment. *Mine Water Environ.* **2008**, *27*, 210–224.
43. Ferreira da Silva, E.; Ávila, P.F.; Salgueiro, A.R.; Candeias, C.; Pereira, H.G. Quantitative–spatial assessment of soil contamination in S. Francisco de Assis due to mining activity of the Panasqueira mine (Portugal). *Environ. Sci. Pollut. Res.* **2013**, *20*, 7534–7549.
44. Candeias, C.; Melo, R.; Ávila, P.F.; Ferreira da Silva, E.; Salgueiro, A.R.; Teixeira, J.P. Heavy metal pollution in mine–soil–plant system in S. Francisco de Assis–Panasqueira mine (Portugal). *Appl. Geochem.* **2014**, *44*, 12–26.
45. Jaques Ribeiro, L.M.; Gonçalves, A.C.R. Contributo para o conhecimento geológico e geomorfológico da área envolvente do Couto Mineiro da Panasqueira. Centro de Estudos de Geografia e Ordenamento do Território. *Revista de Geografia e Ordenamento do Território* **2013**, *3*, 93–116. (In Portuguese)
46. *Atlas do Potencial Eólico para Portugal Continental*, Version 1.0 [CD-ROM]; ISBN 972-676-196-4; Instituto Nacional de Engenharia, Tecnologia e Inovação I.P. (INETI): Lisboa, Portugal, 2004. (In Portuguese)

47. Reis, A.C. As Minas da Panasqueira. *Bol. Minas* **1971**, *8*, 3–34. (In Portuguese)
48. Costa, P.; Estanqueiro, A. Development and Validation of the Portuguese Wind Atlas. In Proceedings of the European Wind Energy Conference, Athens, Greece, 27 February–2 March 2006.
49. Costa, P.; Estanqueiro, A. Building a Wind Atlas for Mainland Portugal Using a Weather Type Classification. In Proceedings of the European Wind Energy Conference, Athens, Greece, 27 February–2 March 2006.
50. Costa, P.A.S. Atlas do Potencial eólico para Portugal Continental. Master's Thesis, University of Lisbon, Lisboa, Portugal, 2004. (In Portuguese)
51. Turner, A.P. The responses of plants to heavy metals. In *Toxic Metals in Soil-Plant Systems*; Sheila, M.R., Ed.; John Wiley & Sons: Hoboken, NJ, USA, 1994.
52. Mcbride, M.B.; Richards, B.; Steenhuis, T.; Russo, J.J.; Sauvé, S. Mobility and solubility of toxic metals and nutrients in soil fifteen years after sludge application. *Soil Sci.* **1997**, *162*, 487–500.
53. Van Reeuwijk, L.P. *Procedures for Soil Analysis*, 6th ed.; International Soil Reference and Information Centre: Wageningen, The Netherlands, 2002.
54. ISO 10390:1994 Soil; In *Soil Quality—Determination of pH*; International Organization for Standardization: Geneva, Switzerland, 1995.
55. Schnitzer, M.; Khan, S.U. *Substances in the Environment*; Marcel Dekker: New York, NY, USA, 1972.
56. Stevenson, F.J. *Humus Chemistry*; Wiley: New York, NY, USA, 1982.
57. Yin, Y.; Allen, H.E.; Huang, C.P.; Sparks, D.L.; Sanders, P.F. Kinetics of mercury (II): Adsorption and desorption on soil. *Environ. Sci. Technol.* **1997**, *31*, 496–503.
58. You, S.J.; Yin, Y.; Allen, H.E. Partitioning of organic matter in soils: Effects of pH and water soil ratio. *Sci. Total Environ.* **1999**, *227*, 155–160.
59. Zar, J.H. *Biostatistical Analysis*; Prentice Hall: New York, NY, USA, 1996.
60. Johnson, R.A.; Wichern, D.W. *Applied Multivariate Statistical Analysis*; Prentice-Hall: New York, NY, USA, 1998.
61. Corwin, D.L.; Lesh, S.M.; Oster, J.D.; Kaffka, S.R. Monitoring management-induced spatio-temporal changes in soil quality through soil sampling direct by apparent electrical conductivity. *Geoderma* **2006**, *131*, 369–387.
62. Hakanson, L. Ecological risk index for aquatic pollution control, a sedimentological approach. *Water Res.* **1980**, *14*, 975–1001.
63. Loska, K.; Wiechula, D.; Korus, I. Metal contamination of farming soils affected by industry. *Environ. Int.* **2004**, *30*, 159–165.
64. Liu, W.H.; Zhao, J.Z.; Ouyang, Z.Y.; Solderland, L.; Liu, G.H. Impacts of sewage irrigation on heavy metal distribution and contamination in Beijing, China. *Environ. Int.* **2005**, *32*, 805–812.
65. Tuckey, J.W. *Exploratory Data Analysis*; Addison Wesley: Boston, MA, USA, 1977.
66. Abrahim, G.M.S.; Parker, R.J. Assessment of heavy metal enrichment factors and the degree of contamination in marine sediments from Tamaki Estuary, Auckland, New Zealand. *Environ. Monit. Assess.* **2008**, *136*, 227–238.
67. Reimann, C.; Caritat, P. *Chemical Elements in the Environment: Factsheets for the Geochemist and Environmental Scientist*; Springer: Berlin, Germany, 1998.
68. Bowen, H.J.M. *Trace Elements in Biochemistry*; Academic Press: London, UK, 1966.

69. U.S. Environmental Protection Agency (USEPA). *Risk Assessment Guidance for Superfund, Volume I: Human Health Evaluation Manual*; EPA 540-1-89-002; U.S. Environmental Protection Agency: Washington, DC, USA, 1989.
70. U.S. Environmental Protection Agency (USEPA). *Soil Screening Guidance: Technical Background Document*; EPA 540-R-95-128; U.S. Environmental Protection Agency: Washington, DC, USA, 1996.
71. Linders, J.B.H.J. Risicobeoordelino voor de mens bij blootstelling aan stoffen: Uitgangspunten en veronderstellingen. In *Rapport/Rijksinstituut voor Volksgezondheid en Milieuhygiene (nr. 725201003)*; RIVM: Bilthoven, The Netherlands, 1990. (In Dutch)
72. Berg, R.V.D. *Human Exposure to Soil Contamination: A Qualitative and Quantitative Analysis towards Proposals for Human Toxicological Intervention Values (Partly Revised Edition)*; Report No. 725201011; National Institute for Public Health and the Environment: Bilthoven, The Netherlands, 1994.
73. U.S. Environmental Protection Agency (USEPA). *Risk Assessment Guidance for Superfund: Volume III–Part A, Process for Conducting Probabilistic Risk Assessment*; EPA 540-R-02-002; U.S. Environmental Protection Agency: Washington, DC, USA, 2001.
74. U.S. Environmental Protection Agency (USEPA). *Integrated Risk Information System (IRIS)*; U.S. Environmental Protection Agency: Washington, DC, USA, 2013.
75. INE. Portal do Instituto Nacional de Estatística—Statistics Portugal. Available online: http://www.ine.pt/ (accessed on 23 September 2014). (In Portuguese)
76. U.S. Environmental Protection Agency (USEPA). *Guidance for Evaluating the Oral Bioavailability of Metals in Soils for Use in Human Health Risk Assessment*; OSWER 9285.7-80; U.S. Environmental Protection Agency: Washington, DC, USA, 2007.
77. Luo, X.S.; Ding, J.; Xu, B.; Wang, Y.J.; Li, H.B.; Yu, S. Incorporating bioaccessibility into human health risk assessments of heavy metals in urban park soils. *Sci. Total Environ.* **2012**, *424*, 88–96.
78. Hu, X.; Zhang, Y.; Luo, J.; Wang, T.; Lian, H.; Ding, Z. Bioaccessibility and health risk of arsenic, mercury and other metals in urban street dusts from a mega-city, Nanjing, China. *Environ. Pollut.* **2011**, *159*, 1215–1221.
79. U.S. Environmental Protection Agency (USEPA). *Screening Levels (RSL) for Chemical Contaminants at Superfund Sites*; U.S. Environmental Protection Agency: Washington, DC, USA, 2013.
80. Luo, X.S.; Yu, S.; Li, X.D. The mobility, bioavailability, and human bioaccessibility of trace metals in urban soils of Hong Kong. *Appl. Geochem.* **2012**, *27*, 995–1004.
81. U.S. Department of Agriculture. Available online: http://www.nrcs.usda.gov (accessed on 23 September 2014).
82. Tidball, R.R.; Ebens, R.J. Regional geochemical baselines in soils of the Powder River Basin, Montana–Wyoming. In *Geology and Energy Resources of the Powder River*; 28th Annual Field Conference Guidebook; American Association of Petroleum Geologists (AAPG): Tulsa, OK, USA, 1976.
83. Ministry of the Environment. *Soil, Ground Water and Sediment Standards for the Use under Part XV.1 of the Environmental Protection Act*; Ministry of the Environment: Ottawa, Canada, 2011.

84. Fiedler, H.J.; Rösler, H.J. *Spurenelemente in der Umwelt*; Gustav Fischer Verlag: Jena, Germany, 2013. (In German)
85. Mench, M. Notions sur les éléments en traces pour une qualité des sols et des produits végétaux. *Purpan* **1993**, *166*, 118–127. (In French)
86. Deschamps, E.; Ciminelli, V.S.T.; Lange, F.T.; Matschullat, J.; Raue, B.; Schmidt, H. Soil and sediment geochemistry of the iron quadrangle, Brazil: The case of arsenic. *J. Soils Sediment.* **2002**, *2*, 216–222.
87. Ferreira, M.M.S.I. Dados Geoquímicos de Base de Solos de Portugal Continental, Utilizando Amostragem de Baixa Densidade. Ph.D. Thesis, University of Aveiro, Aveiro, Portugal, 2004. (In Portuguese)
88. Yuan, G.; Lavkulich, L.M. Sorption behavior of copper, zinc, and cadmium in response to simulated changes in soil properties. *Commun. Soil Sci. Plant Anal.* **1997**, *28*, 571–587.
89. Hettiarachchi, G.M.; Ryan, J.A.; Chaney, R.L.; La Fleur, C.M. Sorption and desorption of cadmium by different fractions of biosolids-amended soils. *J. Environ. Qual.* **2003**, *32*, 1684–1693.
90. Qishlaqi, A.; Moore, F. Statistical analysis of accumulation and sources of heavy metals occurrence in agricultural soils of Khoshk River Banks, Shiraz, Iran. *J. Agric. Environ. Sci.* **2007**, *2*, 565–573.
91. Chabukdhara, M.; Nema, A.K. Heavy metals assessment in urban soil around insutrial clusters in Ghaziabad, India: Probabilistic health risk approach. *Ecotoxicol. Environ. Saf.* **2013**, *87*, 57–64.
92. De Miguel, E.; Iribarren, I.; Chacón, E.; Ordoñez, A.; Charlesworth, S. Risk-based evaluation of the exposure of children to trace elements in playgrounds in Madrid (Spain). *Chemosphere* **2007**, *66*, 505–513.
93. Ferreira-Baptista, L.; de Miguel, E. Geochemistry and risk assessment of street dust in Luanda, Angola: A tropical urban environment. *Atmos. Environ.* **2005**, *39*, 4501–4512.
94. Dudka, S.; Miller, W.P. Permissible concentrations of arsenic and lead in soils based on risk assessment. *Water Air Soil Pollut.* **1999**, *113*, 127–132.
95. De Burbure, C.; Buchet, J.P.; Bernard, A.; Leroyer, A.; Nisse, C.; Haguenoer, J.M.; Bergamaschi, E.; Mutti, A. Biomarkers of renal effects in children and adults with low environmental exposure to heavy metals. *J. Toxicol. Environ. Health* **2003**, *66*, 783–798.
96. Drexler, J.W.; Brattin, W.J. An *in vitro* procedure for estimation of lead relative bioavailability: With validation. *Hum. Ecol. Risk Assess.* **2007**, *13*, 383–401.
97. Coelho, P.; Costa, S.; Costa, C.; Silva, S.; Walter, A.; Ranville, J.; Pastorinho, R.; Harrington, C.; Taylor, A.; Dall'Armi, V.; *et al.* Biomonitoring of several toxic metal(loid)s in different biological matrices from environmentally and occupationally exposed populations from Panasqueira mine area, Portugal. *Environ. Geochem. Health* **2013**, *36*, 255–269.

5

Impacts of Artisanal and Small-Scale Gold Mining (ASGM) on Environment and Human Health of Gorontalo Utara Regency, Gorontalo Province, Indonesia

Yayu Indriati Arifin [1,2,*], Masayuki Sakakibara [1,†] and Koichiro Sera [3,†]

[1] Graduate School of Science & Engineering, Ehime University, 2-5 Bunkyo-cho, Matsuyama 790-8577, Japan; E-Mail: sakakiba@sci.ehime-u.ac.jp

[2] Department of Geology, State University of Gorontalo, Jl. Jend. Sudirman No. 6 Kota Gorontalo, Gorontalo 96128, Indonesia

[3] Cyclotron Research Center, Iwate Medical University, 348-58 Tomegamori, Takizawa, Iwate 020-0173, Japan; E-Mail: ksera@iwate-med.ac.jp

† These authors contributed equally to this work.

* Author to whom correspondence should be addressed; E-Mail: yayu_arifin@ung.ac.id;

Academic Editors: Jose A. Centeno, Robert B. Finkelman and Olle Selinus

---

Abstract: Mercury concentrations in the environment (river sediments and fish) and in the hair of artisanal gold miners and inhabitants of the Gorontalo Utara Regency were determined in order to understand the status of contamination, sources and their impacts on human health. Mercury concentrations in the sediments along the Wubudu and Anggrek rivers are already above the tolerable level declared safe by the World Health Organization (WHO). Meanwhile, commonly consumed fish, such as snapper, have mercury levels above the threshold limit (0.5 μg/g). The mean mercury concentrations in the hair of a group of inhabitants from Anggrek and Sumalata are higher than those in hair from control group (the inhabitants of Monano, Tolinggula and Kwandang). The mean mercury concentration in the hair of female inhabitants is higher than that in the hair of male inhabitants in each group. Neurological examinations were performed on 44 participants of artisanal and small-scale gold mining (ASGM) miners and inhabitants of Anggrek and Sumalata. From the 12 investigated symptoms, four common symptoms were already observed among the participants, namely, bluish gums, Babinski reflex, labial reflex and tremor.

Keywords: mercury; ASGM; Gorontalo Utara Regency

1. Introduction

Indonesia is perhaps the world's second largest mercury emitter from artisanal and small-scale gold mining (ASGM) [1]. It is estimated that about 125 and 145 tons of mercury was emitted in 2000 and 2005, respectively [1,2]. Rapid growth of mercury emission may be related to intensive mining activities in existing ASGM sites and the opening of new ASGM sites. Sulawesi Island is home of ASGM sites with huge mercury emissions per year, with Poboya in Palu of central Sulawesi Province and Talawaan in Minahasa of North Sulawesi Province [3].

The Gorontalo Province of Northern Sulawesi, Indonesia, has several artisanal and small-scale gold mining (ASGM) sites in each Regency: (1) Pohuwato Regency: Gunung Pani and Bulontio; (2) Boalemo Regency: Bilato; (3) Bone Bolango Regency: Tulabolo; and (4) Gorontalo Utara Regency: Hulawa and Ilangata villages. The ASGM activities in the Hulawa village of the Sumalata subdistrict began in the 1970s, while the ASGM activities in Ilangata and the Ilangata Barat villages of the Anggrek subdistrict just started five years ago. Every year, approximately 572 kg of mercury contaminates the environment of the Gorontalo Utara Regency [4]. Yet, there is no report on the status of the environmental pollution related to the ASGM activities in the Gorontalo Utara Regency.

The mercury pollution in the environment (river sediment and fish) related to the ASGM activities in North Sulawesi is reported as baseline information in the subjects [5,6]. For a fish-eating community, such as the Gorontalo Utara inhabitants, data on mercury levels in fish are needed for determining the sources of mercury exposure in the human body [7–9]. Mercury contaminations and health assessments of miners and inhabitants from some ASGM sites in Indonesia, namely, Talawaan, Tatelu, Galangan and Sekotong, have been reported [3,10–13]. Mercury concentration in human hair is often used as a bioindicator of the mercury levels in the human body. Human hair is sampled for the determination of mercury levels in the human body. It has many advantages because it is easy to collect, handle, and analyze and can record the contamination history over a long period [14–16]. In addition to mercury, more than 40 elements have so far been detected in hair [17–19].

The health status of miners is mainly determined by following a standardized protocol performed by medical doctors. The relationships among the mercury in hair, habits, health status and localization of ASGM are often discussed [20,21]. Scalp hair analysis was used as the first step for a risk assessment of heavy metal exposure to the human body for people who are working and living in the vicinity of a mine area, outside of such an area and in a metropolitan city [12,22–26]. The advantages of using hair samples for monitoring the impact of environmental pollution on human health are reported elsewhere [27,28].

This study is aimed at determining the status of mercury contamination in people of the Gorontalo Utara Regency, those living near ASGM sites and others who are living in Gorontalo Utara. The possible sources of contamination will also be investigated. The health conditions of the miners and inhabitants living around the mining sites were investigated using a standard neurological examination protocol.

2. Experimental Section

2.1. Study Area

Samples were collected from five districts in the Gorontalo Utara Regency: Anggrek, Kwandang, Monano, Sumalata and Tolinggula (Figure 1). Geographically, Tolinggula, Sumalata, Monano, Anggrek and Kwandang are situated on hills and mountains along the coastline of the Gorontalo Utara Regency. Inhabitants of the Gorontalo Utara Regency mainly work as farmers and fishermen. Marine fish are commonly part of their diets, along with rice, corn and vegetables, which are also produced on the nearby hills alongside the coastline.

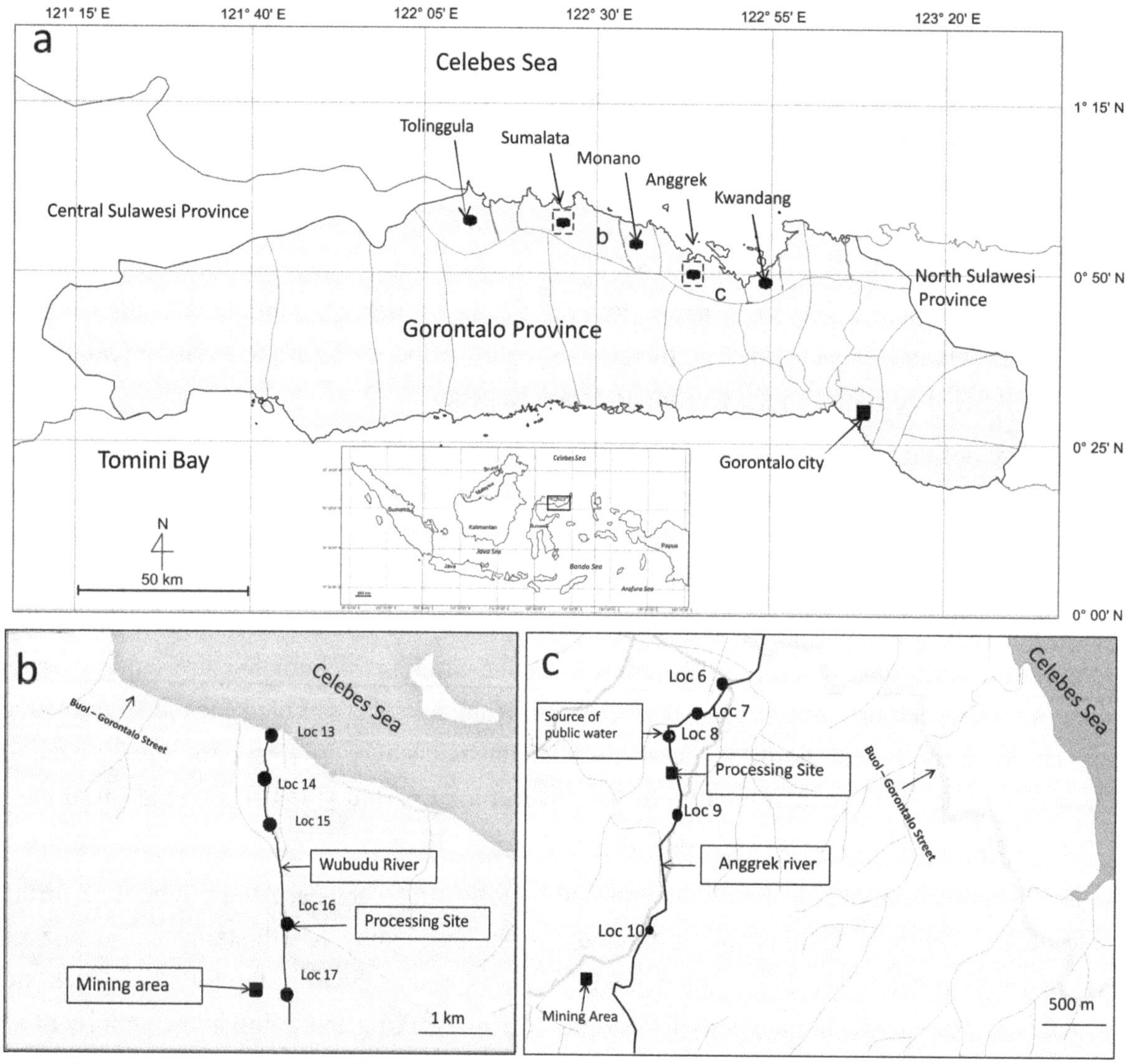

Figure 1. (**a**) Gorontalo Province map showing sampling locations (•) of human hair from Gorontalo Utara Regency, showing Tolinggula Sumalata, Anggrek, Monano and Kwandang districts. Location of Gorontalo Province in Indonesian map is shown (inset). The two rectangular shapes are ASGM locations and sampling sites for sediments and fishes; (**b**) Map of Sumalata gold mining site, showing locations (•) are sediment sampling sites and (**c**) map of Anggrek gold mining site, showing locations (•) are sediment sampling sites. Information on locations of ASGM ore extraction and processing sites are given in the text.

The ASGM activities in the Sumalata and Anggrek districts are located along the Wubudu and Anggrek riverbanks, respectively (Figure 1). Information on the locations, where a sediment sample was collected (locations 6, 7, 8, 9 and 10), is provided below. Some ASGM processing sites are close to locations 6, 7 and 8. There are no ASGM activities close to location 9, but between locations 9 and 10, there is a significant amount of ASGM activities on the river. Meanwhile, an ASGM ore extraction and processing site is close to location 10.

ASGM processing (panning and amalgamation) occurs on the estuary of the Wubudu River, close to location 13. On the Wubudu riverbank between locations 14 and 15, we found many ASGM ore processing sites. Many ASGM processing sites are found around location 16, while there is an ASGM ore extraction and processing site close to location 17. The activities may contaminate the environment, as well as the Wubudu and Anggrek rivers and their estuaries.

The bioaccumulation of mercury, which may occur in living organisms such as paddy rice, corn and marine fish, become agents that spread mercury contamination through the food web of inhabitants of the Gorontalo Utara Regency. The mercury concentration in river sediments and fish will be used as background information about the mercury in the biotic and abiotic environments.

The Sumalata and Anggrek districts are locations with ASGM activities, while Kwandang, Monano and Tolinggula are districts without mining activities. The residents of Anggrek and Sumalata are considered the ASGM miners group, while the residents of Kwandang, Monano and Tolinggula are considered the control group.

2.2. Sampling

2.2.1. Hair

Human scalp hair samples were taken from 95 participants from inhabitants of Anggrek (n = 25), Sumalata (n = 23) and other regions of the Gorontalo Utara Regency (Kwandang (n = 7), Monano (n = 37) and Tolinggula (n = 4)) between 2012 and 2013. Of the 95 participants, 53 were female, and the mean age was 23 years (range: 8 months–63 years). Among the 95 participants, 19 were ASGM workers, 15 were housewives, six were unemployed, one was teacher, one was university student and 38 were children (participants with ages below 18 years old).

The mercury concentrations in the hair samples from Anggrek, Kwandang, Monano, Sumalata and Tolinggula were determined to understand the status of contamination. The distribution of participants according to sex, location and occupation are summarized in Table 1. Approximately 10–20 strands of hair was cut close to skin from the right back side (mastoidal region of the temporal bone) and then labeled and stored in a sample plastic bag [28].

The mercury concentration in hair samples will be used to characterize the risk through a comparison with reference values published by the German Human Biomonitoring Commission in 1999 (Commission Human—Biomonitoring of the Federal Environmental Agency Berlin, 1999) [29]. The German Human Bio Monitoring (HBM) commission established toxicology threshold limits, which can be put into three categories. The first category is normal or HBM I, where the mercury level in hair is below 1 μg/g. The above normal category is an alert level between HBM I and HBM II, where the mercury hair content is from 1 to 5 μg/g. Meanwhile, above 5 μg/g is categorized in the high level or over HBM II.

2.2.2. Sediment

We collected several sediment samples along the Sumalata and Anggrek Rivers, and the locations of the sampling points are shown in Figure 1. Approximately up to 15 cm from the river bed sediment was collected using a shovel and stored in a plastic bag, which was kept in a cool box. The sample was collected from several points at one location, according to the averaging principle [30].

2.2.3. Fish

Several marine fish species anchovy (*Engraulis japonicus*), gray snapper (*Lutjanus griseus*), yellow tail snapper (*Ocyurus chrysurus*), redbelly yellowtail fusilier (*Caesio cuning*), red snapper (*Lutjanus sp.*), and lane snapper (*Lutjanus synagris*) were bought from local fishermen of the Sumalata river estuary area. The samples were placed in plastic bags and stored in a cool box. The mercury concentrations in fish were determined using cold vapor AAS (CVAAS of Varian AA240 FS).

2.3. Analytical Procedure

2.3.1. Particle Induced X-Ray Emission (PIXE)

Elemental analysis for the scalp hair samples was performed by particle induced x-ray emission (PIXE) in the Cyclotron Research Center, Iwate Medical University, Japan. The precision and accuracy of this method have been reported elsewhere [31–35]. Hair samples were washed using Milli-Q water and shaken in an ultrasonic bath for 1 min. Then, the samples were dried by wiping them with a tissue. The dried hair samples were washed again by being stirred in acetone for 5 min. Then, they were washed again using Milli-Q water, wiped well with tissue and left to dry at room temperature. The hair samples (approximately seven hairs per person) were stuck on a target holder. A 2.9 MeV-proton beam hit the target after passing through a beam collimator of graphite, whose diameter was 6 mm. X-rays of energy higher than that of the K-K$_\alpha$ line were detected by a Si(Li) detector (25.4 µm thick Be window; 6 µm active diameter) with a 300 µm-thick Mylar absorber. For measurements of X-rays lower than the K-K$_\alpha$ line, a Si(Li) detector (80 mm Be; 4 mm active diameter), which has a large detection efficiency for low energy X-rays, was used. Descriptions of the data acquisition system and the measuring conditions are reported elsewhere [33]. The typical beam current and integrated beam charge were 100 nA and 40 mC, respectively. The procedure for the standard-free method for untreated hairs is almost the same as that reported in the previous studies [31].

2.3.2. Atomic Absorption Spectroscopy

The mercury concentrations in the sediments and fish species were determined using cold vapors AAS (CVAAS of Varian AA240 FS) in BPPM Gorontalo, since those samples need quick and special treatment compared to human hair samples. Accuracy and Standard procedure used in AAS are certified by Indonesian Government and they used standard procedures.

The threshold limit for mercury in river sediments is 10 µg/kg [36]. The threshold limit for mercury in fish and its product is 0.5 µg/g, according to the Bureau of Food and Drug Supervision of the Ministry of

Health of the Republic of Indonesia, which is consistent with the recommended safety levels of WHO/ICPS [36].

Fish samples were washed with distilled water and dried in tissue paper after defrosting in the laboratory. A portion of the edible muscle tissue was removed from the dorsal part of each fish, homogenized and stored in clean-capped glass vials in a freezer until analysis. The fish samples were digested for total mercury determination by an open flask procedure developed at National Institute for Minamata Disease (NIMD) in Japan by Akagi and Nishimura [37,38].

Sediment samples were dried in oven for 24 h at 40 °C, cleaned from parts dead animal and plants. Sediment samples were powdered using Agate mortar for about two hours. Powdered sediment samples were sent to BPPMHP for AAS measurement.

2.4. Neurological Examination

Neurological examinations were performed on a limited number of participants by a team of medical doctors using a standard protocol. The participants were 27 people from Sumalata and 17 people from Anggrek. The examinations were conducted on site: mining sites for the miners and at home for the inhabitants. A total of 12 symptoms related to mercury poisoning were included in the neurological examination: (1) Signs of bluish discoloration of gums; (2) Rigidity and ataxia (walking or standing); (3) Alternating movements or dysdiadochokinesia; (4) Irregular eye movements or nystagmus; (5) Field of vision; (6) Knee jerk reflex; (7) Biceps reflex; (8) Babinski reflex; (9) Labial reflex; (10) Salivation and dysarthria; (11) Sensory examination; and (12) Tremor: tongue, eyelids, finger to nose, pouring, posture holding and the Romberg test. We used 1 and 0 for positively and negatively observed symptoms, respectively.

2.5. Statistical Analysis

The mercury hair sample and neurological examination data were analyzed statistically with Origin (OriginLab (2007) version 8.0). Kolmogorov-Smirnov tests were used to study the normality of the distribution of inhabitant mercury hair samples. Because the data are log-normally distributed, the Kruskal-Wallis ANOVA test was used to identify differences among the subgroups. The relationship between the mercury concentration and age of participant in both groups is determined using the Spearman correlation coefficient.

3. Results and Discussion

3.1. Mercury in Hairs

The distributions and range of mercury levels in 95 hair samples collected from the five subdistricts are summarized in Table 1. The hair mercury concentrations of all participants are more than 1 mg/g, which indicates the toxicity level is already in alert level according to HBM [29]. The number of subjects with high mercury levels over 10 μg/g was 10 (40%), 7 (30.4%), and 4 (8.5%) in Anggrek, Sumalata, and the control group (Kwandang, Monano and Tolinggula), respectively. According to the Kolmogorov-Smirnov test, the distribution of data of mercury hair from the Gorontalo Utara Regency was not normal; instead, it had a log normal distribution. The geometrical mean is more suitable for log normal distribution data.

Table 1. Geometrical mean, standard deviation and range of hair mercury content of inhabitants of Gorontalo Utara Regency.

Residence	Sex	*N*	Hair Mercury Content (μg/g)		
			Mean ± SD	Min	Max
Anggrek	F	11	14.2 ± 2.9	4.7	144.8
	M	14	7.0 ± 1.9	2.1	17.9
	Total	25	9.6± 2.5	2.1	144.8
Kwandang	F	6	6.7 ± 1.6	4.0	14.6
	M	1	3.5 ±	3.5	3.5
	Total	7	6.1 ± 1.7	3.5	14.6
Monano	F	22	6.2 ± 1.6	2.8	28.1
	M	15	5.0 ± 1.3	3.5	6.9
	Total	37	5.7 ± 1.5	3.8	28.1
Sumalata	F	11	10.0 ± 2.1	3.8	69.8
	M	12	6.6 ± 1.7	2.5	13.7
	Total	23	8.0 ± 2.0	2.5	69.8
Tolinggula	F	3	5.0 ± 1.2	4.4	5.9
	M	0			
	Total	3	5.0 ± 1.2	4.4	5.9
Total	F	53	8.1 ± 2.1	2.8	144.8
	M	42	6.0 ± 1.7	2.1	17.9
	Total	95	7.1 ± 2.0	2.1	144.8

3.1.1. Mercury Concentration for Males and Females

The lognormal distribution of hair mercury levels in males and females is shown in Figure 2. Five females had mercury levels greater than 25 μg/g, and none of them worked as ASGM miners. Those five females may have been exposed to mercury from another source (affecting female inhabitants only). The elevated hair mercury levels that were above average (7.1 μg/g) and even the highest (17.9 μg/g) mercury level were found among the ASGM miners.

The average hair mercury levels for all, male and female inhabitants in the Monano district are 5.7, 5.0 and 6.2 μg/g, respectively. These levels show that there are no significant differences between the mean hair mercury of males and females in that district. While the average of all mercury hair content for females is 8.1 μg/g (more than 30 percent higher than males (6.0 μg/g)), such conditions were also found for the subgroups of Kwandang and Sumalata. The condition in Anggrek is even higher (three times). The large discrepancy of mercury levels between female and male inhabitants suggests that female inhabitants are receiving mercury from another source (e.g., whitening cream).

3.1.2. Relation between Mercury Concentration and Age

The mercury concentration in human hairs depends on several factors, including age. Figure 3 shows the mercury concentrations *vs.* the age of miners and non-miners. There is a positive, strong and significant relationship (r = 0.31; p = 0.01) between the age and mercury content of the group of inhabitants, while there was no significant correlation ($r = -0.16$; $p = 0.44$) for the group of miners. Such conditions imply that the hair mercury concentrations of non-miners are age dependent, while for miners, the correlation remains unknown. Some factors related to the hair mercury concentration were not considered here, including habits, food consumption and drugs.

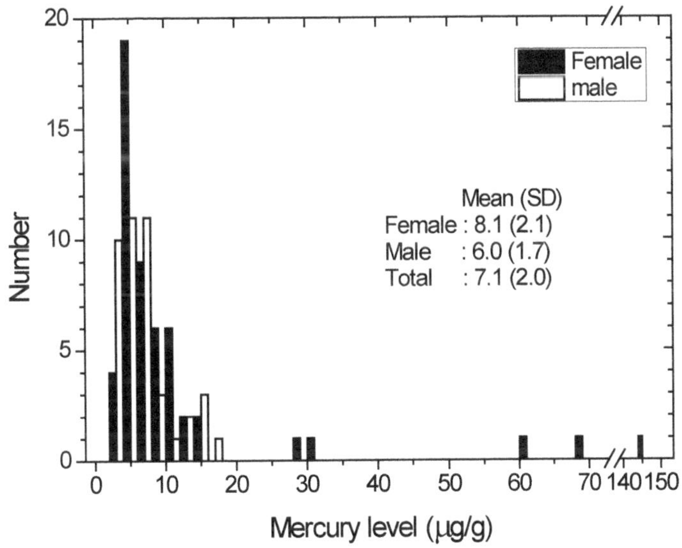

Figure 2. Distribution of the hair mercury among the total population. Open bar and solid bar indicate male and female, respectively. Geometrical mean and Standard Deviation are shown for male, female and total.

The positive correlation of hair mercury levels and age of the non-ASGM miner population is related to the inhabitants; constant consumption of mercury in their diets, which are already contaminated by mercury. Meanwhile, the lack of a significant correlation for the ASGM miners is not as important, given that the majority of ASGM miners have mercury levels above the non-miners.

Children (below 18 years old) had higher mercury hair levels for several reasons: spending more time playing outdoors, hand-to-mouth behavior, lower ability to metabolize certain contaminants, *etc.*

3.1.3. Relation between Mercury Concentration and Localization

A comparison of the hair mercury distribution among inhabitants of the Anggrek and Sumalata districts (ASGM site) and inhabitants of other districts without an ASGM site is shown in Figure 4. The mean hair mercury concentrations (SD) of the ASGM site and non-ASGM site groups are 8.8 (2.2) µg/g and 5.7 (1.5) µg/g, respectively. We used the Kruskal–Wallis test to identify the differences between groups, and there was no significant difference in the 95% level of confidence.

An effect of localization could be observed, as both groups were receiving the same source of mercury in their diet (food and fish from the same source). However, the mean hair mercury level of inhabitants of the ASGM site is higher than that in the non-ASGM site, indicating there is another source of mercury that corresponds to the ASGM activities. The most probable source of the elevated mercury level in inhabitants of the ASGM site is the mercury vapor from smelting processes, which mainly occurs outside, in gold shops and sometimes inside houses. The mercury emissions from gold shops could reach up to 53.4 μg/m^3, whereas the normal atmospheric level in rural areas is approximately 0.002–0.004 μg/m^3 [39].

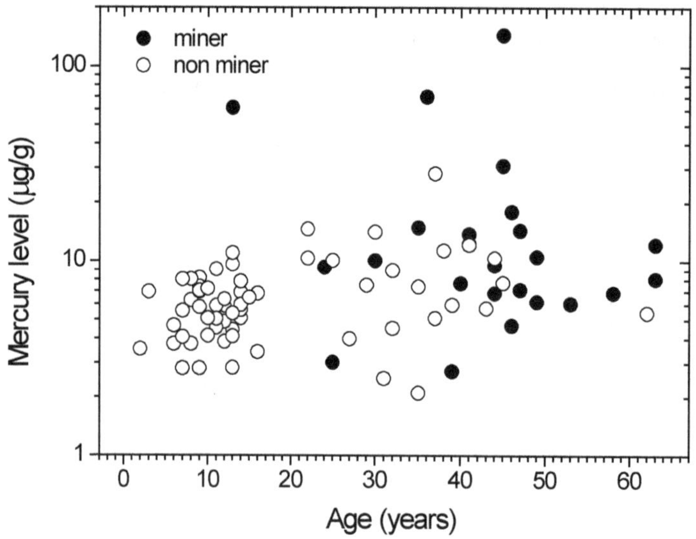

Figure 3. Distribution of mercury level among population of Gorontalo utara Regency. Open (○) and closed (●) symbols denoted for non miner and miner groups, respectively.

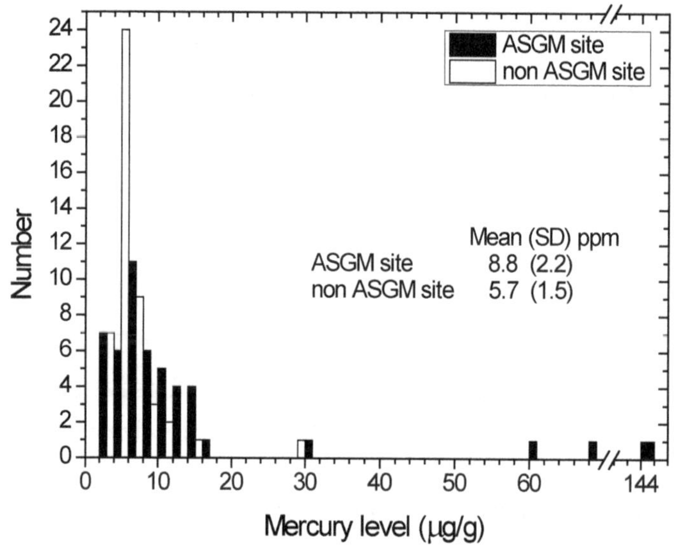

Figure 4. Distribution of the hair mercury among the total population according to their location from ASGM. Black and white bar indicate ASGM site inhabitants and non ASGM site inhabitants, respectively. Mean and standard deviation (SD) for both groups are given on the graph.

3.1.4. Results Comparison with Other Publications

Hair mercury concentrations of inhabitants from control areas (Kwandang, Monano and Tolinggula districts) will be treated as background levels. In the Table 2 mercury in human hairs from control areas of this study is compared with other publications. Elevated background level of hair mercury concentrations in Gorontalo Utara Regency is similar to high fish consumption areas, such as Philippines and Sulawesi; and far above lower fish consumption areas such as Tanzania and Mongolia. The fish consumption is most likely become the only factor determining the background levels of hair mercury concentration [40]. The values of background mercury levels of high fish consumption areas is may depends on mercury content on most eatable fish species and frequency of eating fish.

Table 2. Hair mercury concentrations (μg/g) of inhabitants from control areas of this study compared to other publications [40].

	This Study	Indonesia-Sulawesi	Philippines	Tanzania	Mongolia
Number	47	20	39	24	34
Minimum	2.8	0.83	0.98	0.08	0.03
Mean	5.7	1.64	4.02	0.36	0.1
Maximum	28.1	3.72	34.71	0.68	0.62

3.2. Mercury in River Sediments and Fishes

The mercury concentrations in the Wubudu River sediments are shown in Figure 5. All values are already far above the threshold limits by WHO/ICPS [36]. Locations 15, 16 and 17 have higher mercury concentrations because they are close to the ASGM processing units, and the levels gradually decrease downstream (locations 13 and 14). The mercury concentration in location 16 is lower than that in 15 and 17 because it is located in the junction and then may be diluted by another river branch inlet (Figure 5).

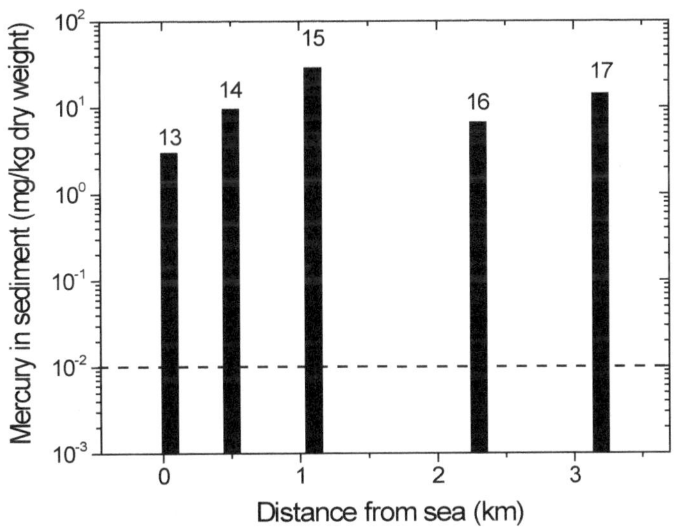

Figure 5. Mercury content in sediment from Wubudu river. Numbers on top of bars corresponds with sampling location. The dotted line indicates the recommended safety level (WHO/ICPS 1990).

The distribution of mercury concentrations in the river sediments is depicted in Figure 6. Locations 8, 9 and 10 are close to the ASGM processing site, while locations 6 and 7 are not (Figure 1). It is evident that the ASGM activities are the source of the elevated mercury levels in the sediments at locations 8, 9 and 10 (Figure 1). Although Figure 6 shows a connection between the branches in the Anggrek river system, our observations showed some river branches are disconnected due to the dry season. Compared to the Wubudu River, the Anggrek River is smaller, and several branches may be cut off during the dry season.

The mercury concentrations in the fish are depicted in Figure 7. The values vary from species to species. Most species have mercury levels below the threshold, but the fish that are commonly consumed, such as snapper (*Lutjanus synagris* and *Ocyurus chrysurus*), already have mercury levels above the threshold limit by WHO/ICPS 1990 [36]. Although some common edible fish have mercury levels below the maximum tolerable limit by WHO/ICPS, the frequency of eating such fish is critical. WHO established provisional tolerable weekly intake (PTWI) about 2.5 g/kg body weight in order to protect the fetus from neurotoxic effects [41].

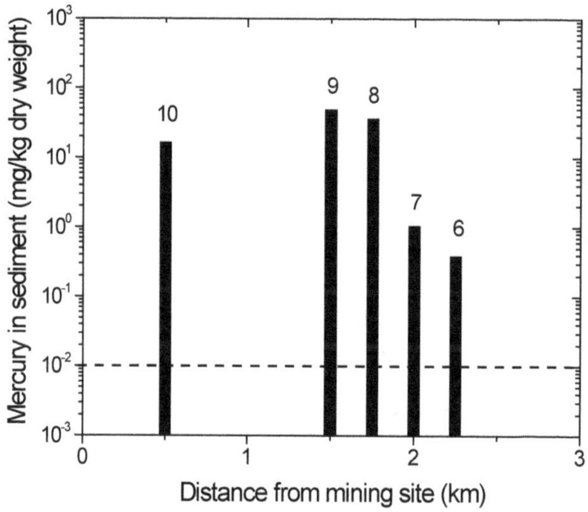

Figure 6. Mercury content in sediment of Anggrek Rivers. Numbers on top of bars correspond with sampling location. The dotted line indicates the recommended safety level (WHO/ICPS 1990).

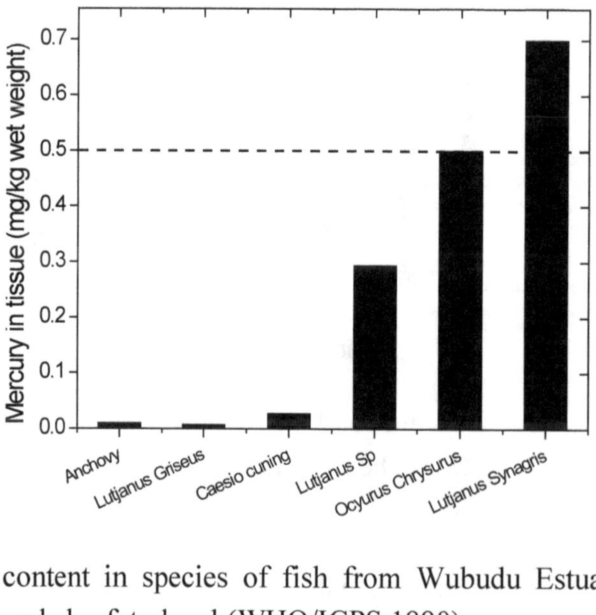

Figure 7. Mercury content in species of fish from Wubudu Estuary. The dashed line indicates the recommended safety level (WHO/ICPS 1990).

3.3. Neurological Examinations

From the 12 objective symptoms that were evaluated (Table 3), some common symptoms (bluish gums (1), Babinski reflex (8), labia reflex (9), and tremor (12)) were observed among the ASGM miners and inhabitants of Anggrek and Sumalata. The miners from Anggrek showed additional symptoms, namely rigidity and ataxia (2), alternating movements (3) and irregular eye movements (4).

No recent study has reported on mercury contamination using scalp hair as a bioindicator and the health effects of inhabitants of Gorontalo Utara Regency related to the ASGM activities in the Anggrek and Sumalata districts. Using scalp hair as a bioindicator of mercury contamination mainly reflects the uptake of the organic mercury compound via fish consumption [42,43].

The mean mercury levels of inhabitants from Anggrek and Sumalata are 14.2 and 10.0 μg/g, respectively. The values are two times higher than the smallest mean value (5.0 μg/g) of the Tolinggula district. Of the 21 subjects that have mercury hair concentrations greater than 10 μg/g, 15 (71.4%) of them are females, and four (26.7%) of those females live outside the ASGM area. Females that have hair mercury concentrations greater than 10 μg/g have the potential to contaminate their fetuses, risking abnormal brain development [44].

The dominant positive symptoms observed in the miners and inhabitants are described in Figure 8. The common neurological disturbances that were observed among the ASGM miners and inhabitants of Anggrek and Sumalata are bluish gums, Babinski reflex, labial reflex and tremor. However, the Anggrek miners showed more positive symptoms, namely rigidity and ataxia (walking or standing), alternating movements or dysdiadochokinesia, irregular eye movements or so called nystagmus. Harari *et al.*, found that tremor was a dominant symptoms among Ecuadorian gold miners, while Tomicic *et al.*, observed that ataxia and tremor are dominant symptoms among Burkina Fassian gold miners [45,46].

Table 3. Objective symptoms observed of the participants.

Groups (Number of Person)	Symptoms											
	1	2	3	4	5	6	7	8	9	10	11	12
Anggrek Miners (4)	3	3	3	3	2	0	0	3	3	1	3	4
Anggrek Inhabitants (13)	3	2	2	2	1	2	2	10	10	3	5	4
Sumalata Miners (4)	4	1	1	1	1	1	1	3	3	0	0	3
SumalataInhabitants (23)	20	2	2	2	5	5	2	20	20	2	2	15

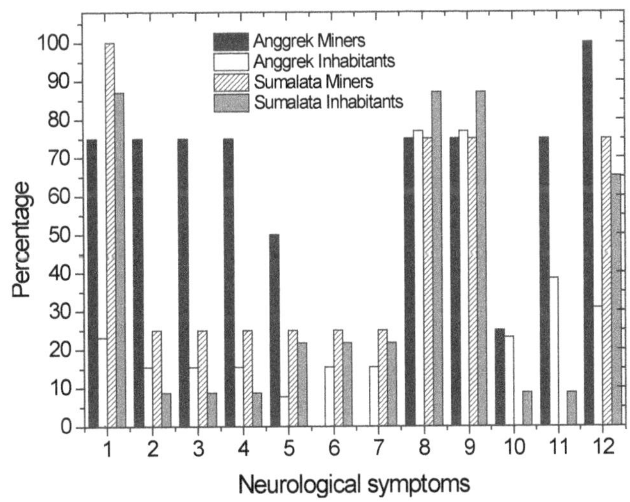

Figure8. Percentage of positive symptoms observed in ASGM miners and inhabitants of Sumalata and Anggrek. Babinski reflex(8)and labial reflex(9) are common symptoms observed in all subgroups.

The relationship between the level of methyl mercury in scalp hair and neurological abnormalities found in adults has been discussed by researchers [47,48]. Although the total hair mercury level found in miners and inhabitants of Anggrek who participated in neurological examinations are between 3.4 and 14.9 μg/g, only Babinski reflex and labial reflex disturbances are dominant. On the other hand, the miners and inhabitants of Sumalata with lower total hair mercury levels (6.1–10.4 μg/g) already showed at least four disturbances (Babinski reflex, labial reflex, bluish gums and tremor). We can assume that the methyl mercury levels of the Sumalata groups are higher than those of the Anggrek group because they were exposed for a longer period of time [49,50]. The high mercury concentrations in the Wubudu estuary sediments and fish (e.g., snapper) are the elevated mercury level sources for the Sumalata inhabitants.

4. Conclusions

The contamination status of groups of inhabitants who are living around the ASGM sites (Anggrek and Sumalata) and outside the sites (Monano, Kwandang and Tolinggula) is very high, according to HBM levels. The higher risk of mercury contamination due to the ASGM activities in ASGM sites is indicated by the higher mean hair mercury levels of inhabitants of the ASGM sites compared to those of inhabitants of the non-ASGM sites. Females have higher mean hair concentrations than males, and this result shows that female inhabitants are more vulnerable to mercury contamination. A significant and positive correlation found for the hair mercury levels and age of non-miner inhabitants suggests that living in ASGM sites potentially leads to mercury contamination.

The mercury concentrations of the Wubudu river sediments of Sumalata are above the threshold limits set by WHO, and the distribution is strongly related to the location of ASGM processing sites along the Wubudu riverbanks. The mercury concentrations of the Anggrek river sediments are already above the threshold limit set by WHO. The mercury levels in commonly consumed fish, which were caught in the Sumalata and Anggrek rivers and estuaries, are also reported. Most commonly consumed fish species (*Lutjanus synagris* and *Ocyurus chrysurus*) in the Regency have mercury levels above the maximum tolerable limits of the WHO [36]. Serious health problems are indicated by the dominant symptoms observed among the ASGM inhabitants, including bluish gums, Babinski reflex, labial reflex and tremor.

The proposed route for mercury to enter the human body is only an indirect way through the food web of the inhabitants, while ASGM miners receive a combination of indirect and direct exposure to mercury vapor including from smelting processes and direct contact with liquid mercury.

Acknowledgments

The authors wish to thank the government of Gorontalo Utara Regency, Indonesia for allowing us to conduct research and its support with sampling. One author (YIA) wishes to thank the Japanese Government for providing a Monbusho Scholarship for graduate studies in Ehime University.

Author Contributions

All authors contributed to the work presented in the manuscript. Yayu Indriati Arifin as principal researcher made substantial contribution to this work which was undertaken in association with her

Ph.D. program. Masayuki Sakakibara as Ph.D. supervisor provided critical analyses and commentary during development of the manuscript. Koichiro Sera provided the PIXE measurement of hair samples, which is also a substantial contribution to the manuscript.

References

1. Veiga, M.M.; Maxson, P.A.; Hylander, L.D. Origin and consumption of mercury in small-scale gold mining. *J. Clean. Prod.* **2006**, *14*, 436–447.
2. Pacyna, E.P.; Pacyna, J.M.; Sundseth, K.; Munthe, J.; Kindborn, K.; Wilson, S.; Steenhuisen, F.; Mason, P. Global emission of mercury to the atmosphere from anthropogenic sources in 2005 and projections to 2020. *Atmos. Environ.***2010**, *44*, 2487–2499.
3. Bose-O'Reilly, S.; Drasch, G.; Beinhoff, C.; Rodrigues-Filho, S.; Roider, G.; Lettmeier, B.; Maydl, A.; Maydl, S.; Siebert, U. Health assessment of artisanal gold miners in Indonesia. *Sci. Total Environ.* **2010**, *208*, 713–725.
4. Arifin, Y.A.; Sakakibara, M.; Takakura, S.; Jahja, M.; Lihawa, F.; Machmud, M. Artisanal and small-scale gold mining in Gorontalo Utara Regency, Indonesia. In Proceedings of the 23rd Symposium on Geo-Environments and Geo-Technics, Tsukuba, Japan, 29–30 November 2013; pp. 105–108.
5. Limbong, D.; Kumampung, J.; Ayhuan, D.; Arai, T.; Miyazaki, N. Mercury pollution related to artisanal gold mining in north Sulawesi Island, Indonesia. *Bull. Envrion. Contam. Toxicol.* **2005**, *75*, 989–996.
6. Agusa, T.; Kunito, T.; Iwata, H.; Monirith, I.; Tana, T.S.; Subramanian, A.; Tanabe, S. Mercury contamination in human hair and fish from Cambodia: Levels, specific accumulation and risk assessment. *Environ. Pollut.* **2005**, *134*, 79–86.
7. Vieira, H.C.; Morgado, A.; Soares, A.M.V.M.; Abreu, S.N. Mercury in scalp hair near the Mid-Atlantic Ridge (MAR) in relation to high fish consumption. *Biol. Trace Elem. Res.* **2013**, *153*, 29–35.
8. Diringer, S.E.; Feingold, B.J.; Ortiz, E.J.; Gallis, J.A.; Araujo-Flores, J.M.; Berky, A.; Pan, W.K.Y.; Hsu-Kim, H. River transport of mercury from artisanal and small-scale gold mining and risks for dietary mercury exposure in Madre de Dios, Peru. *Environ. Sci. Process Impacts.* **2015**, 17, 478–487.
9. Niane, B.; Guédron, S.; Moritz, R.; Cosio, C.; Ngom, P.M.; Deverajan, N.; Pfeifer, H.R.; Poté, J. Human exposure to mercury in artisanal small-scale gold mining areas of Kedougou region, Senegal, as function of occupational activity and fish consumption. *Environ. Sci. Pollut. Res.* **2014**, doi:10.1007/s11356-014-3913-5.
10. Castilhos, Z.C.; Rodrigues-Filho, S.; Rodrigues, A.P.C.; Villas-Boas, R.C.; Veiga, M.; Beinhoff, C. Mercury contamination in fish from gold mining areas in Indonesia and human health risk assessment. *Sci. Total Environ.* **2006**, *368*, 320–325.
11. Bose-O'Reilly, S.; Lettmeier, B.; Gothe, R.M.; Beinhoff, C.; Siebert, U.; Drasch, G. Mercury as a serious health hazard for children in gold mining areas. *Environ. Res.* **2008**, *107*, 89–97.

12. Krisnayanti, B.D.; Anderson, C.W.N.; Utomo, W.H.; Feng, X.; Handayanto, E.; Mudarisna, N.; Ikram, H. Assessment of environmental mercury discharge at a four-year-old artisanal gold mining area on Lombok Island, Indonesia. *J. Environ. Monit.* **2012**, *14*, 2598–2607.
13. Wolowiec, P.; Michalak, I.; Chojnacka, K.; Mikulewicz, M. Hair analysis in health assessment: Invited critical review. *Clin. Chim. Acta.* **2013**, *419*, 139–171.
14. Kempson, I.M.; Lombi, E. Hair analysis as a biomonitor for toxicology, disease and health status: Critical review.*Chem. Soc. Rev.***2011**, *40*, 3915–3940.
15. Laffont, L.; Sonke, J.E.; Maurice, L.; Monrroy, S.L.; Chincheros, J.; Amouroux, D.; Behra, P. Hg speciation and stable isotope signatures in human hair as a tracer for dietary and occupational expossure to mercury. *Environ. Sci. Technol.* **2011**, *45*, 9910–9916.
16. Esteban, M.; Castaño, A. Non-invasive matrices in human biomonitoring: A review.*Environ. Int.* **2009**, *35*, 438–449.
17. Molina-Villalba, I.; Lacasaña, M.; Rodríguez-Barranco, M.; Hernández, A.F.; Gonzalez-Alzaga, B.; Aguilar-Garduño, C.; Gil, F. Biomonitoring of arsenic, cadmium, lead, manganese and mercury in urine and hair of children living near mining and industrial areas. *Chemosphere* **2015**, *124*, 83–91.
18. Król, S.; Zabiegała, B.; Namieśnik, J. Human hair as a biomarker of human exposure to persistent organic pollutants (POPs). *TrAC Trends Analyt. Chem.* **2013**, *47*, 84–98.
19. Li, Y.; Zhang, X.; Yang, L.; Li, H. Levels of Cd, Pb, As, Hg, and Se in hair of residents living in villages around Fenghuang Polymetallic Mine, southwestern China. *Bull. Environ. Contam. Toxicol.* **2012**, *89*, 125–128.
20. Chojnacka, K.; Górecka, H.; Górecki, H.The influence of living habits and family relationships on element concentrations in human hair. *Sci. Total Environ.* **2006**, *366*, 612–620.
21. Chojnacka, K.; Zielinska, A.; Michalak, I.; Gorecki, H. The effect of dietary habits on mineral composition of human scalp hair. *Environ. Toxicol. Pharmacol.* **2010**, *30*, 188–194.
22. Afridi, H.I.; Kazi, T.G.; Brabazon, D.; Naher, S. Assosication between essential trace and toxic elements in scalp hair samples of smokers rheumatoid arthritis subjects. *Sci. Total Environ.* **2011**, *412–413*, 93–100.
23. Olivero-Verbel, J.; Caballero-Gallardo, K.; Negrete-Marrugo, J. Relationship between localization of gold mining areas and hair mercury levels in people from Bolivar, North of Colombia. *Biol. Trace Elem. Res.* **2011**, *144*, 118–132.
24. Castilhos, Z.; Rodrigues-Filho, S.; Cesar, R.; Rodrigues, A.P.; Villas-Bôas, R.; de Jesus, I.; Lima, M. Human exposure and risk assessment associated with mercury contamination in artisanal gold mining areas in the Brazilian Amazon. *Environ. Sci. Pollut. Res.* **2015**, doi:10.1007/s11356-015-4340-y.
25. Huang, M.; Wang, W.; Leung, H.; Chan, C.Y.; Liu, W.K.; Wong, M.H.; Cheung, K.C. Mercury levels in road dust and household TSP/PM 2.5 related to concentrations in hair in Guangzhou, China. *Ecotoxicol. Eenviron. Safety* **2012**, *81*, 27–35.
26. Peng, L.; Feng, X.; Zhang, C.; Zhang, J.; Cao, Y.; You, Q.; Leung, A.O.W.; Wong, M.H.; Wu, S.C. Human exposure to mercury in a compact fluorescent lamp manufacturing area: By food (rice and fish) consumption and occupational exposure. *Environ. Pollut.* **2015**, *198*, 126–132.

27. Castaño, A.; Sánchez-Rodríguez, J.E.; Cañas, A.; Esteban, M.; Navarro, C.; Rodríguez-García, A.C.; Arribas, M.; Díaz, G.; Jiménez-Guerrero, J.A. Mercury, lead and cadmium levels in the urine of 170 Spanish adults: A pilot human biomonitoring study. *Int. J. Hyg. Environ. Health* **2012**, *215*, 191–195.
28. Varrica, D.; Tamburo, E.; Dongarrà, G.; Sposito, F. Trace elements in scalp hair of children chronically exposed to volcanic activity (Mt. Etna, Italy). *Sci. Total Environ.* **2014**, *470*, 117–126.
29. Schulz, C.; Angerer, J.; Ewers, U.; Kolossa-Gehring, M. The german human biomonitoring commission. *Int. J. Hyg. Environ. Health.* **2007**, *210*, 373–382.
30. Ohio Environmental Protection Agency. Sediment Sampling Guide and Methodologies. Available online: http://www.epa.ohio.gov/portals/35/guidance/sedman2001.pdf (accessed on 1 April 2015).
31. Kempson, I.; Skinner, W.M.; Kickbride, K.P. Advanced analysis of metal distribution in human hair. *Environ. Sci. Technol.* **2006**, *40*, 3423–3428.
32. Islam, S.M.D.; Sera, K.; Takatsuji, T.; Hossain, A.M.D.; Nakamura, T. Estimation of hair arsenic and statistical nature of arsenicosis in highly arsenic exposed Banglish village in Comilla district of Bangladesh. *Int. J. PIXE* **2011**, *21*, 101–118.
33. Sera, K.; Futatsugawa, S.; Matsuda, K. Quantitative analysis of untreated bio-samples. *Nuclear Instrum.Method. Phys. Res. B.* **1999**, *150*, 226–233.
34. Sera, K.; Futatsugawa, S.; Murao, S. Quantitative analysis of untreated hair samples for monitoring human exposure to heavy metals. *Nuclear Instrum. Method. Phys. Res. B* **2002**, *189*, 174–179.
35. Clemente, E.; Sera, K.; Futatsugawa, S.; Murao, S. PIXE analysis of hair samples from artisanal mining communities in the Acupan region, Benguet, Philippines. *Nucl. Instrum. Methods. Phys. Res. B* **2004**, *219–220*, 161–165.
36. WHO/IPCS, Environmental Health Criteria 101, Methylmercury. Available online: http://www.who.int/phe/news/Mercury-flyer.pdf (accessed on 1 December 2014).
37. Voegborlo, R.B.; Akagi, H. Determination of mercury in fish by cold vapour atomic absorption spectrometry using an automatic mercury analyzer. *Food Chem.* **2007**, *100*, 853–858.
38. Akagi, H.; Nagamuma, A. Human exposure to mercury and the accumulation of methylmercury that is associated with gold mining in the Amazon Basin, Brazil. *J. Health Sci.* **2000**, *46*, 323–328.
39. Cordy, P.; Veiga, M.; Crawford, B.; Garcia, O.; Gonzalez, V.; Moraga, D.; Roeser, M.; Wip, D. Characterization, mapping, and mitigation of mercury vapour emissions from artisanal mining gold shops. *Environ. Res.* **2013**, *125*, 82–91.
40. Baeuml, J.; Bose-O'Reilly, S.; Gothe, G.M.; Lettmeier, B.; Roider, G.; Drasch, G.; Siebert, U. Human biomonitoring data from mercury exposed miners in six artisanal small-scale gold mining areas in Asia and Africa. *Minerals* **2011**, *1*, 122–143.
41. Gibb, H.; O'Leary, K.G. Mercury exposure and health impacts among individuals in the artisanal and small-scale gold mining community: A comprehensive review. *Environ. Health. Perspect.* **2014**, *122*, 667–672.
42. Barbosa, A.C.; Jardim, W.; Dorea, J.G.; Fosberg, B.; Souza, J. Hair mercury speciation as a function of gender, age, amd body mass index in inhabitants of the Negro River Basin, Amazon, Brazil. *Arch. Environ. Contam. Toxicol.* **2001**, *40*, 439–444.
43. Pesch, A.; Wilhelm, M.; Rostek, U.; Schmitz, N.; Weishoff-Houben, M.; Ranft, U.; Idel, H. Mercury concentration in urine, scalp hair, and saliva in children from Germany. *J. Exposure Analys. Environ. Epidem.* **2002**, *12*, 252–258.

44. Grandjean, P.; Weihe, P.; White, R.F.; Debes, F.; Araki, S.; Yokoyama, K.; Murata, K.; Sorensen, N.; Dahl, R.; Jorgensen, P.J. Cognitive deficit in 7-year old children in prenatal exposure to methyl mercury. *Neurotoxicol. Teratol.* **1997**,*19*, 417–428.
45. Harari, R.; Harari, F.; Gerhardson, L.; Lundh, T.; Skerving, S.; Stroemberg, U.; Broberg, K. Exposure and toxic effects of elemental mercury in gold-mining activities in Ecuador. *Toxicol. Lett.* **2012**, *213*, 75–82.
46. Tomicic, C.; Vernez, D.; Belem, T.; Berode, M. Human mercury exposure associated with small-scale gold mining in Burkina Faso. *Int. Arch. Occup. Environ. Health.* **2011**, *84*, 539–546.
47. Auger, N.; Kofman, O.; Kosatsky, T.; Armstrong, B. Low-level methylmercury exposure as a risk factor for neurologic abnormalities in adults. *Neutoxicology* **2005**,*26*, 149–157.
48. Zahir, F.; Rivai, S.J.; Haq, S.K.; Khan, R.H. Low dose mercury toxicity and human health. *Experiment. Toxicol. Pharmacol.* **2005**, *205*, 351–360.
49. Zillioux, E.J. Mercury in Fish: History, Sources, Pathways, Effects, and Indicator Usage. In *Environmental Indicators*; Springer Netherland: Dordrecht, The Netherlands, 2015; pp. 743–766.
50. Malm, O.; Branches, F.J.P.; Akagi, H.; Castro, M.B.; Pfeiffer, W.C.; Harada, M.; Bastos, W.R.; Kato, H. Mercury and methylmercury in fish and human hair from the Tapajos river basin, Brazil. *Sci. Total Environ.* **1995**, *175*, 141–150.

6

Anthrax and the Geochemistry of Soils in the Contiguous United States

Dale W. Griffin [1,*], Erin E. Silvestri [2], Charlena Y. Bowling [2], Timothy Boe [3], David B. Smith [4] and Tonya L. Nichols [5]

[1] Coastal and Marine Science Center, U.S. Geological Survey, 600 4th Street South, St. Petersburg, FL 33701, USA

[2] National Homeland Security Research Center, U.S. Environmental Protection Agency, 26 W. Martin Luther King Drive, MS NG16, Cincinnati, OH 45268, USA; E-Mails: silvestri.erin@epa.gov (E.S.); bowling.charlena@epa.gov (C.Y.B.)

[3] National Homeland Security Research Center, Oak Ridge Institute for Science and Education, with the U.S. Environmental Protection Agency, 109 T.W. Alexander Drive, Research Triangle Park, NC 27709, USA; E-Mail: boe.timothy@epa.gov

[4] Denver Federal Center, U.S. Geological Survey, Box 25046, MS 973, Denver, CO 80225, USA; E-Mail: dsmith@usgs.gov

[5] National Homeland Security Research Center, Threat and Consequence Assessment Division, U.S. Environmental Protection Agency, Ronald Reagan Building, MC 8801RR, 1200 Pennsylvania Avenue, NW, Washington, DC 20460, USA; E-Mail: nichols.tonya@epa.gov

* Author to whom correspondence should be addressed; E-Mail: dgriffin@usgs.gov;

Abstract: Soil geochemical data from sample sites in counties that reported occurrences of anthrax in wildlife and livestock since 2000 were evaluated against counties within the same states (MN, MT, ND, NV, OR, SD and TX) that did not report occurrences. These data identified the elements, calcium (Ca), manganese (Mn), phosphorus (P) and strontium (Sr), as having statistically significant differences in concentrations between county type (anthrax occurrence *versus* no occurrence). Tentative threshold values of the lowest concentrations of each of these elements (Ca = 0.43 wt %, Mn = 142 mg/kg, P = 180 mg/kg and Sr = 51 mg/kg) and average concentrations (Ca = 1.3 wt %, Mn = 463 mg/kg, P = 580 mg/kg and Sr = 170 mg/kg) were identified from anthrax-positive counties as prospective investigative tools in determining whether an outbreak had "potential" or was "likely" at any given geographic location in the contiguous United States.

Keywords: anthrax; pathogen; soil; microbiology; geology; North America; USA

---

1. Introduction

B. anthracis infections in wildlife and livestock have been recognized as a critically important disease in the United States for over 200 years. Historical data on environmental, weather/climate and geographical factors that influence the occurrence of these infections are well known and include; (1) warm seasons during dry periods that follow moderate to heavy precipitation events (weather/climate); (2) regions containing post-flood organic detritus and/or short dry grazing grasses (environmental); and (3) topological lows, such as waterholes or riverbanks, calcareous and alluvial soils with elevated nutrient content and pH values greater than 6.0 (geology). Other geological factors that may influence *B. anthracis* outbreak occurrence, as noted through *in vivo* or *in vitro* observations, are elevated phosphate (which results in higher protective antigen production), magnesium, sodium, copper, zinc (needed for lethal factor production) and manganese (typically found in very low concentrations in calcareous soils and needed for gene regulation of exotoxins and antibiotics) [1–5].

There are over 140 strains of *Bacillus anthracis*, and all pathogenic strains carry both pX01 and pX02 virulence plasmids [6]. Two separate groups of *B. anthracis*, the "Ames" and Western North America (WNA) clades, are responsible for wildlife and livestock anthrax outbreaks in North America. Animal outbreaks of anthrax are a common occurrence in the contiguous United States, and they are typically constrained to a few geographical regions (e.g., Texas, Minnesota, Montana and the Dakotas). The "Ames" or "Ames-like" clade has caused periodic outbreaks in southern Texas and is believed to have been introduced through the importation of infected livestock during European colonization [7,8]. The WNA clade is genetically most similar to isolates of the Eurasian clade and account for ~89% of non-human cases in North America [7]. It is believed that the WNA clade was introduced to the Americas by human migration across the Bering Strait that occurred prior to ~11,000 years ago when the land bridge between Asia and North America last closed at the end of the Younger Dryas [7,9,10]. Genetic analyses of WNA clade isolates show evidence of a north to south distribution pattern that is rooted in northern Canada [7]. Costs associated with outbreaks can be significant. The 2005 North Dakota outbreak was estimated to have cost ~$650 thousand U.S. dollars (costs associated with activities, such as surveillance, diagnosis, immunization and disposal) [11]. Similarly, the periodic large outbreaks that affect bison and other wildlife in Canada are believed to cost ~$500 thousand Canadian dollars per episode, and various Canadian agencies spend an estimated $15 thousand to $26 thousand per year on aerial carcass surveillance [12]. Even small outbreaks can significantly impact the economic well-being of the livestock industry, where profit margins are based on low expected annual herd losses [13].

Given the geographic restriction of most annually-occurring cases and outbreaks of anthrax in the contiguous United States, geochemical data obtained by the U.S. Geological Survey's (USGS) "North American Soil Geochemical Landscapes Project" were evaluated in collaboration with the Environmental

Protection Agency (EPA) to determine which elements may influence the background distribution of this pathogen. These data may help decision makers better prepare for and mitigate potential or actual outbreak events and provide an accurate graphical representation of areas within the contiguous United States that favor the natural propagation of this species.

2. Experimental Section

2.1. Sample Sites and Geochemical Data

Using a generalized random tessellation stratified design for sample site selection, 4,857 sample sites (~1 site per 1,600 km^2) were utilized for the USGS North American Soil Geochemical Landscapes Project, and 209 of those sites were utilized in this study [14]. In a major geochemical mapping project such as this, the quality of chemical analyses is of utmost importance. Reimann *et al.* (2008) recommend the following five quality control (QC) procedures [15]:

- Collection and analysis of field duplicates;
- Randomization of samples prior to analysis;
- Insertion of international reference materials (RMs);
- Insertion of project standards; and
- Insertion of analytical duplicates of project samples.

In this project, field duplicates were not collected. This approach was evaluated during the pilot studies (Smith *et al.*, 2009) and reported on by Garrett (2009) [16,17]. Based on the results of the pilot studies, it was felt that the additional collection of field duplicates during the national-scale study would not add significantly to the QC analysis and, therefore, was not worth the added expense. The remaining four QC procedures were carried out fully.

To estimate trueness as measured in terms of bias, one or more standards consisting of both international RMs and internal project standards were analyzed with the project samples. In this project, trueness estimation was done on three separate levels. The USGS contract laboratory analyzed an RM with every batch of 48 samples. At the second tier, the USGS QC officer inserted at least one RM between every batch of 20–30 samples. The USGS principal investigator for the project (David B. Smith) initiated the final QC tier, which included the insertion of two blind RMs within each batch of 20–30 samples. Precision was assessed both by repeated analyses of RMs and by replicate analyses of real project samples. Quality control samples (RMs and analytical duplicates) constituted approximately 12% of the total number of samples analyzed. A complete discussion of the QC protocols used in this project, including detailed tables of bias and precision, is given in Smith *et al.* (2013) [14].

In short, the <2-mm fraction of each sample that was collected from a depth of 0 to 5 cm below the soil surface was analyzed for aluminum (Al), arsenic (As), calcium (Ca), iron (Fe), mercury (Hg), potassium (K), magnesium (Mg), sodium (Na), sulfur (S), titanium (Ti), silver (Ag), barium (Ba), beryllium (Be), bismuth (Bi), cadmium (Cd), cerium (Ce), cobalt (Co), chromium (Cr), cesium (Cs), copper (Cu), gallium (Ga), indium (In), lanthanum (La), lithium (Li), manganese (Mn), molybdenum (Mo), niobium (Nb), nickel (Ni), phosphorus (P), lead (Pb), rubidium (Rb), antimony (Sb), scandium (Sc), selenium (Se), tin (Sn), strontium (Sr), tellurium (Te), thorium (Th), thallium (Tl), uranium (U), vanadium (V), tungsten (W), yttrium (Y) and zinc (Zn) [14]. Elemental concentrations were reported as weight percent (wt % = Al, Ca, Fe, K, Mg, Na, Ti and S) or milligrams per kilogram (mg/kg) [14].

2.2. B. Anthracis Case and Outbreak Data by State County, 2000–2013

Figure 1 illustrates state counties reporting outbreaks or cases of anthrax in agricultural animals/wildlife since 2000 (red counties). States utilized for statistical analyses included Minnesota, Montana, North Dakota, Nevada, Oregon, Texas and South Dakota. State county outbreak and case data were compiled from state animal health organizations and the National Animal Health Reporting System [18]. Geochemical sample sites (USGS Geochemical Landscape Project sample site numbers presented in data tables [14]) were chosen within each county (Table 1). The following anthrax-positive counties were utilized for statistical evaluation: (1) Minnesota: Clay, Kittson, Lake of the Woods, Marshall Pennington, Polk and Roseau; (2) Montana: Gallatin, Sheridan and Roosevelt; (3) Nevada: Washoe; (4) North Dakota: Barnes, Cass, Grand Forks, Nelson, Pembina, Stark, Steele and Traill; (5) Oregon: Klamath; (6) South Dakota: Aurora, Brown, Brule, Buffalo, Charles Mix, Corson, Day, Dewey, Hand, Hughes, Hyde, Lyman, Marshall, Mellette, Potter, Spink, Tripp and Walworth; and (7) Texas: Edwards, Irion, Kinney, McCulloch, Real, Sutton, Uvalde and Val Verde. In summary, there were 120 sample sites located within these 46 counties.

Figure 1. Counties (red) in the contiguous United States reporting cases and/or outbreaks of agricultural/wildlife anthrax since 2000. Counties with no reported cases (blue) where sample sites were utilized for geochemical statistical analyses *versus* those sample sites in counties in the same state that reported cases and/or outbreaks.

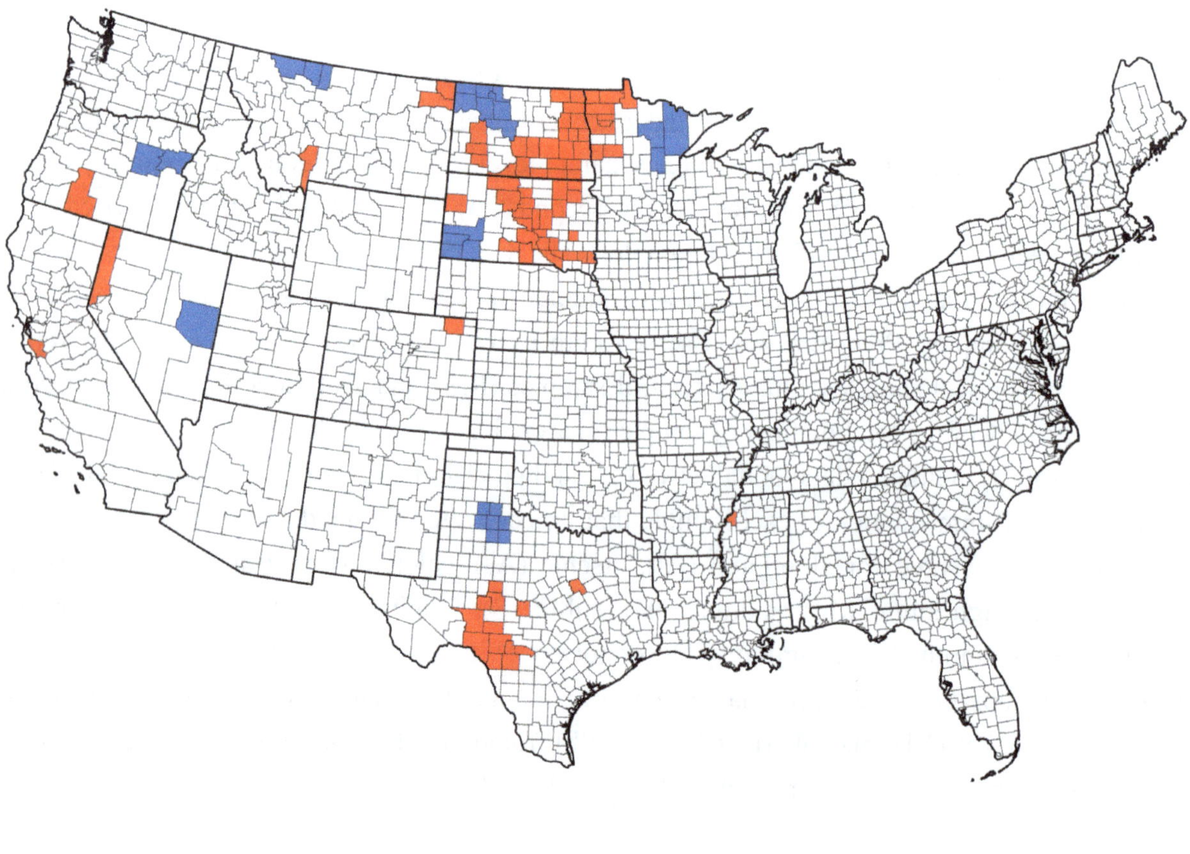

Table 1. State, county and U.S. Geological Survey's (USGS) sample site data [14].

State	Counties (total number)	USGS Geochemical Landscape Project sample site numbers (numbers grouped by county (total number)
State Counties Reporting Outbreaks or Cases of Anthrax in Livestock or Wildlife, 2000–2013 Utilized for Statistical Evaluation		
Minnesota	Clay, Kittson, Lake of the Woods, Marshall, Pennington, Polk and Roseau (7)	2265, 6361, 857, 9094, 7129, 10969, 4825, 4953, 8921, 9177, 12121, 729, 1753, 3545, 6617, 7641 and 2009 (17)
Montana	Gallatin, Sheridan and Roosevelt (3)	2798, 3310, 5246, 6974, 11070, 1854, 7742 and 12414 (8)
Nevada	Washoe (1)	671, 1503, 2719, 3551, 5791, 6815, 8863, 9695, 10719, 11743 and 12447 (11)
North Dakota	Barnes, Cass, Grand Forks, Nelson, Pembina, Stark, Steele and Traill (8)	601, 1177, 4697, 8793, 3417, 7513, 11609, 5273, 8025, 8345, 9369, 1881, 3966, 5310, 8062, 12441, 2201 and 6297 (18)
Oregon	Klamath (1)	14, 927, 1951, 5023, 6047, 7162, 8186, 10143, 11258, 12282 and 13215 (11)
South Dakota	Aurora, Brown, Brule, Buffalo, Charles Mix, Corson, Day Dewey, Hand, Hughes, Hyde, Lyman, Marshall, Mellette, Potter, Spink, Tripp and Walworth (18)	1224, 8648, 10120, 4185, 8985, 3528, 4808, 13000, 4296, 12744, 1662, 9086, 10878, 12926, 3865, 7961, 3275, 4734, 8830, 10443, 7624, 11720, 1736, 5832, 9928, 6347, 8904, 1113, 2137, 12377, 3723, 638, 6937, 11033, 89, 200, 712, 456, 2504, 10891, 11464, 2841 and 10009 (43)
Texas	Edwards, Irion, Kinney, McCulloch, Real, Sutton, Uvalde and Val Verde (8)	4804, 8900, 12095, 7364, 9656, 3356, 6092, 708, 6596, 11716, 7452 and 12996 (12)
State Counties Not Reporting Outbreaks or Cases of Anthrax in Livestock or Wildlife, 2000–2013 Utilized for Statistical Evaluation		
Minnesota	Aitkin, Itasca and St. Louis (3)	1077, 11317, 12341, 473, 1653, 1689, 3289, 2677, 3701, 4725, 6005, 7797 and 8245 (13)
Montana	Glacier, Toole and Liberty (3)	3502, 11694, 2222, 3246, 7342, 10414, 11438, 6318 and 8366 (9)
Nevada	White Pine (1)	271, 1359, 2015, 2063, 3087, 3407, 4367, 8463, 9231, 9551, 10255, 11279, 11375 and 11999 (14)
North Dakota	Burke, Divide, Mclean, Mountrail, Renville, Ward and Williams (7)	7150, 11246, 12270, 3054, 6462, 7486, 10558, 318, 11326, 2030, 62, 5438, 9534, 3134, 7230 and 13118 (16)
Oregon	Baker and Grant (2)	3342, 6926, 8974, 9742, 10510, 13070, 1102, 1550, 2574, 4174, 4622, 5198, 5646, 9294 and 12366 (15)
South Dakota	Custer, Fall River, Pennington and Shannon (4)	1675, 4811, 11147, 3979, 13003, 651, 4123, 4747, 5771, 8395 and 12491 (11)
Texas	Briscoe, Cottle, Dickens, Floyd, Hall, King and Motley (7)	4735, 3967, 7039, 11135, 191, 11391, 8063, 11647, 6015, 10111 and 4287 (11)

The anthrax-negative counties utilized for statistical evaluation (these were chosen randomly without knowledge of site geochemistry from each relevant state after the anthrax positive counties were mapped) included: (1) Minnesota: Aitkin, Itasca and St. Louis; (2) Montana: Glacier, Toole and Liberty; (3) Nevada: White Pine; (4) North Dakota: Burke, Divide, Mclean, Mountrail, Renville, Ward and Williams; (5) Oregon: Baker and Grant; (6) South Dakota: Custer, Fall River, Pennington and Shannon; and (7) Texas: Briscoe, Cottle, Dickens, Floyd, Hall, King and Motley. In summary, there were 89 sample sites located within these 27 counties.

2.3. Statistics

The non-parametric Mann–Whitney U test was utilized to evaluate differences in geochemistry between counties where anthrax outbreaks or cases had been reported since the year 2000 and counties within the same states where no cases were noted for the same time period using SPSS (IBM, Tampa, FL, USA) [19]. In the USGS Geochemical Landscape Project element concentration data set, there are values expressed as below minimum detection limits (MDL) for certain elements (Ag = 189 of 209, Cs = 170/209, Cd = 19/209, S = 2/209, Se 67/209 and Te = 198/209 data points). For statistical analyses, those values were set at the MDL for the respective elements (e.g., <1 is set at 1).

3. Results and Discussion

Comparing 120 sample sites from 46 counties (seven states, MN, MT, NV, ND, OR, TX and SD) that had reported anthrax outbreaks or cases to 89 sites from 27 counties (same states) that did not report outbreaks or cases resulted in the identification of seven elements with statistically significant differences in their respective concentrations (Table 2, all counties, Column 2). These elements included Ca ($p = 0.006$), Nb ($p = 0.035$), Ni ($p = 0.028$), P ($p = 0.028$), S ($p = 0.002$), Sn ($p = 0.024$) and Sr ($p = 0.041$). With the exception of Nb and Sr, the total state average of elemental concentrations was higher in anthrax-positive counties. When the elements were looked at individually, several trends emerged.

3.1. Strontium

When contrasting the elements by each state, only Sr had average concentrations that were higher in all anthrax-positive counties *versus* anthrax-negative counties, and the lowest observed concentration was 116 mg/kg. Strontium data were significantly different in three of the seven states.

3.2. Calcium

These concentrations were similar in both types of counties, with only one instance where average concentrations in negative counties exceeded positive counties, and that was in NV at 5.05 and 3.03 wt %, respectively. This anomaly can be explained in that the average concentrations in both the negative and positive counties were the second and third overall highest average concentrations in comparison to the data obtained from each of the other evaluated states. Overall, calcium data were significantly different between county types in three of the seven states.

Table 2. The significance (Mann–Whitney U test *p*-values; in bold where <0.05) of elemental concentrations (averages in brackets [#/#] where there was an overall or greater than two state significant *p*-values) in counties reporting outbreaks or cases of anthrax in livestock and wildlife *versus* counties that have not reported outbreaks or cases of anthrax since the year 2000.

Element	All Counties 46 (120)/27 (89)	Texas 8 (12)/7 (11)	N. Dakota 8 (18)/7 (16)	S. Dakota 18 (43)/4 (11)	Minnesota 7 (17)/3 (13)	Nevada 1 (11)/1 (14)	Oregon 1 (11)/2 (15)	Montana 3 (8)/3 (9)
Al	0.791 [5.9/5.3]	[4.2/3.9]	[4.6/4.7] *	[5.1/4.8]	[4.5/4.1]	**0.000** [8.4/5.6]	**0.001** [9.6/8.0]	**0.034** * [4.7/5.7]
As		**0.018**						
Ba	0.223 * [582/634]	**0.001** * [283/444]	**0.001** * [556/627]	[691/755] *	**0.021** * [485/520]	**0.001** [928/672]	[528/682] *	[599/740] *
Be								**0.041** *
Bi		**0.002**				**0.015** *		
Ca	**0.006** [3.3/1.8]	**0.000** [10.4/1.1]	[1.8/1.4]	**0.004** [1.3/0.7]	**0.005** [2.2/1.0]	[3.0/5.1] *	[2.6/2.5]	[1.9/0.9]
Co						**0.000**	**0.023** *	
Cr		**0.019**						
Cu								**0.034** *
Fe						**0.000**		
Ga						**0.000**		
K		**0.019***						**0.012** *
La						**0.004** *	**0.023** *	
Li						**0.001** *		
Ln		**0.019**						
Mn	0.072 [761/702]	**0.006** [530/304]	**0.045** [783/602]	**0.01** [1024/530]	**0.004** * [463/1144]	**0.014** [925/569]	[1120/1343]	[487/424]
Mo	0.128 * [0.9/1.0]	**0.001** [1.1/0.6]	[0.8/0.8]	**0.009** * [1.2/1.5]	**0.002** * [0.4/0.8]	[1.3/1.2]	[0.9/1.3] *	[0.7/1.1] *
Na	0.693 [1.2/0.9]	**0.001** * [0.2/0.5]	[0.8/0.9]	**0.001** [0.9/0.6]	[1.1/1.1] *	[2.2/1.0]	**0.02** [2.3/1.6]	[0.9/0.9]
Nb	**0.035** * [7.9/9.0]	**0.021** [10.1/7.5]	[6.8/6.8]	[8.8/9.9]	[5.7/6.1] *	[10.2/12.7] *	**0.000** * [6.2/10.8]	[7.7/9.3] *

Table 2. *Cont.*

Element	All Counties 46 (120)/27 (89)	Texas 8 (12)/7 (11)	N. Dakota 8 (18)/7 (16)	S. Dakota 18 (43)/4 (11)	Minnesota 7 (17)/3 (13)	Nevada 1 (11)/1 (14)	Oregon 1 (11)/2 (15)	Montana 3 (8)/3 (9)
Ni	**0.028** [21/18]	[15/12]	[19/17]	**0.01** [25/15]	[15/14]	[16/14]	[42/30]	[14/20] *
P	**0.028** [761/692]	**0.003** [580/330]	**0.002** [652/518]	**0.01** [737/566]	[675/620]	[818/886] *	[1,203/1,099]	[658/827] *
Pb	0.190 * [16/18]	**0.004** [16/13]	[14/13]	**0.000 *** [16/21]	**0.013 *** [14/18]	**0.023 *** [16/21]	**0.043 *** [11/13]	[14/25] *
Rb	0.21 * [58/70]	[69/64]	[64/64]	[69/67]	[58/60] *	**0.001 *** [61/106]	**0.012 *** [27/43]	**0.034 *** [61/84]
S	**0.002 *** [0.05/0.06]	**0.000** [0.06/0.02]	[0.05/0.04]	[0.05/0.04]	[0.04/0.04]	[0.06/0.03]	[0.03/0.03]	[0.06/0.19] *
Sb		**0.000**					**0.045 ***	
Sn	**0.024** [1.53/1.34]	[3.67/1.19]	[1.03/0.93]	**0.003 *** [1.18/1.40]	[0.89/0.95]	**0.029 *** [1.46/1.81]	[1.39/1.75]	[1.09/1.34]
Sr	**0.041** [250/169]	[116/86]	[165/154]	**0.003** [170/137]	[189/179]	**0.000** [457/262]	**0.000** [495/229]	[157/140]
Th						**0.001 ***	**0.012 ***	
Ti						**0.000**		
Tl	0.498 * [0.4/0.47]	**0.029** [0.46/0.35]	[0.44/0.43]	[0.52/0.55] *	[0.35/0.36] *	**0.002 *** [0.37/0.61]	**0.013 *** [0.23/0.35]	**0.036 *** [0.44/0.62]
U	0.837 * [1.90/1.91]	[1.70/1.71] *	**0.006** [1.92/1.45]	**0.007 *** [1.99/2.40]	[2.11/1.14]	[2.05/2.42] *	[1.42/1.69] *	**0.023 *** [1.80/2.58]
V						**0.000**		**0.014 ***
W		**0.04**		**0.015 ***				
Y		**0.018**					**0.008 ***	
Zn								**0.021 ***

Notes: Numbers under column titles = the number of counties with anthrax cases (the total number of sample sites in those counties used for analyses)/the number of counties with no cases (the total number sample sites in those counties used for analyses). [#/#], [the average concentration in counties with reported cases/average concentration in counties with no reported cases]. * = lower concentration in anthrax-positive counties. Elemental concentrations are reported as weight percent (wt % = Al, Ca, Fe, K, Mg, Na, Ti and S) or mg/kg [14]. Elements Cd, Ce, Hg, Mg and Sc did not show significance in any of the states and were nct included to simplify the table.

3.3. Phosphorus

Phosphorus concentration averages in NV (886 mg/kg) and MT (827 mg/kg) were greatest in negative counties, but these concentrations were the third and fourth highest overall concentrations in comparison to the data obtained from the other states. Overall, P data were significantly different in three of the seven states.

3.4. Nickel

Average Ni concentrations by state, with the exception of MT, were higher in anthrax-positive counties. The Ni concentrations in the MT counties averaged 20 mg/kg, which was the fourth highest overall. The only significant difference in Ni concentrations by state occurred in SD.

3.5. Niobium

Significant differences in total Nb concentrations occurred with only two states showing contrasting data, TX and OR, with average concentrations higher in anthrax-positive counties and in anthrax-negative counties, respectively.

3.6. Manganese

Manganese concentrations, while not significant for the total data set ($p = 0.07$), were significant when contrasting counties in TX, ND, SD, MN and NV. Only in MN was a significant difference noted where the Mn average concentration was greater in negative counties, and in this instance, the negative county average was the second highest observed (1144 mg/kg) across all states. Elevated concentrations such as this may mask a relationship.

3.7. Sulfur

The total S significant difference (high concentrations in negative counties) occurred over a small concentration range (0.02 to 0.19 wt %), and the only state-level significant difference that occurred was with the TX data set, which was opposite (high concentrations in positive counties) of the total.

3.8. Other Elements

Similar to the observation with sulfur, the total Sn significant difference (high concentrations in positive counties) was opposite that observed with the two state-level data sets. Several other elements, such as Al, Ba, Mo, Na, Pb, Rb and Tl, exhibited significant differences in multiple or individual states, but in many cases, one state produced a significant difference in anthrax-positive counties and, in another, in anthrax-negative counties. Cesium data produced a significant p-value below 0.05, but this was dismissed, due to the fact that 170 of the 209 data points were below the MDL. Of the remaining four elements (Ag, Cd, Te and Se) with MDL data, none produced p-values below 0.05.

Figure 1 illustrates the counties used for statistical analyses and the data (Mann–Whitney U p-values and, in relevant cases, the average elemental concentrations) are listed in Table 2. Of the 40 elements screened, seven (Ca, Nb, Ni, P, S, Sn and Sr) gave significant differences when samples from all seven states were evaluated as a whole. Of these, eight were positive (meaning the concentration was higher in anthrax counties) significant differences and one (Nb) was negative (the concentration was lower in anthrax counties). The Nb differences resulted in both negative (OR) and positive (TX) "by state" results, questioning the strength and/or validity of this "total" observation. The overall differences in concentrations of other elements, such as Ni and S, also resulted in both significant negative and positive results, and thus, the overall observation is either weak or not valid. The significant difference with Ni is also considered weak given that this was derived from a single positive difference ($p = 0.01$) that was observed within the SD sample set. This observation was also noted with the S data. It may be that one of these or other elements do contribute to virulence, but further research is needed to determine the potential role and threshold concentrations. The remaining three overall positive differences (Ca, P and Sr) had significant p-values in at least three of the seven states for each element. For Mn, there was one negative (due to the second highest average concentration at 1144 mg/kg, relative to the overall seven-state data set average of 808 mg/kg) and four significant positive state data. Manganese was selected for inclusion in the group of selected relevant elements (Ca, Mn, P and Sr) given the predominance of significantly positive state data and the skew produced by the lone negative. The regional distribution and concentration ranges for these four elements (Ca, Mn, P and Sr) and Zn (an element required for the lethal factor) are illustrated in Figure 2. Calcium, Mn and P have also been recognized as elements influencing the growth and/or virulence of this pathogen [1,5,20,21]. Other elements that have been reported to influence this pathogen include Na and S [2,4], and both of these elements resulted in at least one significantly positive state data set (Table 2). Also of note are elements, such as Ba and Rb (both close neighbors to calcium and strontium in the periodic table), which produced multi-state negative significance data, that may inhibit virulence by mechanisms, such as mimicking a critical virulence element [22]. In this case, the probability of conversion is suppressed in geographic regions where the mimicking element exceeds a given threshold concentration. It is interesting (as can be observed in Figure 3) that the concentrations of both of these elements are relatively low in many of the anthrax-positive counties of ND, SD, MN and TX.

Using concentrations observed at sample sites in the states listed in Table 2 for Ca, Mn, P and Sr, several tentative threshold concentrations can be selected for each element in regard to the likelihood of an outbreak occurring at a given location. As an example, the minimum concentration observed in any of these state counties for Ca is 0.43 wt %, and the lowest significant average listed in Table 2 is 1.3 wt %. These concentrations can be utilized as putative thresholds for an investigative tool to determine the likelihood of a naturally occurring outbreak being "potential" at 0.43 wt % or above and "likely" at 1.3 wt % or above. Similarly, "potential" and "likely" thresholds can also be set for Mn (144 and 463 mg/kg), P (180 and 580 mg/kg) and Sr (51 and 170 mg/kg). Figure 4 illustrates those sample sites where those upper or "likely" concentration levels occurred both individually and in combination.

Figure 2. Calcium, phosphorus, manganese, strontium and zinc soil concentration gradient maps for the contiguous United States. Red counties = cases and/or outbreaks of agricultural/wildlife anthrax since 2000. Blue counties = no reported cases and utilized for geochemical statistical comparisons with red counties.

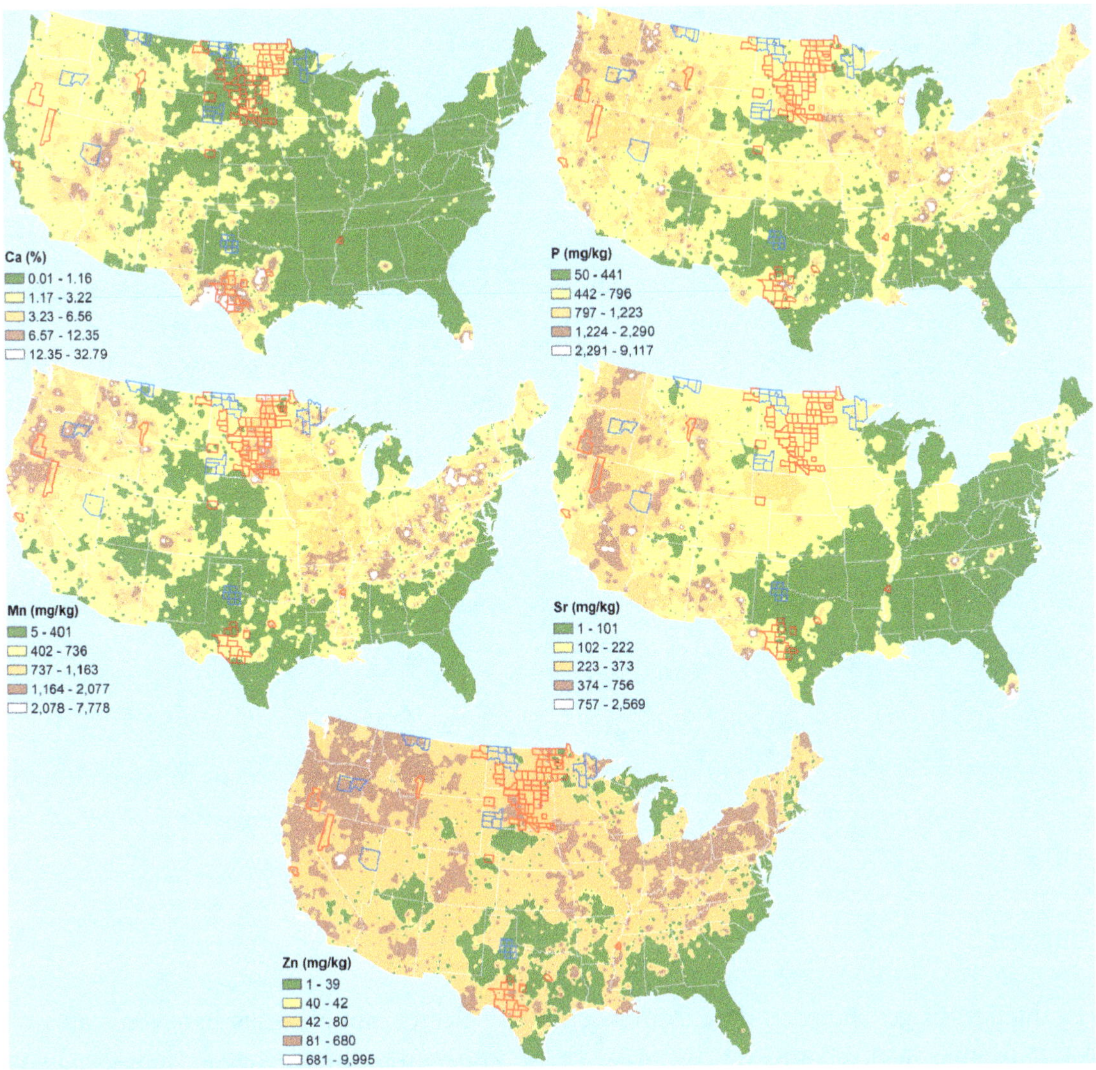

Figure 3. Barium and rubidium soil concentration gradient maps for the contiguous United States. Red counties = cases and/or outbreaks of agricultural/wildlife anthrax since 2000. Blue counties = no reported cases and utilized for geochemical statistical comparisons with red counties.

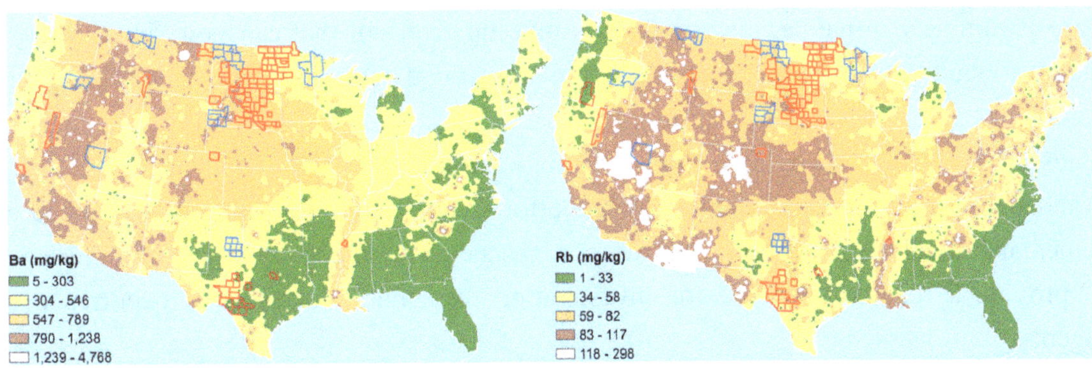

Figure 4. USGS Geochemical Landscape Project sample sites where the average statistically significant concentrations of Ca, Mn, P and Sr were equal to or exceeded 1.3 wt %, 463 mg/kg, 580 mg/kg and 170 mg/kg, respectively. Individual maps and one combined showing the sites where each of these concentrations occurred.

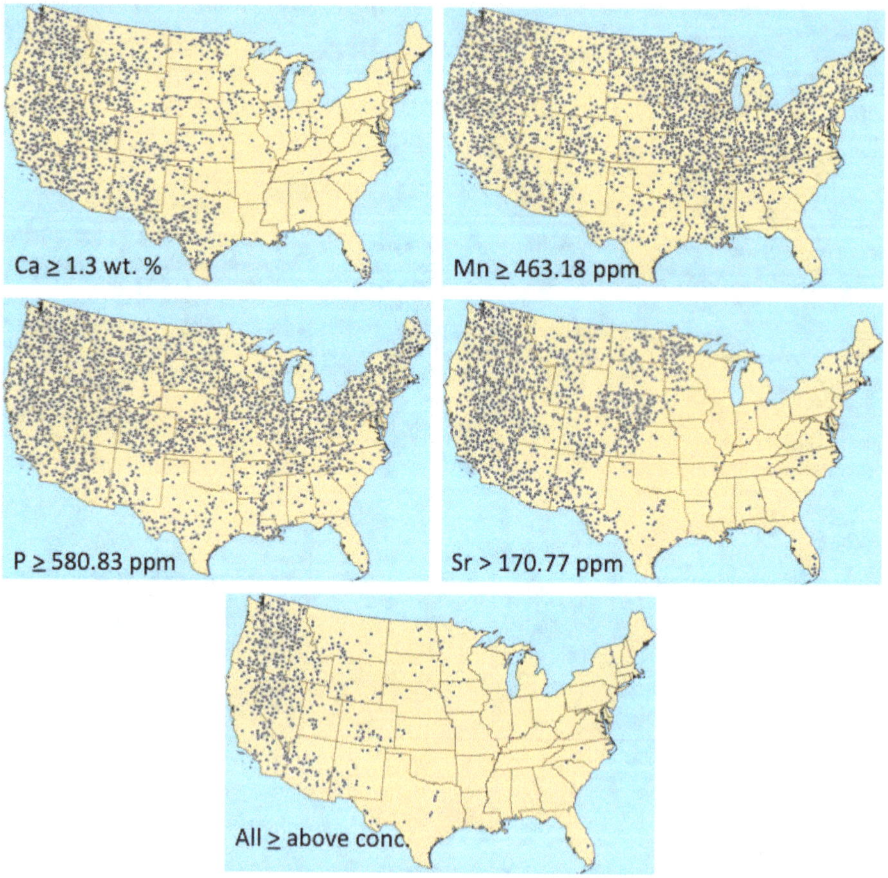

4. Conclusions

The evaluation of geochemical data from a series of selected sample sites in seven states identified four elements that had significant differences in concentrations between anthrax-positive and anthrax-negative counties. The elements were Ca, Mn, P and Sr, which in part match historical observations. Tentative threshold values based on the lowest concentrations and the lowest average concentrations of each of these elements, in the anthrax positive-counties utilized in this study, were identified for use as prospective tools for determining whether or not a naturally occurring outbreak had "potential" or was "likely" at any given geographic location. While these elemental threshold values are preliminary in nature, they present an investigative tool that can be refined through future high-resolution studies that need to be conducted in and around "endemic" areas. The USGS data set is a valuable tool that can be used to determine the background distribution of pathogens in soils of the contiguous United States. Being able to predict the natural occurrence of this agent may help guide animal and public health planning and response efforts. These data also provide insight to assist in environmental remediation decisions following a suspected outbreak or release of this agent and, overall, provide a roadmap forward for investigating the natural background occurrence of other select agents.

Acknowledgments

This project was a joint USGS/USEPA (through its Office of Research and Development) collaboration under EPA IA# DW14957748. The authors would like to thank Sarah Perkins formerly of the USEPA for her help and assistance on this project. This content has been peer and administratively reviewed and has been approved for publication as a joint USGS and USEPA publication. Note that approval does not signify that the contents necessarily reflect the views of the USEPA or the USGS, but rather the authors. The use of trade names is for descriptive purposes only and does not imply endorsement by the U.S. Government.

Author Contributions

All authors contributed equally to this manuscript.

References

1. Weinberg, E.D. The Influence of soil on infectious-disease. *Experientia* **1987**, *43*, 81–87.
2. Griffin, D.W.; Petrosky, T.; Morman, S.A.; Luna, V.A. A survey of the occurrence of *Bacillus anthracis* in North American soils over two long-range transects and within post-Katrina New Orleans. *Appl. Geochem.* **2009**, *24*, 1464–1471.
3. Kochi, S.K.; Schiavo, G.; Mock, M.; Montecucco, C. Zinc content of the *Bacillus anthracis* lethal factor. *Fems Microbiol. Lett.* **1994**, *124*, 343–348.
4. Hugh-Jones, M.; Blackburn, J. The ecology of *Bacillus anthracis*. *Mol. Aspects Med.* **2009**, *30*, 356–367.
5. Wright, G.G.; Angelety, L.H.; Swanson, B. Studies on immunity in anthax. XII. Requirement for phosphate for elaboration of protective antigen and its partial replacement by charcoal. *Infect. Immun.* **1970**, *2*, 772–777.
6. Qi, Y.; Patra, G.; Liang, X.; Williams, L.E.; Rose, S.; Redkar, R.J.; DelVecchio, V.G. Utilization of the rpoB gene as a specific chromosomal marker for real-time PCR detection of *Bacillus anthracis*. *Appl. Environ. Microb.* **2001**, *67*, 3720–3727.
7. Kenefic, L.J.; Pearson, T.; Okinaka, R.T.; Schupp, J.M.; Wagner, D.M.; Ravel, J.; Hoffmaster, A.R.; Trim, C.P.; Chung, W.K.; Beaudry, J.A.; Foster, J.T.; Mead, J.I.; Keim, P. Pre-Columbian origins for North American anthrax. *PLoS One* **2009**, *4*, e4813, doi:10.1371/journal.pone.0004813.
8. Van Ert, M.N.; Easterday, W.R.; Huynh, L.Y.; Okinaka, R.T.; Hugh-Jones, M.E.; Ravel, J.; Zanecki, S.R.; Pearson, T.; Simonson, T.S.; U'Ren, J.M.; *et al.* Global Genetic Population Structure of *Bacillus anthracis*. *PLoS One* **2007**, *2*, e461, doi:10.1371/journal.pone.0000461.
9. Elias, S.A.; Short, S.K.; Nelson, C.H.; Birks, H.H. Life and times of the Bering land bridge. *Nature* **1996**, *382*, 60–63.

10. Williams, R.C.; Steinberg, A.G.; Gershowitz, H.; Bennett, P.H.; Knowler, W.C.; Pettitt, D.J.; Butler, W.; Baird, R.; Dowdarea, L.; Burch, T.A.; *et al.* Gm Allotypes in Native Americans—Evidence for 3 Distinct Migrations across the Bering Land-Bridge. *Am. J. Phys. Anthropol.* **1985**, *66*, 1–19.
11. Mongoh, M.N. Characterization of Anthrax Occurrence in North Dakota: Determinants, Management Strategies, and Economic Impacts. Ph.D. Thesis, North Dakota State University of Agriculture and Applied Sciences, Fargo, North Dakota, USA, September 2007.
12. Salb, A.; Stephen, C.; Ribble, C.; Elkin, B. Descriptive epidemiology of detected anthrax outbreaks in wild wood bison (bison bison athabascae) in northern Canada, 1962–2008. *J. Wildl. Dis.* **2014**, *50*, 459–468.
13. Ramsey, R.; Doye, D.; Ward, C.; McGrann, J.; Falconer, L.; Bevers, S. Factors affecting beef cow-herd costs, production, and profits. *J. Agr. Appl. Econ.* **2005**, *37*, 91–99.
14. Smith, D.B.; Cannon, W.F.; Woodruff, L.G.; Solano, F.; Kilburn, J.E.; Fey, D.L. *Geochemical and Mineralogical Data for Soils of the Conterminous United States*; U.S. Geological Survey Data Series 801; U.S. Geological Survey: Reston, VA, USA, 2013. Available online: http://pubs.usgs.gov/ds/801/ (accessed on 12 May 2014).
15. Reimann, C.; Filzmoser, P.; Garrett, R.G.; Dutter, R. *Statistical Data Analysis Explained*; John Wiley & Sons: Chichester, UK, 2008.
16. Smith, D.B.; Woodruff, L.G.; O'Leary, R.M.; Cannon, W.F.; Garrett, R.G.; Kilburn, J.E.; Goldhaber, M.B. Pilot studies for the North American Soil Geochemical Landscapes Project—Site selection, sampling protocols, analytical methods, and quality control protocols. *Appl. Geochem.* **2009**, *24*, 1357–1368.
17. Garrett, R.G. Relative spatial soil geochemical variability along two transects across the United States and Canada. *Appl. Geochem.* **2009**, *24*, 1405–1415.
18. Animal and Plant Health Inspection Service, United States Department of Agriculture. Available online: http://www.aphis.usda.gov/wps/portal/aphis/home/ (accessed on 8 August 2014).
19. Dytham, C. *Choosing and Using Statistics, A Biologist's Guide*; Blackwell Science: Oxford, UK, 1999.
20. Pasteur, L. On the etiology of anthrax. *Comptes Rendus Seances Acad. Sci.* **1880**, *91*, 86–94.
21. Van Ness, G.; Stein, C.D. Soils of the United States favorable for anthrax. *J. Am. Vet. Med. Assoc.* **1956**, *128*, 7–12.
22. Heldman, E.; Levine, M.; Raveh, L.; Pollard, H.B. Barium ions enter chromaffin cells via voltage-dependent calcium channels and induce secretion by a mechanism independent of calcium. *J. Biol. Chem.* **1989**, *264*, 7914–7920.

7

Risk Factors for *E. coli* O157 and Cryptosporidiosis Infection in Individuals in the Karst Valleys of East Tennessee, USA

Ingrid Luffman [1],* and Liem Tran [2]

[1] Department of Geosciences, East Tennessee State University, Johnson City, TN 37614-1709, USA
[2] Department of Geography, The University of Tennessee, Knoxville, TN 37996-0925, USA;
E-Mail: ltran1@utk.edu

* Author to whom correspondence should be addressed; E-Mail: luffman@etsu.edu;

Abstract: This research examines risk factors for sporadic cryptosporidiosis and *Escherichia coli* (*E. coli*) O157 infection in East Tennessee, using a case-control approach and spatial logistic regression models. The risk factors examined are animal density, land use, geology, surface water impairment, poverty rate and availability of private water supply. Proximity to karst geology, beef cow population density and a high percentage of both developed land and pasture land are positively associated with both diseases. The availability of private water supply is negatively associated with both diseases. Risk maps generated using the model coefficients show areas of elevated risk to identify the communities where background risk is highest, so that limited public health resources can be targeted to the risk factors and communities most at risk. These results can be used as the framework upon which to develop a comprehensive epidemiological study that focuses on risk factors important at the individual level.

Keywords: environmental risk factors; spatial modeling; cryptosporidiosis; *E. coli* O157; spatial epidemiology; spatial logistic regression

---

1. Introduction

The field of medical geology assesses health problems associated with geologic materials with three areas of focus: (1) geology as a source of harmful materials; (2) movement and alteration of harmful materials through the subsurface over time and space; and (3) exposure pathways associated with geologic materials [1]. This research focuses on the third branch, specifically on karst geology and other spatially-distributed risk factors, as pathways for exposure to waterborne diseases.

The aim for epidemiologic research in general is to identify associations between exposures and outcomes to maximize health or to prevent disease [2], and the probability of human infection by pathogens depends on a number of factors, including how well the pathogen survives in the environment and the opportunities for host-pathogen interaction [3].

It is well established that karst regions are at a higher risk for groundwater contamination due to groundwater-surface water interactions and low groundwater residence times [4,5]. Natural and anthropogenic processes impact water quality at karst springs, as surface contamination is quickly carried into the groundwater supply when contaminated surface runoff flows into sinkholes and sinking streams [6,7]. Contaminated groundwater supplies used for public or private water supplies can result in outbreaks of disease that are more prevalent in karst regions [8,9].

Exposure to impaired surface water [10–13], agricultural activity [10,13–16] and karst geology [17] has been linked to outbreaks of cryptosporidiosis and *Escherichia coli* O157 (*E. coli* O157) infection worldwide. Since the first outbreak of cryptosporidiosis related to recreational water in the United States was reported in 1988, *Cryptosporidium* has emerged as the most recognized cause of disease outbreak associated with recreational water [18], as it is pervasive in the environment, resistant to chlorine and has a low infectious dose (10 to 30 oocysts) [19]. From 2006 to 2009, Tennessee reported 315 cryptosporidiosis cases statewide. Forty-nine (15.7%) were from the northeast region, though this region represents only 6% of the state's population. Forty-seven of the forty-nine cases (96%) in the northeast region were in two counties, and while some of these cases were attributed to a specific exposure (such as contaminated food or water), the sources of infection for most of the cases remained unexplained.

E. coli O157 is a pathogen first identified in 1982 as the cause of two outbreaks of disease in Oregon and Michigan, USA [18]. Since that time, the disease has become widely distributed throughout the United States and the rest of the world because of the high survival rate of the pathogen and low infectious dose (between 10 and 100 organisms) [11]. *E. coli* O157 infection is associated with consumption of contaminated water or food, such as undercooked beef, dairy products and salads; however, a connection between environmental exposure and *E. coli* O157 outbreaks has also been established [11,14,18,20,21]. *E. coli* O157 infection causes an estimated 96,534 illnesses in the United States each year, 3268 of which can require hospitalization [22]. From 2000 to 2010, 903 cases of *E. coli* O157 infection were reported in Tennessee. In 21 cases, the onset of symptoms was preceded by international travel, and only two cases were associated with a known outbreak. Therefore, in the majority of the Tennessee cases, the cause of illness is unknown.

Because known risk factors for cryptosporidiosis and *E. coli* O157 infection are associated with an individual's environment (apart from exposure through food and human contact), an analysis of these datasets would benefit from explicitly including space and spatial relationships between potential risk factors and disease. Proximity to a known risk factor may increase the incidence of cryptosporidiosis or *E. coli* O157 infection in a population, and therefore, epidemiologic research should take into account the spatial relationship between the individual, the environment and other individuals, keeping in mind the relationship between and among cases of these diseases. A geographic approach to the assessment of risk for cryptosporidiosis and *E. coli* O157 infection that includes the use of GIS and spatial statistical modeling can be a powerful method to infer associations between the environment and health [23].

Much of East Tennessee falls within the Valley and Ridge physiographic province of North America, characterized by folded Paleozoic sedimentary rocks (limestone, shale and sandstone) with flat-lying sedimentary rocks to the west and Precambrian metamorphic rocks of the Blue Ridge province to the east [24]. Building on the established link between karst geology, water quality and health, this research examines the role of karst geology and other environmental risk factors for cryptosporidiosis and *E. coli* O157 infection in East Tennessee.

2. Methods

The research was accomplished in two steps. First, spatial databases of disease data and explanatory variables were assembled, and exploratory mapping was done. In this step, the cases were geocoded, rates were calculated and standardized for each zip code and explanatory variables were extracted for each case and zip code and overlaid with the disease data. In the second step, regression models were developed using a case-control approach to examine the risk for disease in the individual.

2.1. Data

For this study, a dataset of patient records for 903 *E. coli* O157 infection and 555 cryptosporidiosis cases occurring in Tennessee from 2000 to 2010 was extracted from the Foodborne Diseases Active Surveillance Network (FoodNet) database, USA Department of Health and Human Services. The patient records consisted of patient age, gender, date of specimen, address, recent travel history and whether the infection was associated with an outbreak. Appropriate safeguards were taken to protect patient privacy and confidentiality. Case records for East Tennessee addresses were extracted and examined for duplicates, recent travel, association with a known outbreak and incomplete records, and geocoding was completed using the University of South California WebGIS Services batch geocoder [25]. After cleaning, the datasets contained 247 cryptosporidiosis and 250 *E. coli* O157 infection records (Figure 1).

The environmental risk factors selected as explanatory variables were geology, surface water impairment, agricultural animal population density by zip code, land use, groundwater well permit density by county and poverty rate at the block group level (Table 1). Each explanatory variable was extracted at the best resolution available. These data are publicly available as spatially-referenced spreadsheet data (related to a geographic unit such as a county or census unit) or as shapefiles that were directly imported into ArcGIS 10.0 [26].

Karst regions were delineated by selecting polygons classified as limestone or dolomite in the 1:250,000 Geology of Tennessee shapefile [27] and creating a new layer of the karst-prone regions of Tennessee. Surface water shapefiles and attribute data for the Year 2008 305(b) Report [28] and Year 2008 303(d) Report [29] were downloaded from the Environmental Protection Agency Reach Address Database [30]. Using the near tool in ArcGIS, two raster files containing values for the distance in kilometers to the nearest karst area (KARST) and distance to the nearest impaired stream segment (STREAM) were constructed.

Agricultural animal population densities were calculated for each zip code tabulation area (ZCTA) using the USDA Agricultural Census Data from 2007 [31] for dairy cows (MILK), beef cows (BEEF), hogs (HOG) and sheep (SHEEP). The 2006 National Land Cover Dataset [32] was reclassified and smoothed to construct three 500 m × 500 m rasters of percent cover for each of three land use classes (PASTURE, FOREST and DEVELOPED). A database of well permits was obtained from the Tennessee Department of Environment and Conservation, summed by county and joined to the 2010 Tiger/Line county layer (WELLS). Poverty rates at the block group level (POVRATE) were obtained from USA Census data [33]. Raster layers for each variable were constructed in ArcGIS for input as spatial explanatory variables in the spatial logistic regression model (Figure 2).

Figure 1. Study area and approximate locations of disease cases from 2000 to 2010.

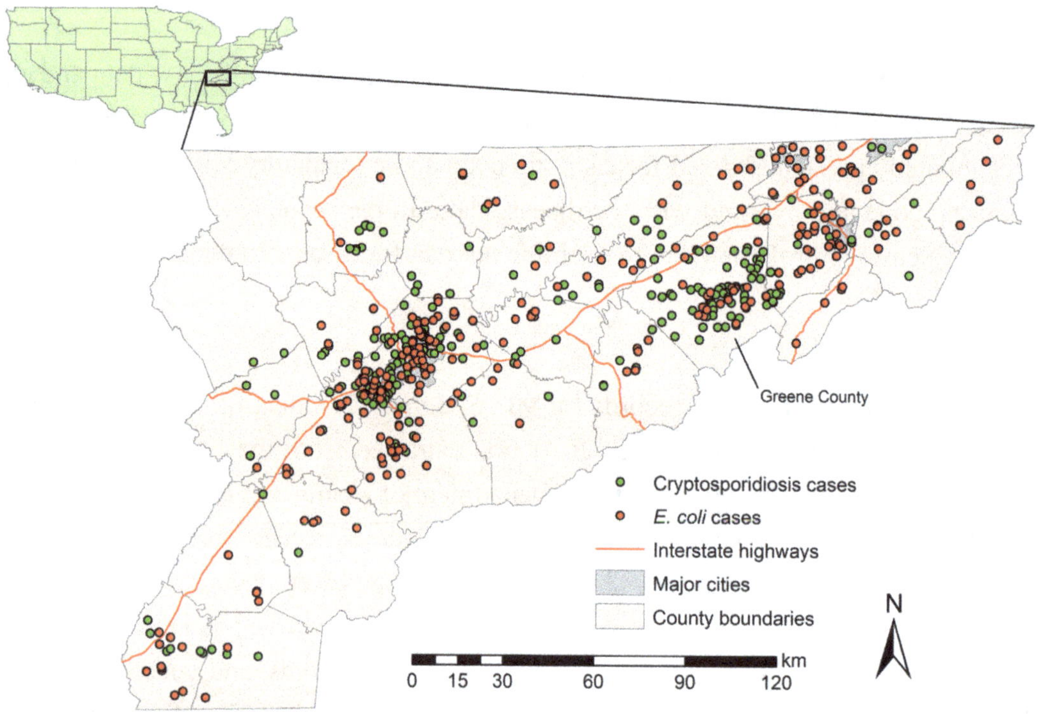

Table 1. Candidate explanatory variables for cryptosporidiosis and *E. coli* O157 infection.

Variable	Description	Units
KARST [1]	Distance to nearest karst geology	Kilometers (Euclidean distance)
STREAM [2]	Distance to nearest *E. coli* contaminated stream segment	Kilometers (Euclidean distance)
BEEF [3]	Beef cow population density (zip code level data)	Animals/km^2
MILK [3]	Dairy cow population density (zip code level data)	Animals/km^2
HOG [3]	Hog population density (zip code level data)	Animals/km^2
SHEEP [3]	Sheep population density (zip code level data)	Animals/km^2
DEVELOPED [4]	Percent cover in a 500 m × 500 m raster cell	Percent, expressed as decimal
FOREST [4]	Percent cover in a 500 m × 500 m raster cell	Percent, expressed as decimal
PASTURE [4]	Percent cover in a 500 m × 500 m raster cell	Percent, expressed as decimal
WELLS [5]	Number of well permits by population (county level data)	Permits/10,000 population
POVRATE [6]	Poverty rate (block group level data)	Percent, expressed as decimal

Data Sources: [1] [27]; [2] [28,29]; [3] [30]; [4] [31]; [5] TDEC Well permit database; [6] [33].

Figure 2. Environmental risk factors used as covariates in the spatial logistic regression model.

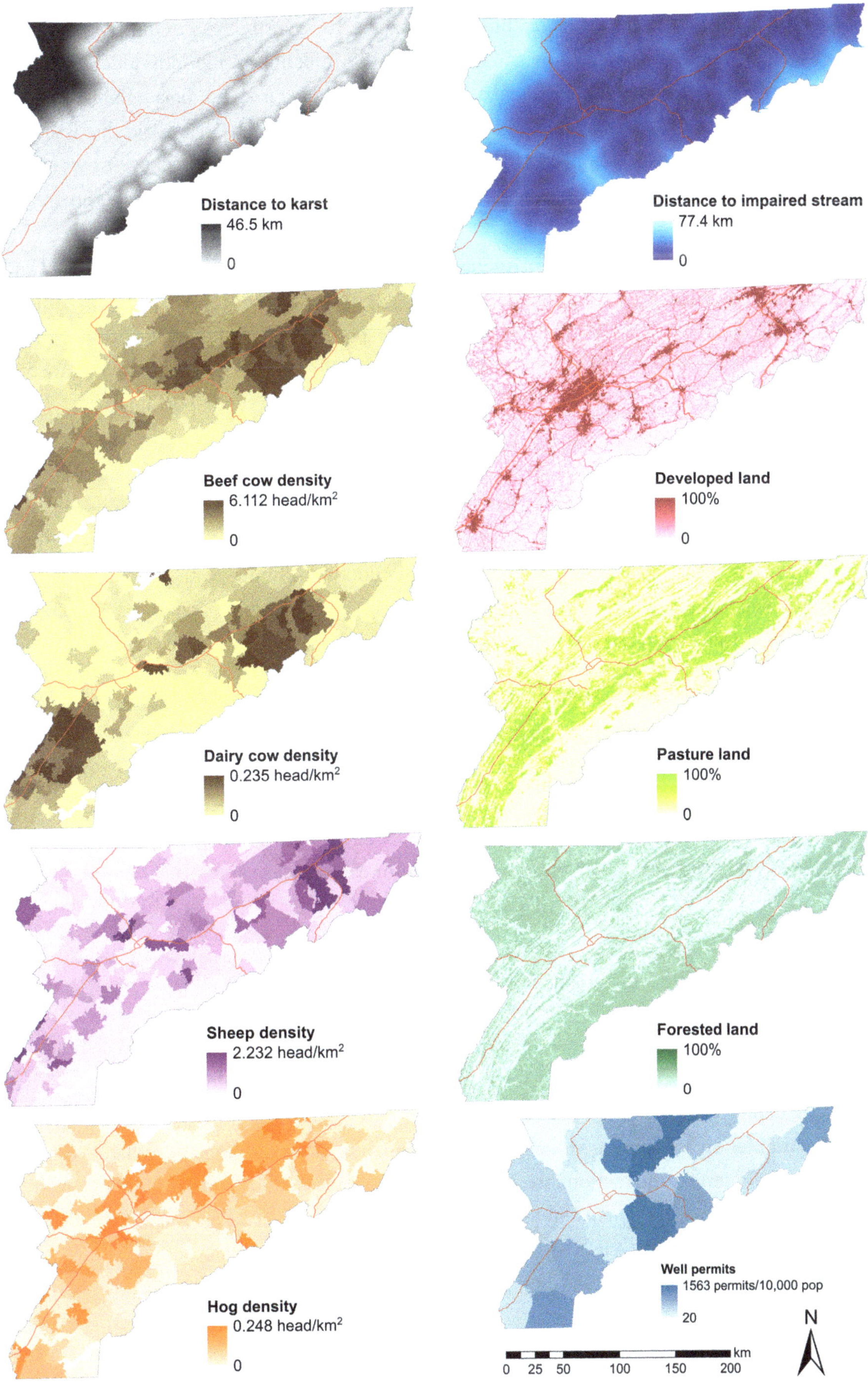

2.2. *Spatial Logistic Regression Model*

The objective of a case-control modeling approach is to identify and quantify the relationship between risk factors and cryptosporidiosis and *E. coli* O157 infection in the individual. One limitation of a case-control study using an existing database is that control data may not be available, in which case random absence data can be generated and used as the control dataset [34]. To avoid this issue, a spatial logistic regression model was developed in R [35], using the `slrm` function (R package `spatstat`) [36]. The case data were entered as a point process, and the covariate data were input as image files that span the area of interest.

The explanatory variables selected for inclusion in cryptosporidiosis models were: beef and dairy cow population density; sheep population density; percent of developed, forested and agricultural land; distance to karst geology; distance to impaired stream; poverty rate; and well permit density. Hog population density was not included in the model, because exploratory analyses indicated there was no significant statistical correlation between hog population density and cryptosporidiosis.

Explanatory variables selected for inclusion in the *E. coli* O157 models were: beef and dairy cow population density; hog population density; percent of developed, forested and agricultural land; distance to karst geology; distance to impaired stream; poverty rate; and well permit density. Sheep population density was not included in the model, because there was no significant statistical correlation between sheep density and *E. coli* O157 infection in preliminary analyses.

Risk maps were generated in ArcGIS 10.0 for both cryptosporidiosis and *E. coli* O157 infection from the model coefficients using the raster calculator tool and the equation:

$$P = [1 + \exp(-\log a - BX)]^{-1} \tag{1}$$

where P is the risk for disease at any given raster cell, log a is an offset term representing log-transformed population, B is the vector of model coefficients and X is the vector of covariate values. The Akaike information criterion (AIC), a diagnostic tool to quantify the trade-off between increased explanatory power and information loss associated with the use of additional explanatory variables in a model, was used to select the best model for each disease.

3. Results

3.1. *Cryptosporidiosis*

Multiple spatial logistic regression models were generated in R using the `slrm` function, with different combinations of covariates and interaction terms (Table 2). Model C1 includes all candidate covariates, except HOG, which showed no relationship with cryptosporidiosis. Model C2 includes only those variables significant in Model C1, and C3 includes all variables significant in C1 plus all possible interaction terms. Interactions were examined, but were not statistically significant ($p > 0.05$). Model results were generally consistent between models, and Model C1 was the best model, using the Akaike information criterion (AIC) as a diagnostic tool. Given the order of the AIC, the range of 8957–8968 between the three models is not large, indicating minimal additional loss of information with increased model complexity.

Table 2. Spatial logistic regression model (SLRM) coefficients (*p*-values in parentheses) for cryptosporidiosis individual models. Shaded cells represent excluded variables. Model diagnostics (AIC) are shown on the bottom row.

Covariates	SLRM Coefficients (*p*-values)		
	C1	**C2**	**C3**
(Intercept)	−18.58868	−19.28357	−19.54150
BEEF	0.1899209 (0.000)	0.415818 (0.000)	0.384648 (0.000)
MILK	9.700272 (0.599)		
SHEEP	−6.439952 (0.973)		
DEVELOPED	0.02983753 (0.000)	0.034451 (0.000)	0.041139 (0.000)
PASTURE	0.01080318 (0.000)	0.016177 (0.000)	0.012557 (0.000)
FOREST	−0.0055259 (0.761)		
WELLS	−0.001641 (0.000)	−0.001450 (0.000)	−0.000690 (0.000)
KARST	−0.0001505 (0.000)	−0.0001545 (0.000)	−0.000518 (0.000)
STREAM	−0.0000237 (0.004)	−0.0000198 (0.014)	−0.0000029 (0.014)
POVRATE	−0.3994621 (0.538)		
Model Diagnostics			
AIC	8957.298	8961.791	8968.142

The factors most significant for increased risk for cryptosporidiosis are proximity to karst geology (KARST), proximity to *E. coli* impaired streams (STREAM), higher beef cow population density (BEEF), residence within developed (DEVELOPED) or agricultural (PASTURE) land and a lower well density by population (WELLS).

A map showing background environmental risk generated using Model C1 (Figure 3) and Equation (1) using an offset of log(population density) [37] shows elevated risk (as the probability of disease) along developed corridors, in urban centers and in one predominantly rural area (Greene County area). Faint northeast-southwest trending linear areas of high risk show the contribution to risk from karst geology.

Figure 3. Spatial logistic regression model (C1) risk map for cryptosporidiosis (see Table 2 for the coefficients).

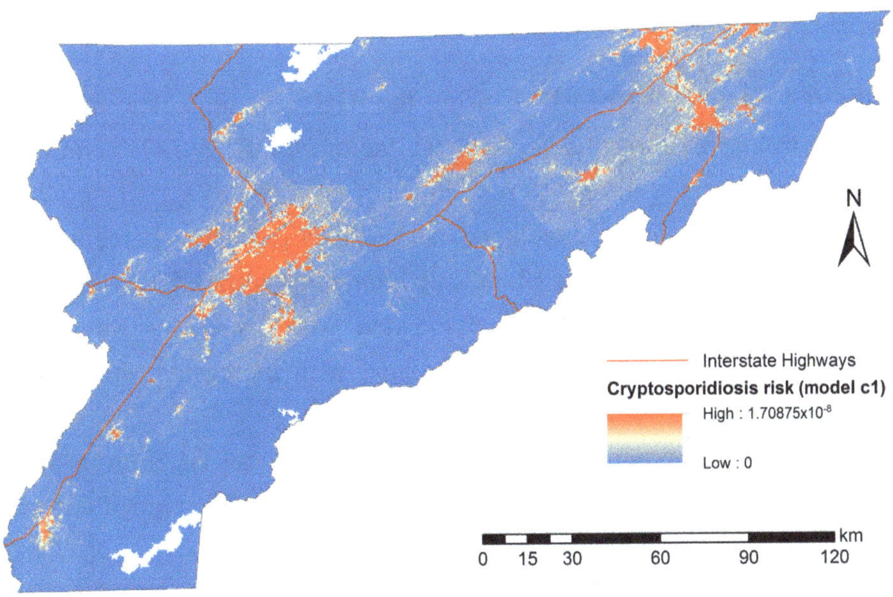

3.2. E. coli O157

Spatial logistic regression models for *E. coli* O157 infection were developed in R for various combinations of covariates and interaction terms (Table 3). Results were generally consistent between models. Model E1 included all candidate variables, with no interaction terms. Model E2 included only the significant variables from E1, and a comparison of AIC shows that E2 is a slight improvement over E1. Model E3 was constructed using only the variables in E2 plus all possible interaction terms. Only two interaction terms (DEVELOPED × PASTURE and HOG × KARST) emerged as significant, and the AIC increased due to the increased complexity in the model.

Table 3. Spatial logistic regression model coefficients (*p*-values in parentheses) for *E. coli* O157 individual models. Shaded cells represent excluded variables. Model diagnostics (AIC) are shown in the bottom row.

Covariates	SLRM Coefficient (*p*-values)			
	E1	E2	E3 †	E4
Constant	−19.43082	−19.27842	−19.56200	−19.14675
BEEF	0.3765216 (0.000)	0.3863660 (0.000)	1.633936 (0.000)	0.3046392 (0.000)
MILK	−2.96153 (0.001)	−0.299347 (0.001)	−20.07985 (0.001)	−1.319051 (0.001)
HOG	3.016985 (0.023)	2.954141 (0.023)	4.032882 (0.023)	1.794563 (0.023)
DEVELOPED	0.0322240 (0.000)	0.0307588 (0.000)	0.0320371 (0.000)	0.0282152 (0.000)
PASTURE	0.0166063 (0.000)	0.0150557 (0.000)	0.0093708 (0.000)	0.0103302 (0.000)
FOREST	0.0187083 (0.737)			
WELLS	−0.00122612 (0.000)	−0.00122976 (0.000)	−0.000922645 (0.000)	−0.00128114 (0.000)
KARST	−0.000219501 (0.000)	−0.000216085 (0.000)	−0.000380838 (0.000)	−0.000336388 (0.000)
STREAM	0.0000023 (0.721)			
POVRATE	0.184116 (0.774)			
HOG*KARST			0.00698929 (0.036)	0.00518194 (0.064)
DEVELOPED*PASTURE			0.000405056 (0.005)	0.000354069 (0.003)
Model Diagnostics				
AIC	9190.348	9184.642	9194.744	9176.378

† Model E3 included all possible interactions between explanatory variables, but only coefficients for significant interactions are presented in the table to conserve space. Model E4 included only the two interaction terms listed.

The final model (E4) was the best SLRM (using the AIC as a diagnostic tool) and included only significant covariates from previous models. The risk factors for *E. coli* O157 infection identified in Model E4 are: distance to karst geology (KARST); beef cow (BEEF), dairy cow (MILK) and hog (HOG) population density; percent of developed land (DEVELOPED); percent of agricultural land (PASTURE); and well permit density (WELLS). The interaction term DEVELOPED*PASTURE was significant ($p < 0.05$). Disease is positively associated with increasing values of BEEF, HOG, DEVELOPED and PASTURE and negatively associated with increasing values of MILK, WELLS and KARST.

A map of background environmental risk generated using Model E4 (Figure 4) and Equation (1) with an offset of log(population density) shows elevated risk along developed corridors and in urban centers, in areas of agricultural land use and in areas of karst.

Figure 4. Spatial logistic regression model (E4) risk map for *E. coli* O157 infection (see Table 3 for the coefficients).

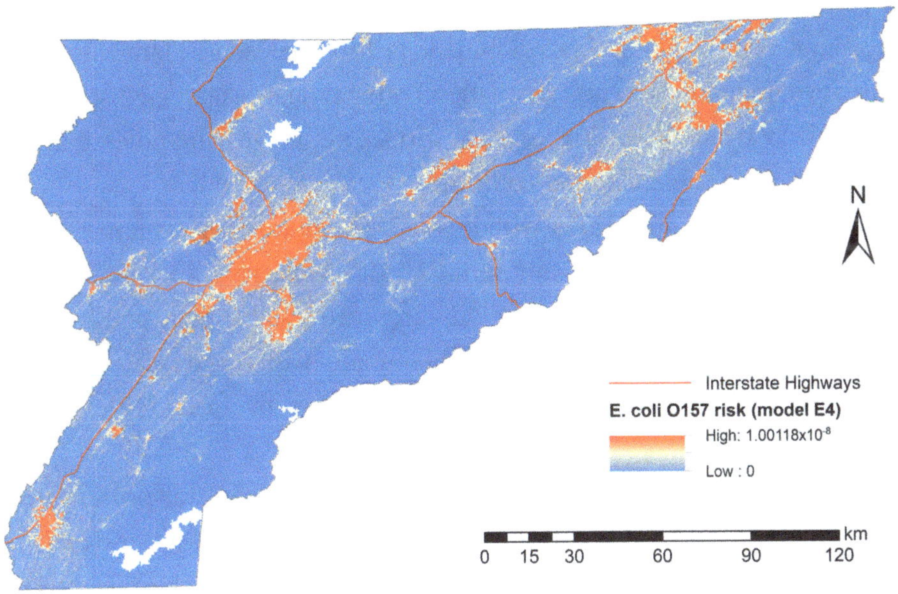

4. Discussion

Both cryptosporidiosis and *E. coli* O157 infection are waterborne diseases with low infectious doses and high survivability in the environment. It is reasonable therefore to see similar environmental risk factors for both diseases. However, there are also notable differences, which will be discussed in the sections that follow.

4.1. Karst Geology

Proximity to karst geology was a small, but consistently significant, risk factor for both diseases. This finding is in agreement with previous research for cryptosporidiosis [17] and is not surprising for a number of reasons. First, karst areas are underlain by limestone that is less resistant to weathering and erosion. Karst areas therefore coincide with valley bottoms in East Tennessee, which is where development is concentrated due to the ease of construction and access to transportation corridors (roads and rivers). This may lead to increased opportunities for human-to-human transmission. Second, and perhaps more importantly, in karst areas, surface water and groundwater are well connected through sinkholes and springs, and so, surface contamination readily enters the groundwater system and can emerge elsewhere as a spring, having had little opportunity for the natural attenuation typical of non-karst regions. Patients may unwittingly become infected through contact with an impaired spring. Proximity to karst geology is therefore an important risk factor and should be included in future studies of environmental risk factors for cryptosporidiosis and *E. coli* O157 infection.

4.2. Surface Water Quality

For cryptosporidiosis, proximity to an *E. coli*-impaired stream (STREAM) was associated with increased risk for disease, which is in agreement with risk factors reported in other studies [38–40]. Contact with contaminated water may be more likely the closer the patient resides to the stream, although it is important to note that proximity to a stream does not necessarily mean that contact occurs between an individual and the contaminant, and no data were available to determine whether individuals with either disease had physical contact with recreational water. Nevertheless, in East Tennessee, the general pattern of land development is for forested lands at higher elevations along ridge tops and for developed lands to hug the valley bottoms near established streams. The fluviokarst hydrology, characterized by both surface and subsurface drainage, sinkholes and abundant springs, provides ample opportunity for recreational contact.

Public water suppliers in the study area withdraw 82.2% of water by volume from surface lakes or streams, 15.9% from wells and 10.5% from springs [41]. Moreover, in karst areas with fluviokarst hydrology, groundwater-surface water interactions are well established, and surface contamination may quickly enter groundwater supplies and contaminate wells and springs. Spring response to precipitation includes increased flow and suspended sediment load [42], further evidence for groundwater-surface water interactions.

For *E. coli* O157 infection, proximity to an *E. coli*-impaired stream was not an important risk factor for disease, which contrasts previous studies that associated recreational water exposure with increased risk for *E. coli* O157 infection. [13,14]. A study of 350 *E. coli* O157 outbreaks in the United States from 1982 to 2002 determined that in 9.5% of the cases, the transmission route was related to recreational water contact, 4.5% was related to contaminated water supply, 3% was attributed to cattle contact and 21% was of unknown transmission (the remainder of cases were attributed to foodborne or person-to-person transmission) [10]. Surface water streams that are recognized by the state and by the Environmental Protection Agency as impaired due to the presence of *E. coli* are considered a public health threat, because *E. coli* is an indicator organism for the presence of both cryptosporidiosis and *E. coli* O157 in surface water. Environmental contamination of surface water supplies, resulting in the presence of fecal bacteria in streams and lakes, is known to increase the risk for bacteria-related sickness and death in humans [2,18,38,42]. Nevertheless, research that employs surface water quality spatial databases in spatial disease models is not well represented in the literature. The spatial models developed in this research associate proximity to an *E. coli*-impaired surface water stream with cryptosporidiosis, but not with *E. coli* O157 infection. While *E. coli* is the standard indicator for fecal pollution used by the state of Tennessee for the presence of both *E. coli* O157 and *Cryptosporidium* in surface water, prior research has shown that it is a poor indicator for the presence of *E. coli* O157 (in one study, the pathogen was detected in less than 1% of samples testing positive for *E. coli* [43]), but it is a reasonable indicator for *Cryptosporidium* oocysts (in the same study, oocysts were detected in 40% of samples testing positive for *E. coli*). Similarly, *E. coli* and turbidity were positively correlated in surface water samples, but *E. coli* O157 was not significantly correlated with turbidity [44]. The findings of the research presented here support the questioning of the use of *E. coli* as an appropriate indicator bacteria for *E. coli* O157 and as an indicator for the public health threat.

4.3. Land Use

The percent of agricultural land (PASTURE) and the percent of developed land (DEVELOPED) were associated with increased risk for both diseases, suggesting multiple pathways of transmission. A high percentage of developed land can be thought of as a proxy for high population density, and a higher number of cases of disease would be expected in these areas, due to the number of residents and consequent opportunities for human-to-human transmission. Agricultural land was also associated with increased disease in the individual and in the population, likely due to the presence of agricultural animals and opportunities for animal-to-human transmission [40,45].

The data used in this study were not sufficiently detailed to speciate the cryptosporidiosis cases into *C. hominis* and *C. parvum*, which are the two species commonly associated with human-to-human contact and animal-to-human contact, respectively. Others have found a positive association between developed land and *C. hominis* and between agricultural land and with *C. parvum* [46], but there is no way to test this using the cryptosporidiosis case data available for this study.

The association of developed land with *E. coli* O157 infection contrasts two other studies that positively associated disease with rural areas [14] and [47] farm density. Their findings agree, however, with the positive association between disease and agricultural land found in this study. The significance of contrasting land use variables as risk factors for both diseases suggests multiple pathways for infection. In developed land, transmission may be by human-to-human contact, foodborne transmission or through direct animal contact during farm visits. In pasture and forested lands, transmission may be through environmental contamination, foodborne transmission or through animal-to-human contact. No data about the patient's occupation was available in the dataset; however, it is reasonable to recognize that farmers, farm families and farm workers will have different exposures and immunity to both diseases, which may influence model results. The significance of the interaction term between developed land and agricultural land for *E. coli* O157 infection can be thought of as a variable expressing the proximity of development to agriculture (*i.e.*, locations where developed land and agricultural land are both dominant), providing increased opportunity for contact between residents and agricultural activity, which has been related to increased risk for *E. coli* O157 infection [13,14].

4.4. Agricultural Animal Population Densities

The positive association of beef cow population density (BEEF) with increased risk for disease agrees with other studies that have linked cattle populations with cryptosporidiosis [46,48] and *E. coli* O157 infection [14,20,21]. Although beef cow population density was positively associated with both diseases, dairy cow population density was not significantly associated with cryptosporidiosis and was negatively associated with *E. coli* O157 infection. Because of the differences in how their populations are associated with the two diseases, it is therefore important to differentiate between beef and dairy cattle in similar studies. All cattle-related studies reviewed for this research treated cattle as one group, but this research suggests that the cattle population should be partitioned into beef and dairy. The protective effect of dairy cow population density may result from the regulation of farming practices in dairy farms, specifically the controls required to capture and treat runoff, which reduce the pathogen load in the environment. In contrast, beef cattle are more common in East Tennessee, and no environmental regulations exist to control runoff from pasture land nor to control access to streams by cattle. Consequently, runoff from agricultural fields is a non-point source of surface water pollution, which increases the environmental pollution load. Interpreting the negative association between dairy cattle and *E. coli* O157 infection as a protective effect is a plausible hypothesis, but cannot be confirmed at this point.

The positive association found between hog population density (HOG) and *E. coli* O157 infection contrasts with two other studies that found a negative association [15] and no association [21].

4.5. Poverty Rate

Poverty rate was not retained as an explanatory variable for either disease, which may indicate that poverty rate at the block group level is not a good indicator of risk for disease in the individual. A better variable to include in the individual model may be the socioeconomic status of the individual, rather than the individual's block group, because the aggregate variable smoothes out variability, and there is no way to know the actual socioeconomic status of the individual when using aggregate data.

4.6. Well Permits

Well permit density was positively related to cryptosporidiosis and *E. coli* O157 infection. While not indicative of drinking water source for a given case of disease, well permit density can indicate whether private water supply is more or less common in a county, so it is a measure of the availability of a private water supply. The finding that increased disease risk in the individual is associated with decreased well density indicates that the availability of private water supplies has a protective effect. Wells in the study area have an average depth of 309 feet, which easily bottom within the karst limestone bedrock unit that underlies much of the study area. In fact, one eighth of the deepest caves in the USA are found within karst areas of Tennessee, and because these caves regularly descend beyond the average depth of the private wells, the depth of the wells is not a compelling explanation for their apparent protective effect. Note, however, that this finding agrees with a recent Tennessee Department of Health clinical epidemiological study on cryptosporidiosis conducted in the Greene County, Tennessee, region from 2009 to 2011. This study used a supplemental form to gather drinking water source, recreational water exposure, food, travel and animal exposures at the individual level. No association with private water supplies was found. This result, however, contrasts with other studies that associated private water supply with increased risk for *E. coli* O157 infection [14] and cryptosporidiosis [17,48].

4.7. Limitations

This study examines environmental risk factors for two diseases that can also be transmitted through other exposures related to an individual's behavior or lifestyle. These variables may include consumption of undercooked beef or unpasteurized dairy products, visits to farms, contact with infected persons and playing or swimming in contaminated surface water [3,11,14,45,46,49–51]. The individual models developed here do not capture this individual behavior, but instead, can capture potential exposure to risk for the individual by inclusion of environmental variables at the local scale. Proximity to contaminated surface water or to agricultural activity can increase the likelihood that a person will come in contact with an environmental reservoir of cryptosporidiosis or *E. coli* O157 and in this way can increase background risk. The individual model, therefore, can be thought of as the environmental background risk at the individual level (large-scale environmental risk).

Selection of a "best" model is secondary to identifying risk factors for *E. coli* O157 infection and cryptosporidiosis from a set of potential environmental and socioeconomic explanatory variables. An understanding of the environmental and socioeconomic variables that emerge as significant risk factors for disease can help to inform policies to combat disease prevalence. Often, these relationships can be discerned by exploratory mapping of disease cases overlaid with risk factors; however, the modeling process is important to statistically quantify the risk and the important risk factors. Risk maps, such as those displayed in Figures 2 and 3, can visually communicate the environmental background risk for disease within the study area. Because cryptosporidiosis and *E. coli* O157 infection are rare diseases, the probabilities are low, but differences in high *versus* low risk are apparent.

Care must be taken in interpreting maps such as these, because individual behavior has not been factored in. Background risk maps may therefore be most useful in developing the framework for a public education campaign to combat a disease endemic within a population or in developing a more in-depth epidemiological study. Knowledge of the explanatory variables used by the model to generate the risk map can be useful to identify the behaviors to target in such a campaign, for example warning residents of the risks associated with agricultural animal contact or playing in or around an impaired stream. In this way, limited public health resources can be targeted at the locations and the behaviors most associated with disease.

While geospatial analysis and the explicit inclusion of space when assessing disease risk can be a valuable tool to identify populations at risk, any model is only as good as the data and assumptions used to generate the model. Non-reporting of diseases because a patient does not seek medical attention, because a sample is not taken during the medical examination or due to incomplete reporting of disease incidence can erode the quality of a dataset. Patterns in non-reporting can also affect results if members of one socioeconomic group are less likely (or more likely) to be exposed or to seek treatment [46]. Care must be taken, therefore, in the interpretation of model results, because spatial differences in reporting rates may introduce bias into the modeled relationship between disease and environmental risk factors.

5. Conclusions

This research has shown that environmental variables are important risk factors for cryptosporidiosis and *E. coli* O157 infection in the individual. Proximity to karst geology was associated with both diseases, indicating that geology, specifically limestone and dolomite formations that are prone to karst weathering, should be incorporated as a proximity measure in waterborne disease risk models. Proximity to impaired surface water was a risk factor for cryptosporidiosis, but not *E. coli* O157 infection, likely related to the utility of *E. coli* as an indicator for *E. coli* O157.

Beef cow population density was positively associated with both diseases, while dairy cow population density was negatively associated with *E. coli* O157 infection. Because of the different results for cattle, populations should be partitioned into dairy and beef cattle when included as risk factors in a model for cryptosporidiosis and *E. coli* O157 infection.

Multiple transmission sources for both diseases are indicated by the positive association between percent agricultural land and percent developed land. Because both developed land and pasture land are associated with increased risk for cryptosporidiosis, future studies of environmental risk factors for cryptosporidiosis should partition the cases by species (*C. hominis* and *C. parvum*) to examine the role of pasture and land use. To accomplish this, diagnostic methods must identify *Cryptosporidium* at the species level.

Models such as these can be useful to identify important risk factors for disease and to generate a background risk model. These results can then be used to develop a public education campaign to target limited public health resources to address behaviors associated with the most important risk factors in the communities where opportunities for those behaviors are most likely. These results can also be used as the framework upon which to develop a more comprehensive epidemiological or microbiological study to examine specific pathways for disease that focus on individual level risk factors.

Acknowledgments

The authors express thanks to Agricola Odoi (Department of Comparative Medicine, University of Tennessee) for assistance with epidemiology, to Nicholas Nagle and Yingkui Li (Department of Geography, University of Tennessee) for assistance with statistics and methodology and to Judy Manners (Tennessee Department of Health).

Author Contributions

Ingrid Luffman and Liem Tran conceived and designed the models; Ingrid Luffman performed the modeling; Ingrid Luffman and Liem Tran analyzed and interpreted the results; Ingrid Luffman wrote the paper.

References

1. Bunnell, J.E. Medical geology: Emerging discipline on the ecosystem-human health interface. *EcoHealth* **2004**, *1*, 15–18.
2. Dohoo, I.W.; Martin, W.; Stryhn, H. *Veterinary Epidemiologic Research*; AVC: Charlottetown, Canada, 2003.
3. Robertson, W.; Yasvinski, G. Exposure. In *Animal Waste, Water Quality and Human Health*; Dufour, A.P., Dufour, A., Eds.; IWA Publishing: London, UK, 2012; pp. 257–282.
4. Dura, G.; Pándics, T.; Kádár, M.; Krisztalovics, K.; Kiss, Z.; Bodnár, J.; Asztalos, A.; Papp, E. Environmental health aspects of drinking water-borne outbreak due to karst flooding: Case study. *J. Water Health* **2010**, *8*, 513–520.
5. Jiang, Y.; Wu, Y.; Groves, C.; Yuan, D.; Kambesis, P. Natural and anthropogenic factors affecting the groundwater quality in the Nandong karst underground river system in Yunan, China. *J. Contam. Hydrol.* **2009**, *109*, 49–61.
6. Boyer, D.G.; Pasquarell, G.C. *Agricultural Land Use Impacts on Bacterial Water Quality in a Karst Groundwater Aquifer*; Wiley Online Library: Hoboken, NJ, USA, 1999.

7. Kelly, W.R.; Panno, S.V.; Hackley, K.C.; Martinsek, A.T.; Krapac, I.G.; Weibel, C.P.; Storment, E.C. Bacteria contamination of groundwater in a mixed land-use karst region. *Water Qual. Expo. Health* **2009**, *1*, 69–78.
8. O'Reilly, C.E.; Bowen, A.B.; Perez, N.E.; Sarisky, J.P.; Shepherd, C.A.; Miller, M.D.; Hubbard, B.C.; Herring, M.; Buchanan, S.D.; Fitzgerald, C.C.; *et al.* A waterborne outbreak of gastroenteritis with multiple etiologies among resort island visitors and residents: Ohio, 2004. *Clin. Infect. Dis.* **2007**, *44*, 506–512.
9. Dong, B.-Q.; Yang, J.; Wang, X.-Y.; Gong, Y.; von Seidlein, L.; Wang, M.-L.; Lin, M.; Liao, H.-Z.; Ochiai, R.L.; Xu, Z.-Y.; *et al.* Trends and disease burden of enteric fever in Guangxi Province, China, 1994–2004. *Bull. World Health Organ.* **2010**, *88*, 689–696.
10. Rangel, J.M.; Sparling, P.H.; Crowe, C.; Griffin, P.M.; Swerdlow, D.L. Epidemiology of *Escherichia coli* O157:H7 outbreaks, United States, 1982–2002. *Emerg. Infect. Dis.* **2005**, *11*, 603–609.
11. Chalmers, R.M.; Aird, H.; Boldton, F.J. Waterborne *Escherichia coli* O157. *J. Aplied Microbiol. Symp. Suppl.* **2000**, *88*, 124S–132S.
12. Muniesa, M.; Jofre, J.; García-Aljaro, C.; Blanch, A.R. Occurrence of Escherichia coli O157:H7 and other enterohemorrhagic *Escherichia coli* in the environment. *Environ. Sci. Technol.* **2006**, *40*, 7141–7149.
13. O'Brien, S.J.; Goutam, K.A.; Gilham, C. Contact with farming environment as a major risk factor for Shiga Toxin (Vero Cytotoxin)-producing *Escherichia coli* O157 infection in humans. *Emerg. Infect. Dis.* **2001**, *7*, 1049–1051.
14. Strachan, N.J.; Dunn, G.M.; Locking, M.E.; Reid, T.M.; Ogden, I.D. *Escherichia coli* O157: Burger bug or environmental pathogen? *Int. J. Food Microbiol.* **2006**, *112*, 129–137.
15. Friesema, I.H.; van de Kassteele, J.; de Jager, C.M.; Heuvelink, A.E.; van Pelt, W. Geographical association between livestock density and human Shiga toxin-producing *Escherichia coli* O157 infections. *Epidemiol. Infect.* **2011**, *139*, 1081–1087.
16. Kassenborg, H.D.; Hedberg, C.W.; Hoekstra, M.; Evans, M.C.; Chin, A.E.; Marcus, R.; Vugia, D.J.; Smith, K.; Ahuja, S.D.; Slutsker, L.; *et al.* Farm visits and undercooked hamburgers as major risk factors for sporadic *Escherichia coli* O157:H7 infection: Data from a case-control study in 5 FoodNet sites. *Clin. Infect. Dis.* **2004**, *38*, S271–S278.
17. Klumb, C.; Robinson, T.; Cebelinski, E.; Alexander, B.H.; Smith, K. Evaluation of relationships between private well water, geologic sensitivity, cattle density, and *Cryptosporidium parvum* infection in Minnesota, 2000–2008. In Proceedings of the International Conference on Emerging Infectious Diseases, Minneapolis, MN, USA, 11–17 November 2010; pp. 669–670.
18. Hlavsa, M.C.; Brunkard, J.M. *Surveillance for Waterborne Disease Outbreaks and Other Health Events Associated with Recreational Water—United States, 2007–2008*; U.S. Department of Health and Human Services, Centers for Disease Control and Prevention: Atlanta, GA, USA, 2011.
19. Hlavsa, M.C.; Watson, J.C.; Beach, M.J. Cryptosporidiosis surveillance—United States 1999–2002. *MMWR Surveill. Summ.* **2005**, *54*, 1–8.
20. Michel, P.; Wilson, J.B.; Martin, S.W.; Clarke, R.C.; Mcewen, S.A.; Gyles, C.L. Temporal and geographical distributions of reported cases of *Escherichia coli* O157:H7 infection in Ontario. *Epidemiol. Infect.* **1999**, *122*, 193–200.

21. Valcour, J.E.; Michel, P.; McEwen, S.A.; Wilson, J.B. Associations between indicators of livestock farming intensity and incidence of human Shiga toxin-producing *Escherichia coli* infection. *Emerg. Infect. Dis.* **2002**, *8*, 252–257.
22. Scallan, E.; Hoekstra, R.M.; Angulo, F.J.; Tauxe, R.V.; Widdowson, M.-A.; Roy, S.-L.; Jones, J.L.; Griffin, P.M. Foodborne illness acquired in the United States—Major pathogens. *Emerg. Infect. Dis.* **2011**, *17*, 7–15.
23. Jarup, L. The Role of Geographical Studies in Risk Assessment. In *Spatial Epidemiology Methods and Applications*; Elliott, P., Wakefield, J., Best, N., Briggs, D., Eds.; Oxford University Press: New York, NY, USA, 2000; pp. 415–433.
24. Barton, K.E.; Howell, D.G.; Vigil, J.F. *The North America Tapestry of Time and Terrain*; Geologic Investigations Series I-2781; U.S. Geological Survey: Reston, VA, USA, 2003.
25. Godlberg, D.W.; Wilson, J.P. USC WebGIS Services. Available online: http://webgis.usc.edu/Services/Geocode/BatchProcess/Default.aspx (accessed on 22 November 2011).
26. Environmental Systems Research Institute, Inc. *ArcView 10.0 Desktop*; Environmental Systems Research Institute, Inc.: Redlands, CA, USA, 2011.
27. Greene, D.C.; Wolfe, W.J. 1:250,000 Geology of Tennessee. Available online: http://water.usgs.gov/GIS/metadata/usgswrd/XML/geo250k.xml#stdorder (accessed on 2 April 2011).
28. Denton, G.M.; Brame, C.J.; Arnwine, D.H.; Cartwright, L.K.; Graf, M.H. 2008 305(b) Report The Status of Water Quality in Tennessee. Available online: http://www.tn.gov/environment/water/docs/wpc/2008_305b.pdf (accessed on 2 April 2011).
29. Tennessee Department of Environment and Conservation. Final Year 2008 303(d) List. Available online: http://www.tn.gov/environment/water/docs/wpc/2008_303d.pdf (accessed on 2 April 2011).
30. EPA RADims. Available online: http://epamap32.epa.gov/radims/ (accessed on 17 October 2011).
31. United States Department of Agriculture. 2007 Census of Agriculture. Available online: http://quickstats.nass.usda.gov/?agg_level_desc=ZIP%20CODE (accessed on 2 April 2011).
32. Fry, J.; Xian, A.J.; Jin, S.; Dewitz, J.A.; Homer, C.G.; Yang, L.; Barnes, C.A.; Herold, N.D.; Wickham, J.D. Completion of the 2006 national land cover database for the conterminous United States. *Photogramm. Eng. Remote Sens.* **2011**, *77*, 858–864.
33. United States Census. 2010 Census Table B17017. Available online: http://www.census.gov/acs/www/data_documentation/summary_file/ (accessed on 19 April 2012).
34. Bivand, R.S.; Pebesma, E.J.; Gomez-Rubio, V. *Applied Spatial Data Analysis with R*; Gentleman, R., Hornik, K., Parmigiani, G., Eds.; Springer: New York, NY, USA, 2008.
35. R Core Team. *R: A Language and Environment for Statistical Computing Version 2.15.1*; R Foundation for Statistical Computing: Vienna, Austria, 2012.
36. Baddeley, A.; Turner, R. Spatstat: An R package for analyzing spatial point patterns. *J. Stat. Softw.* **2005**, *12*, 1–42.
37. Baddeley, A.; Berman, M.; Fisher, N.I.; Hardegen, A.; Milne, R.K.; Shah, S.R.; Turner, R. Spatial logistic regression and change-of-support in poisson point process. *Electron. J. Stat.* **2010**, *4*, 1151–1201.
38. Beach, M.J. *Waterborne: Recreational water*. In *Cryptosporidium and Cryptosporidiosis*, 2nd ed.; Fayer, R., Xiao, L., Eds.; CRC Press: Boca Raton, FL, USA, 2008; pp.329–362.

39. Hoek, M.R.; Oliver, I.; Barlow, M.; Heard, L.; Chalmers, R.; Paynter, S. Outbreak of *Cryptosporidium parvum* among children after a school excursion to an adventure farm, South West England. *J. Water Health* **2008**, *6*, 333–338.
40. Centers for Disease Control and Prevention. Cryptosporidiosis outbreak at a summer camp—North Carolina, 2009. *Morb. Mortal. Wkly. Rep.* **2011**, *60*, 918–922.
41. Robinson, J.A.; Brooks, J.M. *Public Water-Supply Systems and Associated Water Use in Tennessee*; Open-File Report 2010–1226; United States Geologic Survey: Reston, VA, USA, 2005.
42. Vesper, D.J.; White, W.B. Metal transport to karst springs during storm flow: An example from Fort Campbell, Kentucky/Tennessee, USA. *J. Hydrol.* **2003**, *276*, 20–36.
43. Wilkes, G.E.; Edge, T.; Gannon, V.; Jokinen, C.; Lyautey, E.; Medeiros, D.; Neumann, N.; Ruecker, N.; Topp, E.; Lapen, D.R. Seasonal relationships among indicator bacteria, pathogenic bacteria, *Cryptosporidium* oocysts, *Giardia* cysts, and hydrological indices for surface waters within an agricultural landscape. *Water Res.* **2009**, *43*, 2209–2223.
44. Dorner, S.M.; Anderson, W.B.; Gaulin, T.; Candon, H.L.; Slawson, R.M.; Payment, P.; Huck, P.M. Pathogen and indicator variability in a heavily impacted watershed. *J. Water Health* **2007**, *5*, 241–257.
45. Hunter, P.R.; Hadfield, S.J.; Wilkinson, D.; Lake, I.R.; Harrison, F.C.; Chalmers, R.M. Subtypes of *Cryptosporidium parvum* in humans and disease risk. *Emerg. Infect. Dis.* **2007**, *13*, 82–88.
46. Lake, I.R.; Harrison, F.C.; Chalmers, R.M.; Bentham, G.; Nichols, G.; Hunter, P.R.; Kovats, R.S.; Grundy, C. Case-control study of environmental and social factors influencing cryptosporidiosis. *Eur. J. Epidemiol.* **2007**, *22*, 805–811.
47. Kistemann, T.; Zimmer, S.; Vågsholm, I.; Andersson, Y. GIS-supported investigation of human EHEC and cattle VTEC O157 infections in Sweden: Geographical distribution, spatial variation and possible risk factors. *Epidemiol. Infect.* **2004**, *132*, 495–505.
48. Said, B.; Wright, F.; Nichols, G.L.; Reacher, M.; Rutter, M. Outbreaks of infectious disease associated with private drinking water supplies in England and Wales 1970–2000. *Epidemiol. Infect.* **2003**, *130*, 469–479.
49. Benham, B.L.; Affaut, C.; Zeckoski, R.W.; Mankin, K.R.; Pachepsky, Y.A.; Adeghi, A.M.; Rannan, K.M.; Oupir, M.L.; Habersack, M.J. Modeling bacteria fate and transport in watersheds to support TMDLs. *Am. Soc. Agric. Biol. Eng.* **2006**, *49*, 987–1002.
50. Dietz, V.J.; Roberts, J.M. National surveillance for infection with *Cryptosporidium parvum*, 1995–1998: What have we learned? *Public Health Rep.* **2000**, *115*, 358–363.
51. Suresh, K.G.; Toranzos, G.A.; Faycr, R.; Nissaparton, V.; Olvcda, R.; Ashbolt, N.; Gannon, V. Assessing the importance of zoonotic waterborne pathogens. In *Animal Waste, Water Quality and Human Health*; Dufour, A.I., Bartram, J., Bos, R., Gannon, V., Eds.; IWA Publishing: London, UK, 2012; pp. 17–72.

8

Environmental Risk Assessment Based on High-Resolution Spatial Maps of Potentially Toxic Elements Sampled on Stream Sediments of Santiago, Cape Verde

Marina M. S. Cabral Pinto [1,2,3,*], Eduardo A. Ferreira da Silva [1], Maria M. V. G. Silva [3], Paulo Melo-Gonçalves [4] and Carla Candeias [1]

1 GeoBioTec—Geobiosciences, Geotechnologies e Geoengineering Research Center, Geosciences Department, University of Aveiro, Campus de Santiago, 3810-193 Aveiro, Portugal; E-Mails: eafsilva@ua.pt (E.A.F.S.); candeias@ua.pt (C.C.)

2 CNC Centre-Centre for Neuroscience and Cell Biology, College of Medicine, University of Coimbra, 3004-517 Coimbra, Portugal

3 Department of Geosciences, Geosciences Centre, University of Coimbra, 3000-272 Coimbra, Portugal; E-Mail: mmvslva@ci.uc.pt

4 Department of Physics and Centre for Environmental and Marine Studies (CESAM), University of Aveiro, 3810-193 Aveiro, Portugal; E-Mail: pmg@ua.pt

* Author to whom correspondence should be addressed; E-Mail: marinacp@ci.uc.pt;

External Editors: Jose A. Centeno, Robert B. Finkelman and Olle Selinus

---

Abstract: Geochemical mapping is the base knowledge to identify the regions of the planet with critical contents of potentially toxic elements from either natural or anthropogenic sources. Sediments, soils and waters are the vehicles which link the inorganic environment to life through the supply of essential macro and micro nutrients. The chemical composition of surface geological materials may cause metabolic changes which may favor the occurrence of endemic diseases in humans. In order to better understand the relationships between environmental geochemistry and public health, we present environmental risk maps of some harmful elements (As, Cd, Co, Cr, Cu, Hg, Mn, Ni, Pb, V, and Zn) in the stream sediments of Santiago, Cape Verde, identifying the potentially harmful areas in this island. The Estimated Background Values (EBV) of Cd, Co, Cr, Ni and V were found to be above the Canadian guidelines for any type of use of stream sediments and also above the target values of the Dutch and United States guidelines. The Probably Effect Concentrations (PEC), above which harmful effects are likely in sediment dwelling organisms, were found for Cr and Ni. Some associations between the geological formations of the island and the composition of stream sediments were identified and confirmed by descriptive statistics and by Principal Component Analysis (PCA). The EBV spatial distribution of the metals and the results of PCA allowed us to establish relationships between the EBV maps and the geological formations. The first two PCA modes indicate that heavy metals in Santiago stream sediments are mainly originated from weathering of underlying bedrocks. The first metal association (Co, V, Cr, and Mn; first PCA mode) consists of elements enriched in basic rocks and compatible elements. The second association of variables (Zn and Cd as opposed to Ni; second PCA mode) appears to be strongly controlled by the composition of alkaline volcanic rocks and pyroclastic rocks. So, the second PCA mode is also considered as a natural lithogenic mode. The third association (Cu and Pb; third PCA mode) consists of elements of anthropogenic origin.

Keywords: potentially harmful elements; stream sediments; Estimated Background Value (EBV); Environmental Risk Index (ERI); Principal Component Analysis (PCA); Santiago Island; Cape Verde

---

1. Introduction

The study of the effects of the geological environment on human health is the main area of Geomedicine. Natural processes (e.g., weathering, escape of gases and fluids along major fractures in the Earth's crust, and volcanic related activity) release to the environment large amounts of elements. Some elements are macro and micro nutrients for the human alimentary (digestive) supply, and some of these can be harmful to humans, even in small concentrations, e.g., Hg, As, Pb, Sb, Bi, Cd, Ag, Al, Be, Sn [1]. Besides natural factors, human activities, such as agriculture industry, and specifically mining [2,3], enhance the introduction of these elements in the human food chain.

The dispersion of chemical elements in the environment is carried out by sediments, soils and waters, which are the vehicles which link the inorganic environment to life. Variations in its natural chemical composition may cause metabolic changes favouring the occurrence of endemic diseases, such as gout, fluorosis, arsenicosis and Keshan's disease, or conversely may be health promoting [4]. No more than 10%–12% of neurologic diseases have a strict genetic etiology, while the majority of cases has unknown origin [5]. According to Gorell *et al.* [6], environmental and occupational exposure to Mn, Cu, Pb, Fe, Zn, Al, appears to be a risk factor for Parkinson's and Alzheimer's diseases. Several authors [7–13] suggest a correlation between the inhalation and ingestion of Mn and disorders of the nervous central system in rats, primates and humans. The International Agency for Research on Cancer shows that the occupational exposure to chromium [VI] is carcinogenic to humans [14]. This agency also concluded that nickel compounds are carcinogenic to humans and that metallic nickel is possibly carcinogenic to humans.

Environmental exposure to cadmium and lead is associated with alterations in renal function [15] and cadmium and chromium also are related to hypertension and atherosclerosis [16].

Knowledge of the geochemistry of sediments, soils and waters is essential to understand the causes of some endemic diseases and, therefore, contribute to the improvement of the nutritional status of the population living on areas where excess or deficiency of some elements occur, e.g., [17,18]. The determination of geochemical baselines and the geochemical cartography are of major importance because they provide a base framework required by objective and effective methods for addressing environmental concerns [19].

Understanding the abundance and spatial distribution of chemical elements in the near-surface environment of the Earth is critical for fields such as risk-based assessment of contaminated land, agriculture, animal and human health, water quality, land use planning, mineral exploration, industrial pollution, and environmental regulation [20]. National geochemical surveys have been a priority in many countries given the importance and applicability of the resulting geochemical databases, e.g., [21–24]. These surveys provide the natural state of the environment [20,21,25–29] and allow the discrimination between geogenic sources and anthropogenic pollution [19,30–32], which is useful for the determination of environmental impacts of mines [33,34], agriculture [35], geomedicine [4,7], and other fields. Initially, geochemical maps were used for mineral exploration and, therefore, were elaborated at high sample densities (from 1/1 km^2 to 1/25 km^2). Latter, in the late 1960s, the first national low-density geochemical survey was conducted in Africa with a sampling density of 1/200 km^2. Also in this decade, the U.S. Geological Survey project began a national-scale geochemical database, with a density of approximately one site per 6000 km^2 [20]. National and even continental surveys conducted in various parts of the world had, generally, sample densities ranging from 1/300 km^2 to 1/18,000 km^2 [24]. Maps of baseline values are especially important in countries like Cape Verde, where intervention limits for near-surface environment are not yet established. Recently, a high-density (approximately 1/3 km^2) geochemical survey was conducted in Santiago Island, Cape Verde archipelago, and the first environmental geochemical atlas was compiled for that region [36]. The field work occurred from 2005 until the beginning of 2008, over six campaigns.

A reliable geochemical baseline can only be established if uncontaminated sites are sampled, e.g., [31,35]. The input of elements into stream sediments resulting from human activities has been growing worldwide, making the finding of uncontaminated stream sediment samples more difficult. Fortunately, the human influence was negligible in Santiago before the sampling survey was conducted for this study (2005–2008), compared to that in developed countries.

In order to better understand the relationships between environmental geochemistry and public health, we conducted an environmental risk assessment using the stream sediments sampling medium in the Santiago Island, Cape Verde, following the guidelines proposed by the International Project IGCP 259 [31]. It is important to highlight that this environmental risk is inferred and not calculated on the basis of possible direct or indirect ingestion pathways (pica, airborne dust, transfer through consumption of plants, *etc.*).

Stream sediments are often a preferred medium for sampling in regional and national geochemical surveys [37] because they provide a composite sample of the catchment area upstream of the sampling point [23], which defines the geochemical background, and tends to integrate all sources of sediment (primary rock and soil) [20]. Therefore, stream sediments are an effective medium to represent the geochemical background.

Environmental risk maps of some potentially harmful metal and metalloids (As, Cd, Co, Cr, Cu, Hg, Mn, Ni, Pb, V, and Zn) are presented in this study, identifying the areas of the island which are potentially problematic concerning human health issues. These risk maps were drawn after an estimation of the geochemical background values of the studied elements.

2. Cape Verde Archipelago and Santiago Island: Location and Geology

2.1. Settings of the Archipelago of Cape Verde and Santiago Island

The archipelago of Cape Verde composed of 10 islands (Figure 1) is located at the eastern shore of the Atlantic Ocean, 500 km west from Senegal's Cape Verde, in the African western shore, between the latitudes 17°13′ N (Santo Antão Island) and 14°48′ N (Brava Island) and the longitude 22°42′ W (Boavista Island) and 25°22′ W (Santo Antão Island) (Figure 1). The biggest island is Santiago Island (991 km^2), located in the southern part of the archipelago and with about half of the country's population [38].

Figure 1. The Cape Verde Archipelago and its location in Africa's western coast and Geological cartography of Santiago Island, Cape Verde, modified from [39].

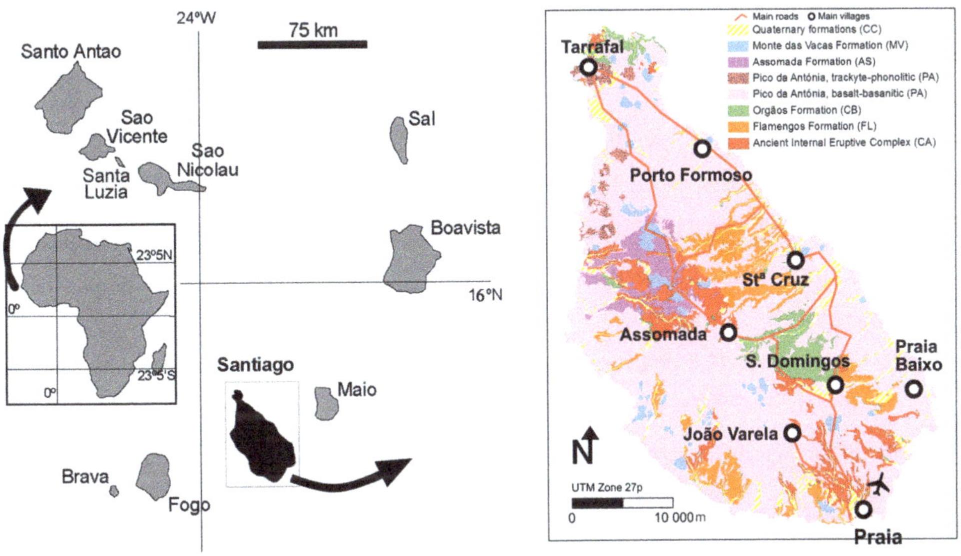

Santiago Island is an elongated NNW-SSE shield-volcano with a maximum length of 54.9 km and a maximum width of 29 km and its maximum altitude reaches 1394 m. The climate is semi-arid, with strong winds during the dry season, and a mean annual precipitation of 321 mm, mainly due to torrential rains, in the wet season [40]. It has 215 km^2 of arable area and estimated water resources of 56.6 × 100 m^3/year at the surface, and 42.4 × 100 m^3/year underground [41].

2.2. Geological Setting of Santiago Island

The major lithological formations of Santiago Island were defined by [39] and [42] (Figure 1), and they show variable geochemistry [36]. The oldest formation, the Ancient Internal Eruptive Complex (CA), is constituted by strongly weathered submarine volcanic products and a dyke complex, which probably represent the submarine edifice-building phase of the island [39,43]. The outcrops of CA are scattered throughout the island (Figure 1), occupying depressions and valleys. There is a wide range of rock types in the CA, mainly basalts and basanites, but gabbros, alkaline syenites, phonolites, trachytes, breccias and carbonatites also occur.

The Flamengos Formation (FL), with 4.57 ± 0.31 Ma [44], is composed of submarine basaltic mantles, with minor hyaloclastic breccias, tuffs, dykes and chimneys. The rocks are limburgites, basanites and basanitoids, with zeolites and carbonates.

The Orgãos Formation (CB) outcrops mostly in the central part of the island but also in the north (Figure 1), and reaches thicknesses of more than 100 m [45]. It is a subaerial and submarine breccia/conglomerate with a sandstone matrix, carbonate and zeolitic cement [39], and probably represents lahars.

The Eruptive Complex of Pico da Antónia (PA) outcrops along more than half of the surface of Santiago Island (Figure 1) and its radiometric age is between 3.25 ± 0.4 and 2.25 ± 0.09 Ma [44]. It corresponds to the main shield-building stage [43] and is essentially formed by thick sequences of basaltic, submarine and subaerial lava flows [46], with intercalated pyroclastic material. The PA formation also contains dikes, chimneys and endogenous domes of phonolites and trachytes [39]. The lithotypes are essentially ankaratrites, limburgites and basanites, but also nephelinites and olivine-melilitite [42] also occur.

The Assomada Formation (AS) occupies a large depression, is constituted by subaerial almost horizontal, basaltic mantles and some basaltic pyroclastes (Figure 1). The rocks are essentially basanites [42], with gray and reddish colours when weathered.

In Santiago Island, there are 50 scoria cones (the highest reaches 230 m), aligned in the NW-SE direction (Figure 1), constituted by basaltic pyroclastic material and small subordinated flows (1.13 ± 0.03 Ma) [44]. They mark the last volcanic episodes in Santiago Island and were named by Serralheiro (1976) as the Monte das Vacas Formation (MV). The loosely aggregated pyroclasts are exploited for construction, promoting gullies and landslides on the flanks due to erosive action of the water during intense rainfall episodes.

The Quaternary Formations (CC) have a small spatial representation (Figure 1), outcropping in the valleys and close to the shore. They are ancient and modern alluvium, torrent deposits, sand dunes and marine beaches deposits. The terraces reach altitudes of about 100 m.

3. Materials and Methods

3.1. Sample Collection and Treatment

Between 2005 and 2008, 337 stream sediments composite samples were collected (0–15 cm) across the Santiago Island at a density of ~1 site per 3 km^2. Sampling locations were identified using a global positioning system (GPS) and the sampling sites were chosen to be as uncontaminated as possible. Therefore, locations affected by pollution, such as locations near factories or heavy traffic roads and arable soils, were avoided. Given the mountainous topography of Santiago Island and its poor road network, sampling sites are somewhat unevenly distributed.

On each site the composite sample (~1 kg) was obtained by collecting five points, spaced approximately 50 m along the water course. Fresh samples were contained in plastic bags and taken to a laboratory for posterior analyses. Field duplicate samples were taken at every 10 sites, yielding field duplicates for 26 locations evenly distributed over the island, which will be used in the Analysis of Variance described in Section 3.3.

All samples were air-dried at ~20 °C and visible pebbles were removed. Stream sediments were then sieved to <2 mm, being this fraction used for all analyses. A 10 g split of the retained stream sediments was milled in an agate mill to <0.074 mm for chemical analysis.

3.2. Chemical Analysis

The chemical analysis was performed at ACME Analytical Laboratories, Ltd., Vancouver, Canada and according to the laboratory standards methods and QA/QC and protocols. Sample duplicates were analyzed to access precision. Individual samples were digested in *aqua regia* and analysed by inductively coupled plasma-mass spectrometry (ICP-MS) for As, Cd, Co, Cr, Cu, Hg, Mn, Ni, Pb, V, and Zn. Digestion with *aqua regia* is a method of chemical attack more commonly used in environmental studies, than mixtures with HF acid or $HClO_4$ [31]. This type of attack is effective in removing the more mobile elements normally associated with clay minerals, organic matter and other secondary minerals [47–49]. It completely dissolves most of the sulphides, oxides, clay minerals and secondary minerals formed during pedogenesis and other exogenous processes, but most silicate minerals are not dissolved. The samples sent for analysis were randomly numbered in order to remove any systematic relationship between the analysis order and the geographic location, following the recommendations of [31].

3.3. Analytical Quality Control

The data resulting from the chemical analysis of the elements was subjected to several data quality tests in order to determine which elements have reliable data to be interpreted by subsequent statistical analysis. The criteria used were: (i) at least 70% of the observations with content greater than the detection limit; (ii) accuracy and precision, quantified by analytical duplicates, having relative standard deviation lower than 10%; and (iii) spatial geochemical variance (σ_G^2) significantly representative, at a 0.01 significance level, of the spatial total observed variance (σ_T^2) quantified by an Analysis of Variance using field duplicates sampled at 26 locations evenly distributed over the island.

This Analysis of Variance consists of partitioning the spatial total observed variance (σ_T^2) into the spatial geochemical variance (σ_G^2) and the variance associated to errors due to field sampling and chemical analysis (σ_{SA}^2):

$$\sigma_T^2 = \sigma_G^2 + \sigma_{SA}^2 \tag{1}$$

Each population variance, σ^2, is estimated by the corresponding sample variance s^2:

$$s_T^2 = s_G^2 + s_{SA}^2 \tag{2}$$

where

$$s_T^2 = \frac{1}{N-1}\sum_{n=1}^{N}(X_{1i} - \overline{X}_1)^2 \tag{3}$$

and

$$s_{SA}^2 = \frac{1}{N}\sum_{n=1}^{N}\frac{(X_{1i} - X_{2i})^2}{2} \tag{4}$$

Here, X_{1i} is the concentration observed at the ith sampling point and X_{2i} is the concentration at the corresponding field duplicate; $N = 26$ is the number of sampling points (degrees of freedom) and the overbars represent spatial average operators.

Note that the variability of the observed data is s_T^2, thus the spatial geochemical variability, s_G^2, can only be represented by the total variability, s_T^2, if $s_{SA}^2 << s_T^2$. To address this issue the following hypothesis test is performed:

$$H_0{:}\sigma_{SA}^2 = 0 \ vs. \ H_1{:}\sigma_{SA}^2 > 0 \tag{5}$$

with the following test statistic

$$F = \frac{s_{SA}^2}{s_T^2} \tag{6}$$

which has a Fisher distribution with N and $N-1$ degrees of freedom, *i.e.*, $F \sim F_{(N, N-1)} = F_{(26, 25)}$. Thus, for each geochemical element, the null hypothesis is rejected at a 1% significance level if $F > 2.589$. The null hypothesis was not rejected for all elements used in this work, meaning that the spatial geochemical variance can be estimated by the observed spatial variance. Moreover, criteria (i) and (ii) were also respected by all these elements.

3.4. Estimated Background Value and Statistical Analysis

The methodology followed in this work to determine the Estimated Background Value (EBV) of each metal at each sampling site ($n = 337$) followed the guidelines of the IGCP 259 project, which state that the stream sediments of these sites must be as uncontaminated as possible. The mapping of the EBVs was performed by ordinary kriging using a theoretical model of spatial continuity fitted to the experimental variograms calculated for each element. Cross validation was carried out for each interpolated variable to assess if the fitted model was suitable for the experimental variogram. The root-mean-square error (RMSE) was used to measure the differences between values predicted by the model and the actual values. RMSE ranges from 0 to infinity, with 0 corresponding to the ideal model. Another measure of error, the mean absolute error (MAD) which is less affected by the presence of outliers, is also presented in Table 1.

Please note that the EBV maps are not shown in this work because of space constraints. Nevertheless, the variographic model of each element used for the mapping of the associated Environmental Risk Index (ERI) is described in Section 3.5.

The Estimated Background Value (EBV) at each sampling site was calculated as the median of the data set limited by the Tukey Range: ($P_{25} - 1.5 \times (P_{75} - P_{25})$, $P_{75} + 1.5 \times (P_{75} - P_{25})$) [50]. The Tukey Range filters out possible outliers and is sometimes referred to as the Non-Anomalous Range.

Table 1. Parameters of the theoretical models of spatial continuity fitted to the experimental variogram of Co, Cr, Cu, Ni, V, PC1, and PC2.

ID	Model	Main Direction	C_0	C_1	Length	Anisotropy Ratio	RMSE	MAD
Co	exponential	0	30	150	4,000	1.27	2.38	1.58
Cr	exponential	45	2,100	1,900	2,000	1.64	3.45	2.01
Cu	exponential	0	160	200	5,000	1.22	1.05	0.98
Ni	exponential	30	2,600	2,800	3,500	1.83	4.82	2.99
V	exponential	0	1,200	600	4,000	1.98	3.56	2.33
PC1	exponential	90	7,000,000	9,000,000	5,000	1.36	2.53	1.87
PC2	exponential	90	1,000,000	7,500,000	2,000	1.23	1.95	1.54

Notes: ID: Variable; Model: theoretical model fitted to the experimental variogram; C_0: nugget effect; C_1: sill for the structure; Length: major range in meters; Anisotropy ratio: Geometrical Anisotropy = major axis/minor axis; RMSE: root-mean-square error; MAD: mean absolute deviation.

A Principal Component Analysis (PCA) was also performed using the correlation matrix, and the number of retained Principal Components (PCs) was objectively determined using the scree graph as follows: the retained modes are those whose eigenvalues decrease sharply. The retained PCs were mapped using the same methodology used in the EBVs' mapping.

Some authors address the question of closure and non-normality when performing a PCA on compositional data [51]. The dataset used in this work is a compositional dataset but it is not a closed one since the data is expressed in its original units and it was not normalized to a constant. Therefore, any logarithmic transformation was performed prior to PCA. The distribution of the data was considered to be approximately Normal due to the Central Limit Theorem and the fact that the concentration of each element at a particular sampling point was computed as the average of the concentrations at five near points. A correlation-based PCA was performed (*i.e.*, the eigenvalues and eigenvectors were computed from the correlation matrix of the original data) instead of a covariance-based PCA because the variables are concentrations of different geochemical elements.

The EBVs' and the PCs' maps were prepared following the recommendations of [31]. The color maps were interpolated by ordinary kriging, based on 337 sites and using a theoretical model of spatial continuity fitted to the experimental variogram calculated for each variable (metal EBV or PC). The parameters of the theoretical models of spatial continuity fitted to the experimental variogram, and the RMSE and MAD values are presented in Table 1.

The color maps were plotted using a color scale classified in eight classes, according to percentiles: [Minimum–P_{10}]; [P_{10}–P_{25}]; [P_{25}–P_{50}]; [P_{50}–P_{75}]; [P_{75}–P_{90}]; [P_{90}–P_{95}]; [P_{95}–$P_{97.5}$]; [$P_{97.5}$–Maximum], where P_x is the *x*th percentile value.

Although the EBV of an element may have a considerable spatial variability, and can, thus, be presented by distribution maps, policy makers usually prefer a single value representative of an entire country or region. Because of this, we determined an EBV representative of the entire Santiago Island (EBV-S) and one EBV representative of each one of its geological formations (EBV-XX where XX are the initials of a particular geological formation). The EBV-S was calculated as the median of the data set limited by the Tukey Range. Each EBV-XX was calculated as the EBV-S, with the difference that the dataset used in the calculations consists of only those sampling points that are located in the XX geological formation.

3.5. Environmental Risk Assessment

The concentration of some metals in some areas of the island may be too high for "all types of property uses", according to the Canadian legislation. Therefore, this issue is assessed in this section by means of numeric measures of these environmental risks. For each element, the Environmental Risk Index (ERI) for all types of property uses is quantified by ERI(s) = C(s)/P, where C(s) is the element content observed at sampling site s, and P represents the legislated permissive level of that element, according the Canadian Legislation [52]. The permissible level is, by definition, the element concentration in the stream sediment medium above which the stream sediment is considered to be unsafe for some purpose. We choose the Canadian Guidelines for all types of property uses as the permissible level. Note that the Canadian legislation provides no values for V. So, we used the target value of the Italian guidelines for public/private green areas and residential sites [53].

The procedure used to interpolate and map the ERI fields was the same used for either the EBV or the PC fields. Particularly, the variographic model used for the ERI of an element is the same determined for that element. For the PCs, a new variographic model was determined using the same procedure. These ERI fields indicate where a particular element is above the permissible level, according to the legislation for its use purposes.

4. Results and Discussion

4.1. Estimated Background Values

Descriptive statistics including the standard deviation (SD), skewness (Skew), kurtosis (Kurt), coefficient of variation percent (CV%), minimum (Min), maximum (Max) and the range of the analyzed metals concentrations along with the EBV-S of Santiago Island were calculated and listed in Table 2.

In order to further explore the relationships between the spatial distribution of the metal contents and the geological formations, the EBV-XX values were calculated. Please remember that an EBV-XX is the estimated background value of a particular metal in the stream sediments collected from a XX geological formation of the Santiago Island (Table 3).

According to Table 3, stream sediments from the Ancient Complex (CA) show high Cr, V, and also Mn. Stream sediments from Flamengos Formation (FL) have high Cu and low Pb concentrations. Órgãos Formation (CB) shown stream sediments with high values of Cu, and low values of Mn and Zn. Stream sediments from Pico da Antónia Formation (PA) have high Co, Cr, Ni and V, and low Zn concentrations. The stream sediments from Assomada Formation (AS) presented high Cd, Mn, Pb and Zn, and low Co, Cr, Cu and Ni (and also V), while the samples collected from the MV formation stands out from the other stream sediment samples by its higher Cd, Hg, As, Pb and Zn concentrations. The sediments of this geological formation are scarce in Cu and V. The Quaternary Formation stream sediments samples are also enriched in As but have low Zn contents. Alluvium samples have high Cr and Ni contents. All these results are in line with those obtained from the comparison of the EBV maps with the geological cartography.

Table 2. Statistical As, Cd, Co, Cr, Cu, Hg, Mn, Ni, Pb, V, and Zn variables analysed, interval ranges, and the baseline values (EBV-S) of metals from the stream sediments of Santiago Island ($n = 337$). Values expressed in $mg \cdot kg^{-1}$.

Var	Min	Med	Me	Max	SD	CV	Sk	Krt	P5–P95	Tukey Range	EBV-S
As	0.3	0.3	0.6	7.2	0.62	1.07	5.18	43.79	0.3–1.6	0.3–1.4	0.25
Cd	0.05	0.10	0.14	1.00	0.09	0.64	3.82	30.16	0.05–0.30	0.05–0.35	0.10
Co	3.1	44.7	45.1	139.9	13.86	0.31	1.21	7.79	26.4–66.1	15.8–73.4	44.65
Cr	8.0	114.0	123.7	463.1	68.03	0.55	1.49	4.48	20.0–251.5	8.0–264.0	111.00
Cu	3.2	48.8	48.6	141.6	17.99	0.37	0.52	2.38	17.6–77.8	9.4–87.6	48.70
Hg	0.01	0.01	0.01	0.08	0.01	0.74	2.13	7.24	0.15–0.54	0.07–0.61	0.26
Mn	197.0	1191.0	1259.9	4210.0	441.65	0.35	2.07	8.87	737.1–2043.5	255.1–2162.1	1182.00
Ni	6.8	155.2	160.5	477.0	76.02	0.47	0.50	1.13	21.3–286.2	6.8–337.5	152.85
Pb	1.4	3.9	5.2	81.4	6.61	1.26	7.53	70.27	2.0–10.1	1.4–10.1	3.80
V	24.0	160.0	161.0	372.0	45.68	0.28	0.64	2.57	92.4–237.3	50.5–262.5	159.00
Zn	15.0	81.0	82.7	189.0	19.14	0.23	1.23	5.35	57.0–111.0	34.0–130.0	81.00

Notes: Min: minimum; Med: median; Me: Mean; Max: maximum; SD: standard deviation; Sk: skewness; Krt: kurtosis; CV: variation coefficient; P5–P95: the interval limited by the 5th and 95th percentile values; Tukey Range [50] or Non-Anomalous range: $P_{25} - 1.5 \times (P_{75} - P_{25}) - P_{75} + 1.5 \times (P_{75} - P_{25})$; EBV-S (Estimated Background Value for Santiago): the median of the data limited by the Tukey Range.

Table 3. Estimated Background Values (EBV-XX) of As, Cd, Co, Cr, Cu, Hg, Mn, Ni, Pb, V, and Zn in the stream sediments of different geological formations in Santiago Island, Cape Verde.

Variable	EBV-CA ($n = 41$)	EBV-FL ($n = 21$)	EBV-CB ($n = 28$)	EBV-PA ($n = 118$)	EB-AS ($n = 15$)	EBV-MV ($n = 18$)	EBV-CC ($n = 9$)	EBV-AL ($n = 87$)
As	0.3	0.3	0.3	0.3	0.3	0.6	0.7	0.3
Cd	0.10	0.10	0.10	0.10	0.20	0.20	0.10	0.10
Co	43.6	41.3	40.3	48.8	35.8	42.6	42.2	44.9
Cr	116.0	112.5	99.0	122.5	20.5	76.0	93.5	119.3
Cu	53.8	57.6	56.7	46.6	26.4	34.2	47.4	48.9
Hg	0.01	0.01	0.01	0.02	0.02	0.03	0.01	0.02
Mn	1199	1036	980	1328	1612	1423	1027	1157
Ni	126.7	139.1	145.1	168.1	20.1	104.1	148.9	164.1
Pb	3.6	2.5	3.3	4.7	6.6	6.0	4.1	3.4
V	166.0	157.5	148.0	167.0	153.0	131.0	147.0	156.0
Zn	86.5	80.0	76.5	76.0	99.0	88.0	73.5	81.0

Notes: CA: Ancient Intern Eruptive Complex; FL: Flamengos Formation; CB: Órgãos Formation; PA: Pico da Antónia Formation; AS: Assomada Formation; MV: Monte das Vacas Formation; CC: Quaternary Formations; AL: Alluvium. Highest chemical element contents in bold and lowest chemical elements contents with gray highlight.

4.2. Multivariate Statistical Analysis

In order to confirm the link between the EBV classes with the geological spatial distribution, a correlation-based PCA was also conducted (see Section 3.4). Using the scree graph (Figure 2a) it was decided to retain three modes, accounting for 61.02% of the total variance (Figure 2b). Based on the biplots show in Figure 2c, the elements can be assembled into the first three principal vectors (PVs), as follows:

Figure 2. (**a**) Scree graph and (**b**) Cumulative Explained Variance of the first 11 PCA (Principal Component Analysis) modes. Red circles are drawn for the three retained components; (**c**) Biplot of PV2 *vs.* PV1 and (**d**) PV3 *vs.* PV1.

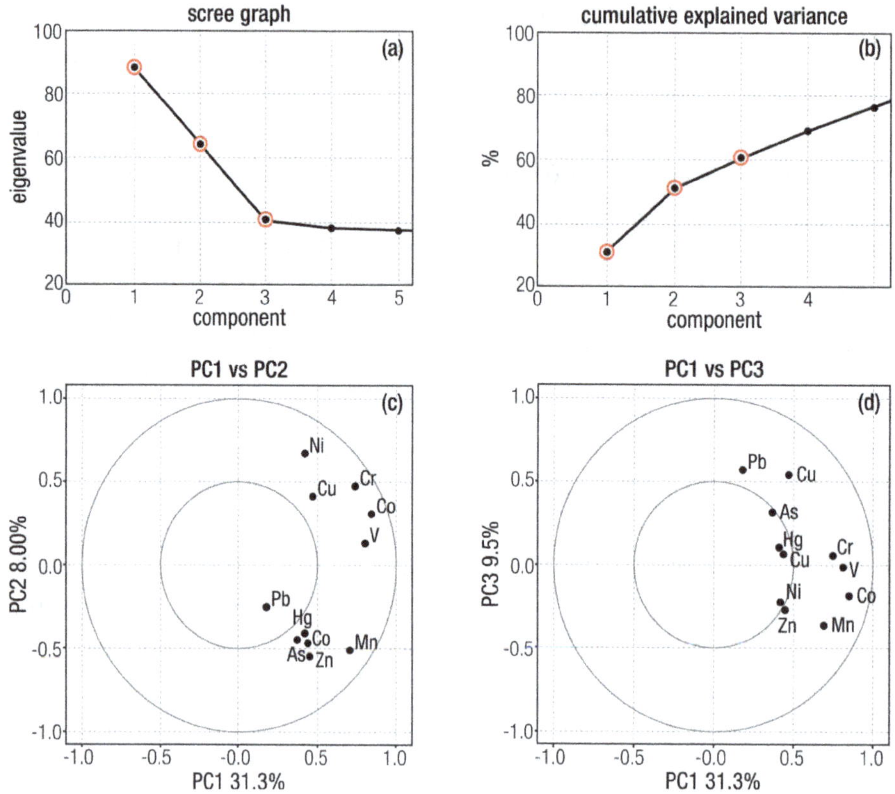

PV1: association of Co, V, Cr, and Mn, displaying high loadings: 0.839, 0.798, 0.732, and 0.686, respectively. The metal association in first PCA mode clearly shows the influence of a lithology rich in siderophile elements (Co, Cr), typical of basic rocks and also the presence of its typical minerals [36], such as pyroxene (V), olivine and serpentine (Co, Cr, Ni). These four elements may exist together in soil and also in stream sediment parent materials, as the weathering products of the exposed bedrocks. Soils (and stream sediments) developed from basic and ultramafic rocks are usually enriched in Ni, Cr and Co [54]. This first factor is then assumed as a natural lithogenic factor.

PV2: Zinc and Cd are associated in the second mode (PV2/PC2), with high negative loadings, −0.558 and −0.513, respectively, in opposition to the element Ni with a strong high positive loading, 0.675. Zinc and Cd are highly associated with pyroclastic deposits of Monte das Vacas Formation. Niquel also shows a positive high value, 0.675, in PC2, leading to the assumption that this metal association primarily shares a natural source feature.

PV3: consists of Cu and Pb association, with the loadings of 0.546 and 0.583, respectively. This mode apparently reflects the influence of anthropogenic sources, namely the possible use of fertilizers and/or pesticides containing Cu and Pb, and/or batteries, particularly at the relatively populous regions, such as Praia, Assomada, Tarrafal and corresponding riversides that can result in the high element loading. These areas pose a potential health risk. Also, the lack of a relationship between these metals and the geological formations induces a link to an anthropogenic source. In fact, the geological formations where Pb concentrations are higher correspond to the geological formations where Cu contents are lower and *vice versa* (e.g., Assomada and Monte das Vacas formations).

The PV1, PV2 and PV3 loadings (Figure 2) account for 31.28%, 20.28% and 9.47% of the total variability, respectively.

When comparing the spatial distribution of the PCs with the geological formations (Figure 3), it is possible to identify a light relationship between them. The association in PC1 displays the influence of a rich lithology in siderofile elements, typical of basic rocks and the presence of minerals such as pyroxene, amphibole, olivine and serpentine, as referred to previously. PC1 is linked with the basaltic-basanite rocks from the PA Formation, contrarily to the Flamengos (FL) and AS Formations; The metal association in PC2, with Zn and Cd (and As), is associated mainly to the pyroclastic rocks of Monte das Vacas, opposed in sign to Ni, which enters in the structure of the basaltic rocks typical minerals, such as serpentine (Co, Cr, Ni). PC3 apparently reflect the influence of the anthropogenic sources, having no relation with the geological cartography.

Figure 3. Spatial distribution of PC1 and PC2. The geological map of Figure 1 is shown in the last panel for easier comparison with the PC spatial fields.

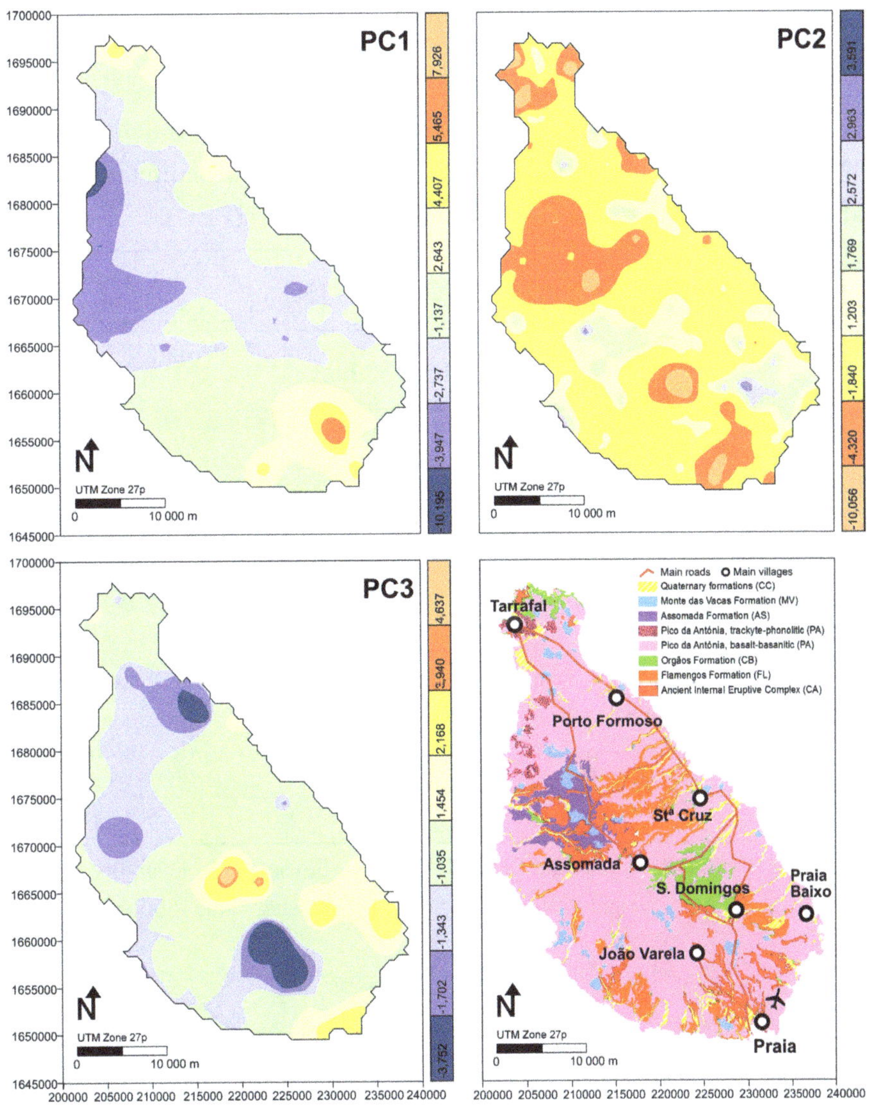

4.3. Environmental Risk Assessment

Before analysing the ERI fields, the comparison of the EBV-S of each studied metal in the stream sediments of Santiago Island and the international values legislated as dangerous for certain uses (guideline values), is given in Table 4.

The EBV-S of Cd, Co, Cr, Ni and V are above the Canadian guidelines for stream sediments (for any use) and above the target values of Dutch [55] and United States [56] guidelines. Numerical sediment quality guidelines for freshwater [57] are commonly used to identify sediments that are likely to be toxic to sediment-dwelling organisms. The Probable Effect Concentrations (PEC) quotients allowed to assess the sediments that contain complex mixtures of chemical contaminants (Table 4). The PEC, above which harmful effects are likely in sediment dwelling organisms were compared for As, Cd, Cr, Cu, Hg, Ni, Pb, and Zn. The EBV-S of Cr and Ni were found to be above the Probable effect level (PEL) [58], the Severe effect level (SEL) [59] and the Toxic effect threshold (TET) [60], as shown in Table 4.

Figure 4 shows the ERI maps each element for all types of property uses. Only the ERI maps of the elements that present regions with values above the unit (*i.e.*, above the legislated permissible values) are shown (Figure 4). These elements are Co, Cr, Cu, Ni and V. The Zn map is not shown because it has ERI > 1 only at six sample locations. These metals are precisely those with higher loadings in PV1 and PV2 (Ni), which revealed to be of natural origin in Santiago island.

Table 4. Estimated Background Values of harmful elements from the stream sediments of Santiago (EBV-S), admissible levels (in mg·kg^{-1}) in stream sediments according to the Ontario, Dutch and United States guidelines, and the numerical sediment quality guidelines for freshwater, including their probable effect concentrations (PEC).

EBV-S		Canadian Guidelines	Dutch Guidelines	United States [56]	Numerical Sediment Quality Guidelines for Freshwater Ecosystems
		All Types of Property Uses	Target Values	Mean Values	Probable Effect Concentrations: PEL; SEL; TET
As	0.60	6	29	3.9	17; 33; 17
Cd	0.91	0.6	0.8	-	3.53; 10; 3
Co	46.4	50	9	9.1	-; -; -
Cr	118	26	100	-	90; 110; 100
Cu	50.8	16	36	14.2	197; 110;86
Hg	0.02	0.2	0.3	-	0.486; 2; -
Mn	1293	-	-	760	-; -; -
Ni	136.1	16	36	15.1	36; 75; 61
Pb	5.00	31	85	14.1	91.3; 250; 170
V	169	90 *	-	81.1	-; -; -
Zn	79	120	140	62.9	315; 820; 540

Notes: PEL: Probable effect level; dry weight [58], in [57]. SEL: Severe effect level; dry weight [59], in [57]. TET: Toxic effect threshold; dry weight [60], in [57]. * Italian legislated value for public/private greens areas and residential sites [53].

Figure 4. Environmental Risk Index (ERI) of some metals for all types of property uses. The geological map of Figure 1 is shown in the last panel for easier comparison with the ERI spatial fields.

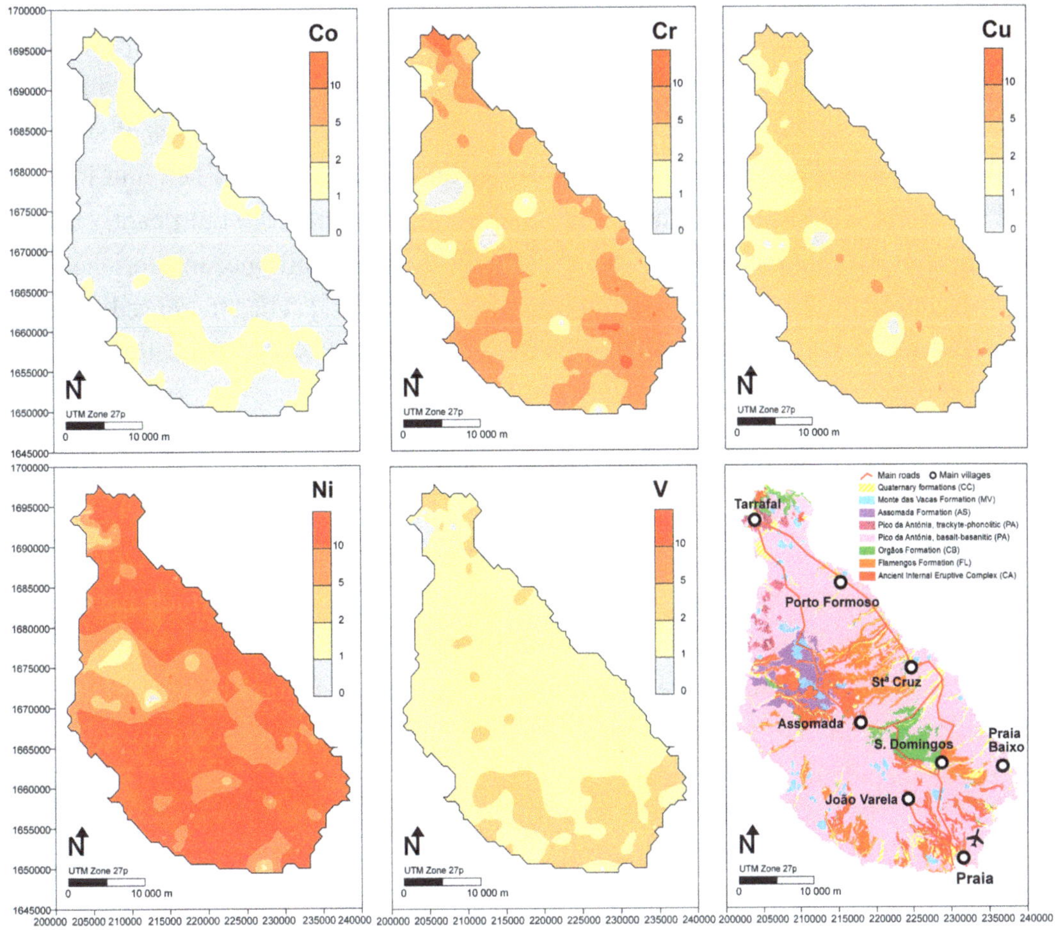

5. Conclusions

A clear chemical characterization of the stream sediments in different geological formations is difficult, since the chemical composition of each sampling point represents the chemical composition of the entire area upstream, covering different geological formations. Despite this constraint, the EBV spatial distribution of the metals and the results of PCA allowed establishing relationships between the EBV maps and the geological formations. Furthermore, it is important to emphasize that the stream lines in Santiago have a negligible water flow.

The first two PCA modes indicate that heavy metals in Santiago stream sediments are mainly originated from weathering of underlying bedrocks. The first metal association (Co, V, Cr, and Mn; first PCA mode) consists of elements enriched in basic rocks and compatible elements. These elements are related to pyroxene, amphibole, and olivine minerals that were found in Santiago stream sediments [61].

The second association of variables, Zn and Cd as opposed to Ni (second PCA mode), appears to be strongly controlled by the composition of alkaline volcanic rocks and pyroclastic rocks. The K-feldspar, zircon, pyroxene, amphibole, and olivine are examples of minerals responsible for this association [36,61]. So, the second PCA mode is also considered as a natural lithogenic mode. The third association (third PCA mode: Cu and Pb) consists of elements that may have an anthropogenic origin.

In terms of the relationship between the stream sediments' composition and the geological formations it can be concluded that the stream sediments associated to the PA formation have the highest background values (EBVs) of the variables Co, Cr, Mn, Ni, and V (first PCA mode), which explains the enrichment seen in association Co-Cr-V-Mn, which is consistent with the mineralogical analysis that consists mainly of pyroxene, plagioclase, potassium feldspar, and phyllosilicates [36,61]; the stream sediments collected associated with the CB formation show depletion in Mn and Zn, which is consistent with the results obtained for the analysis of rocks [36]; the majority of the samples of stream sediments that occur associated with the AS formation is enriched in As, Cd, Hg, and Mn and impoverished in Co-Cr-Cu-Ni association, probably because this geological formation is significantly weathered and consequently impoverished in primary minerals such as pyroxene and olivine, and enriched in secondary minerals, such as hematite, phyllosilicates, serpentine and zeolite [61]. The stream sediments associated with the Monte das Vacas formation are impoverished in Co-Cr-Ni-V. The alluvium samples are particularly enriched in Ni.

The high values of ERIs for some elements demonstrate that the Santiago stream sediments may have higher Co, Cr, Ni, Mn and V risks which are caused by its higher natural origin. Nickel has the highest ERI values. The occurrence of values greater than 1 in the ERI maps shows that, on average, the contents of the respective metals are above the permissive levels. The PEC, above which harmful effects are likely in sediment dwelling organisms, was found for Cr and Ni.

So, this study shows that Santiago stream sediments present high natural heavy metals concentration levels, and are a potential risk to human health, which should be of concern to scientists and the government, needing epidemiologic studies.

Acknowledgments

The authors would like to thank the funding provided by the Portuguese Foundation for Science and Technology (FCT), Geobiotec, Geosciences, and CNC Centres. Oliveira Cruz, Jorge Brito and Luís Filipe Tavares are acknowledged for the logistic support provided in Santiago Island by the Jean Piaget University of Cape Verde. We also appreciated the support given by Regla Hernandez, António Querido, Isildo Gonçalves Gomes, and Isaurinda Baptista from the National Institute of Agricultural Research and Development. The authors also acknowledge with great affection the field support provided by Ricardo Ramos. The authors would also like to acknowledge two anonymous reviewers for conducting thorough peer reviews of this manuscript.

Author Contributions

Marina Cabral Pinto performed the sampling, the pre-analytical treatment of samples, and the statistical analysis. Maria M. V. G. Silva participated in the field work. Eduardo Ferreira da Silva, Paulo Melo-Gonçalves, and Carla Candeias participated in data analysis. Marina Cabral Pinto drafted the manuscript with collaboration of all authors and it was revised by all. All authors read and approved the final manuscript.

References

1. Siegel, F.R. *Environmental Geochemistry of Potentially Toxic Metals*; Springer: Berlin, Germany, 2002.
2. Pinto, M.M.S.C.; Silva, M.M.V.G.; Neiva, A.M.R. Pollution of water and stream sediments associated with the Vale de Abrutiga Uranium Mine, Central Portugal. *Mine Water Environ.* **2004**, *23*, 66–75.
3. Pinto, M.M.S.C.; Silva, M.M.V.G. Contemporary reviews of mine water studies in Europe—Portugal. In *Mine Water and the Environment*; Wolkersdorfer, C., Bowell, R., Eds.; Springer: Berlin, Germany, 2005; pp. 50–53.
4. Komatina, M.M. *Medical Geology: Effects of Geological Environments on Human Health*; Developments in Earth and Environmental Sciences 2; Elsevier Science: Amsterdam, The Netherlands, 2004.
5. Kozlowski, H.; JanickaKlosb, A.; Brasunb, J.; Gaggelli, E.; Valensinc, D.; Valensinc, J. Copper, iron, and zinc ions homeostasis and their role in neurodegenerativedisorders (metal uptake, transport, distribution and regulation). *Coord. Chem. Rev.* **2009**, *253*, 2665–2685.
6. Gorell, J.M.; Johnson, C.C.; Rybicki, B.A.; Peterson, E.L.; Kortsha, G.X.; Kortsha, G.G.; Richardson, R.J. Occupational exposure to manganese, copper, lead, iron, mercury and zinc and the risk of Parkinson's disease. *Neurotoxicology* **1999**, *20*, 239–248.
7. Zatta, P.; Lucchini, R.; van Rensburg, S.J.; Taylor, A. The role of metals in neurodegenerative processes: aluminum, manganese, and zinc. *Brain Res. Bull.* **2003**, *62*, 15–28.
8. Elsner, R.; Spangler, J. Neurotoxicity of inhaled manganese: Public health danger in the shower? *Med. Hypotheses* **2005**, *65*, 607–616.
9. Erikson, K.M.; Syversen, T.; Aschner, J.L.; Aschner, M. Interactions between excessive manganese exposures and dietary iron-deficiency in neurodegeneration. *Environ. Toxicol. Pharmacol.* **2005**, *19*, 415–421.
10. Schneider, J.S.; Decamp, E.; Koser, A.J.; Fritz, S.; Gonczi, H.; Syversen, T.; Guilarte, T.R. Effects of chronic manganese exposure on cognitive and motor functioning in non-human primates. *Brain Res.* **2006**, *1118*, 222–231.
11. Cersosimo, M.G.; Koller, W.C. The diagnosis of manganese-induced parkinsonism. *NeuroToxicology* **2006**, *27*, 340–346.
12. Santamaria, A.B.; Cushing, C.A.; Antonini, J.M.; Finley, B.L.; Mowat, F.S. State-of-the-science review: Does manganese exposure during welding pose a neurological risk? *J. Toxicol. Environ. Health* **2007**, *10*, 417–465.
13. Flyn, M.R.; Susi, P. Neurological risks associated with manganese exposure from welding operations—A literature review. *Int. J. Hyg. Environ. Health* **2009**, *212*, 459–469.
14. International Agency for Research on Cancer. *Chromium, Nickel and Welding*; IARC Monographs on the Evaluation of Carcinogenic Risks to Humans Volume 49; International Agency for Research on Cancer: Lyon, France, 1990.

15. Staessen, J.A.; Buchet, J.P.; Ginucchio, G.; Lauwerys, R.R.; Lijnen, P.; Roels, H.; Fagard, R. Public health implications of environmental exposure to Cadmium and Lead: An overview of epidemiological studies in Belgium. *J. Cardiovasc. Risk* **2007**, *3*, 26–41.
16. Schroeder, H.A. Cadmium, chromium, and cardiovascular disease. *Circulation* **1967**, *35*, 570–582.
17. Panaullah, G.M.; Alam, T.; Baktear Hossain, M.; Loeppert, R.H.; Lauren, J.G.; Meisner, C.A.; Ahmed, Z.U.; Duxbury, J.M. Arsenic toxicity to rice (*Oryza sativa* L.) in Bangladesh. *Plant Soil* **2009**, *317*, 31–39.
18. Yao, Y.; Pei, F.; Kang, P. Selenium, iodine, and the relation with Kashin-Beck disease. *Nutrition* **2011**, *27*, 1095–1100.
19. Plant, J.A.; Smith, D.; Smith, B.; Williams, L. Environmental geochemistry at the global scale. *Appl. Geochem.* **2001**, *16*, 1291–1308.
20. Smith, D.B.; Smith, S.M.; Horton, J.D. History and evaluation of national-scale geochemical data sets for the United States. *Geosci. Front.* **2013**, *4*, 167–183.
21. Salminen, R.; Batista, M.J.; Bidovec, M.; Demetriades, A.; de Vivo, B.; de Vos, W.; Duris, M.; Gilucis, A.; Gregorauskiene, V.; Halamic, J.; *et al. Geochemical Atlas of Europe, Part 1: Background Information, Methodology and Maps*; Geological Survey of Finland: Espoo, Finland, 2005.
22. Johnson, C.C.; Breward, N.; Ander, E.L.; Ault, L. G-BASE: Baseline geochemical mapping of Great Britain and Northern Ireland. *Geochem. Explor. Environ. Anal.* **2005**, *5*, 347–357.
23. Garret, R.G.; Reimann, C.; Smith, D.B.; Xie, X. From geochemical prospecting to international geochemical mapping: A historical overview. *Geochem. Explor. Environ. Anal.* **2008**, *8*, 205–217.
24. Smith, D.B.; Reimann, C. Low-Density geochemical mapping and the robustness of geochemical patterns. *Geochem. Explor. Environ. Anal.* **2008**, *8*, 219–227.
25. Appleton, J.D.; Ridgway, J. Regional geochemical mapping in developing countries and its application to environmental studies. *Appl. Geochem.* **1993**, *2*, 103–110.
26. Xuejing, X.; Xuzhan, M.; Tianxiang, R. Geochemical mapping in China. *J. Geochem. Explor.* **1997**, *60*, 99–113.
27. Reimann, C.; Caritat, P. *Chemical Elements in the Environment—Factsheets for the Geochemist and Environmental Scientist*; Springer-Verlag: Berlin, Germany, 2008.
28. Lech, M.E.; Caritat, P. Regional Geochemical Study Paves Way for National Survey—Geochemistry of Near-Surface Regolith Points to New Resources. Available online: http://www.ga.gov.au/ausgeonews/ausgeonews200706/geochemical.jsp (accessed on 1 June 2007).
29. Inácio, M.; Pereira, V.; Pinto, M. The soil geochemical Atlas of Portugal: Overview and applications. *J. Geochem. Explor.* **2008**, *98*, 22–33.
30. Darnley, A. International geochemical mapping special issue. *J. Geochem. Explor.* **1990**, *39*, 1–13.
31. Darnley, A.G.; Björklund, A.; Bølviken, B.; Gustavsson, N.; Koval, P.V.; Plant, J.A.; Steenfelt, A.; Tauchid, M.; Xie, X. *A Global Geochemical Database for Environmental and Resource Management: Recommendations for International Geochemical Mapping*; Final Report of IGCP Project 259; UNESCO: Paris, France, 1995.
32. Albanese, S.; de Vivo, B.; Lima, A.; Cicchella, D. Geochemical background and baseline values of toxic elements in stream sediments of Campania region (Italy). *J. Geochem. Explor.* **2007**, *93*, 21–34.

33. Levinson, A.A. *Introduction to Exploration Geochemistry*; Applied Publishing Ltd.: Maywood, CA, USA, 1974.
34. Beus, A.A.; Grigorian, V. *Geochemical Exploration Methods for Mineral Deposits*; Applied Publishing Ltd.: Wilmette, IL, USA, 1977.
35. Reimann, C.; Siewers, U.; Tarvainen, T.; Bityukova, L.; Eriksson, J.; Gilucis, A.; Gregorauskiene, V.; Lukashev, V.K.; Matinian, N.N.; Pasieczna, A.; *et al. Agricultural Soils in Northern Europe: A Geochemical Atlas*; Schweizerbart Science Publishers: Stuttgart, Germany, 2003.
36. Cabral Pinto, M.M.S. Geochemical Cartography, with a Low To-Median Density, of Santiago Island, Cape Verde. Ph.D. Thesis, University of Aveiro, Aveiro, Portugal, 2010.
37. Desenfant, F.; Petrovský, E.; Rochette, P. Magnetic signature of industrial pollution of stream sediments and correlation with heavymetals: Case study from south France. *Water Air Soil Pollut.* **2004**, *152*, 297–312.
38. INE 2010. Censo 2010. Available online: http://www.ine.cv (accessed on 21 March 2013).
39. Serralheiro, A. A Geologia da ilha de Santiago (Cabo Verde). *Boletim Museu Laboratório Mineralógico Geológico Faculdade de Ciências de Lisboa* **1976**, *14*, 157–372. (In Portuguese)
40. Instituto Nacional de Meteorologia e Geofisica (INMG). *Climatologic Data of Some Stations in Santiago Island, Praia, Cabo Verde*; Internal Report; INMG: Praia, Santiago Island, Cabo Verde, 2005.
41. *United Nations Development Program for Cape Verde*; PNUD: New York, NY, USA, 1993.
42. Matos Alves, C.A.; Macedo, J.R.; Celestino Silva, L.; Serralheiro, A.; Peixoto Faria, A.F. Estudo geológico, petrológico e vulcanológico da ilha de Santiago (Cabo Verde). *Garcia de Orta Serviços Geológicos* **1979**, *3*, 47–74. (In Portuguese)
43. Ramalho, R.A.S. Building the Cape Verde Islands. Ph.D. Thesis, University of Bristol, Bristol, UK, 2011.
44. Holm, P.M.; Grandvuinet, T.; Friis, J.; Wilson, J.R.; Barker, A.K.; Plesner, P. An ^{40}Ar-^{39}Ar study of the Cape Verde hot spot: Temporal evolution in a semistationary plate environment. *J. Geophys. Res.* **2008**, *113*, doi:10.1029/2007JB005339.
45. Pina, A.F.L. Hydrochemistry and groundwater quality of the island of Santiago, Cape Verde (Hidroquímica e qualidade das águas subterrâneas da ilha de Santiago, Cabo Verde). Ph.D. Thesis, University of Aveiro, Aveiro, Portugal, 2009. (In Portuguese)
46. Martins, S.; Mata, J.; Munhá, J.; Madeira, J.; Moreira, M. Evidências geológicas e geoquímicas para a existência de duas unidades estratigráficas distintas na Formação do Pico da Antónia (Ilha de Santiago, República de Cabo Verde). *Memórias e Notícias Universidade de Coimbra* **2008**, *3*, 123–128. (In Portuguese)
47. Rose, A.W.; Hawkes, E.H.; Webb, J.S. *Geochemistry in Mineral Exploration*, 2nd ed.; Academic Press: London, UK, 1979.
48. Thompson, M. Analytical methods in applied environmental geochemistry. In *Applied Environmental Geochemistry*; Thornton, I., Ed.; Academic Press: London, UK, 1983.
49. Chao, T.T.; Sanzolone, R.F. Decomposition techniques. *J. Geochem. Explor.* **1992**, *44*, 65–106.
50. Tukey, J.W. *Exploratory Data Analysis*; Addison-Wesley: Reading, UK, 1977.

51. Reimann, C.; Filzmoser, P.; Garret, R.G.; Dutter, R. *Statistical Data Analysis Explaned: Applied Environmental Statistics with R*, 1st ed.; John Wiley & Sons: Chichester, UK, 2008.
52. Minister of the Environment (Canada). Soil, Ground Water and Sediment Standards for Use under Part XV.1 of the *Environmental Protection Act*. Available online: http://www.mah.gov.on.ca/AssetFactory.aspx?did=8993 (accessed on 15 April 2011).
53. Italian Legislation: Decreto Ministeriale, n°471, 1999. Regolamento Recante Criteri, Procedure e Modalità per la Messa in Sicurezza, la Bonifica e il Ripristino Ambientale dei Siti Inquinati, ai Sensi Dell'artocolo 17 del Decreto Legislativo 5 Febbraio 1997, n.22, e Successive Modificazioni e Integrazioni; Gazzetta Ufficiale n°293 de 15 December 1999, Supplemento Ordinario n°218. Available online: http://www.eugris.info/FurtherDescription.asp?e=550&Ca=1&Cy=8&DocID=E&DocTitle=Management_administration&T=Italy (accessed on 15 October 2014). (In Italian)
54. Sheng, J.; Wang, X.; Gong, P.; Tian, L.; Yao, T. Heavy metals of the Tibetan top soils—Level, source, spatial distribution, temporal variation and risk assessment. *Environ. Sci. Pollut. Res.* **2012**, *19*, 3362–3370.
55. Ministry of Housing, Spatial Planning and the Environment (VROM). Circular on Target Values and Intervention Values for Soil Remediation. The Netherlands Government Gazette, No. 39, Ministry of Housing, Spatial Planning and Environment, Directorate General for Environmental Protection, Department of Soil Protection. Available online: http://www.esdat.net/Environmental%20Standards/Dutch/annexS_I2000Dutch%20Environmental%20Standards.pdf (accessed on 16 October 2014).
56. Cannon, W.F.; Woodruff, L.G.; Pimley, S. Some statistical relationships between stream sediment and soil geochemistry in northwestern Wisconsin—Can stream sediment compositions be used to predict compositions of soils in glaciated terranes? *J. Geochem. Explor.* **2004**, *81*, 29–46.
57. MacDonald, D.D.; Ingersoll, C.G.; Berger, T.A. Development and evaluation of consensus-based sediment quality guidelines for freshwater ecosystems. *Arch. Environ. Contam. Toxicol.* **2000**, *39*, 20–31.
58. Smith, S.L.; MacDonald, D.D.; Keenleyside, K.A.; Ingersoll, C.G.; Field, J. A preliminary evaluation of sediment quality assessment values for freshwater ecosystems. *J. Gt. Lakes Res.* **1996**, *22*, 624–638.
59. Persaud, D.; Jaagumagi, R.; Hayton, A. *Guidelines for the Protection and Management of Aquatic Sediment Quality in Ontario*; Water Resources Branch, Ontario Ministry of the Environment: Toronto, Canada, 1993.
60. Environment Canada. *EC, MENVIQ (Environment Canada and Ministere de l'Envionnement du Quebec) Interim Criteria for Quality Assessment of St. Lawrence River Sediment*; Environment Canada: Ottawa, Canada, 1992.
61. Cabral Pinto, M.M.S.; da Silva, E.A.F.; Silva, M.M.V.G.; Melo-Gonçalves, P. Estimated background values of some harmful metals in stream sediments of Santiago Island (Cape Verde). In *Geochemistry: Earth's System Processes*; Dionisios, P., Ed.; InTech: Rijeka, Croatia, 2012; pp. 61–80.

9

Health Effects Associated with Inhalation of Airborne Arsenic Arising from Mining Operations

Rachael Martin [1,*], Kim Dowling [1], Dora Pearce [1,2], James Sillitoe [3] and Singarayer Florentine [1]

[1] Faculty of Science, Federation University Australia, University Drive, Mt Helen, VIC 3350, Australia; E-Mails: k.dowling@federation.edu.au (K.D.); dpearce@unimelb.edu.au (D.P.); s.florentine@federation.edu.au (S.F.)

[2] Centre for Epidemiology and Biostatistics, Melbourne School of Population and Global Health, Faculty of Medicine, Dentistry and Health Sciences, The University of Melbourne, Level 3, 207 Bouverie Street, Melbourne, VIC 3010, Australia

[3] Research and Innovation, Federation University Australia, University Drive, Mt Helen, VIC 3350, Australia; E-Mail: j.sillitoe@federation.edu.au

* Author to whom correspondence should be addressed; E-Mail: r.martin@federation.edu.au;

Abstract: Arsenic in dust and aerosol generated by mining, mineral processing and metallurgical extraction industries, is a serious threat to human populations throughout the world. Major sources of contamination include smelting operations, coal combustion, hard rock mining, as well as their associated waste products, including fly ash, mine wastes and tailings. The number of uncontained arsenic-rich mine waste sites throughout the world is of growing concern, as is the number of people at risk of exposure. Inhalation exposures to arsenic-bearing dusts and aerosol, in both occupational and environmental settings, have been definitively linked to increased systemic uptake, as well as carcinogenic and non-carcinogenic health outcomes. It is therefore becoming increasingly important to identify human populations and sensitive sub-populations at risk of exposure, and to better understand the modes of action for pulmonary arsenic toxicity and carcinogenesis. In this paper we explore the contribution of smelting, coal combustion, hard rock mining and their associated waste products to atmospheric arsenic. We also report on the current understanding of the health effects of inhaled arsenic, citing results from various toxicological, biomedical and epidemiological studies. This review is particularly aimed at those researchers engaged in the distinct, but complementary areas of arsenic research within the multidisciplinary field of medical geology.

Keywords: aerosol; arsenic; coal; dust; epidemiology; cancer; mining; smelting; tailings

1. Introduction

Arsenic is the 20th most abundant element in the earth's crust and may be released into the atmosphere as a result of natural processes and anthropogenic activities [1]. Environmental arsenic is released via chemical and physical weathering processes, biological activity and volcanic emissions, while anthropogenic sources include mining, metal smelting and burning of coal. Annual global arsenic emissions are estimated to be 24,000 t [2], with around 60% originating from copper smelting and coal combustion alone [3]. In some urban and highly industrialized areas, less than 2% of the atmospheric arsenic inputs originate from natural sources [3].

Emissions of arsenic-bearing particulate matter (PM) are of particular concern for human populations living in proximity to an emission source. Arsenic and inorganic arsenic compounds are classified as Group 1 carcinogens and are associated with cancers of the lung, bladder, kidney, skin, liver and prostate [2]. It should be noted that within the general population, inhalation is only considered a minor exposure pathway for inorganic arsenic compounds, and ingestion is considered the primary exposure pathway [2]. However, populations living in the vicinity of an arsenic emission source have an increased risk of additional exposure through inhalation of arsenic-contaminated particulates [4–9].

Despite their substantial contribution to global atmospheric arsenic species, mining operations play an understudied role in the generation of contaminated dust and aerosols [10]. To identify some of the emerging issues associated with arsenic in particulate matter this review presents key findings from a range of distinct but complimentary areas of research within the multidisciplinary field of medical geology, including geochemistry, toxicology, biomedicine and epidemiology. We will discuss two key themes: (i) the origin, occurrence and current monitoring of mining-related arsenic in the atmosphere; and (ii) the current understanding of the health effects of inhaled arsenic, citing results from various toxicological, biomedical and epidemiological studies.

2. Mining Operations as a Source of Airborne Arsenic

For brevity, the term "mining operations" is utilized throughout this paper to include all mining and mining-related activities including extraction, mechanical and high temperature processing, transportation, and storage of mine waste products. To compare or describe the impacts of different types of mining operations, specific mining terms are used.

2.1. Generation of Dust and Aerosol: An Overview

Mining operations release arsenic into the atmosphere via wind-borne dispersal of arsenic-laden particulates [11], with dust being the dominant transport medium for these emissions [3]. Active mining operations produce and/or mobilize dust to varying degrees in all stages of the mining process:

during the removal of overburden; in all aspects of the handling of ore, including its extraction, transportation and further processing; as part of waste disposal operations; and as a result of wind erosion of exposed areas [12–15]. Mining operations associated with an opencut coal mining operation in India, for example, generate 9.4 t of dust per day [16]. Active and abandoned mine tailings, mine sites and processing facilities also represent important sources of dust [17–22].

To demonstrate the potential for mine tailings to generate dust emissions, Figure 1 compares the total mass distribution (%) by particle size fraction of four different types of arsenic-bearing gold mine tailings in an historical mining region in regional Victoria, Australia. Comparable with the findings of a Californian-based study [21], our data suggest that mine tailings in this locality may contain up to 45% dust (particles ≤ 100 μm), as recorded in the fine-grained battery sand (Figure 1C). Future analysis may reveal the relationship between total arsenic concentration and particle size in these mine tailings samples.

Figure 1. Percentage mass distribution by particle size fraction for historical mine tailings including: (**A**) coarse battery sand; (**B**) red calcine sand; (**C**) fine battery sand; (**D**) composite coarse/fine battery sand. Size fractions Size fractions 1: >2000 μm; 2: 1000–2000 μm; 3: 500–1000 μm; 4: 250–500 μm; 5: 100–250 μm; 6: 53–100 μm; 7: ≤53 μm. Total arsenic (TAs) concentration (ppm) of each mine waste sample is also shown. (Our results obtained using a modified sieving method protocol described by Kim *et al.* [21]).

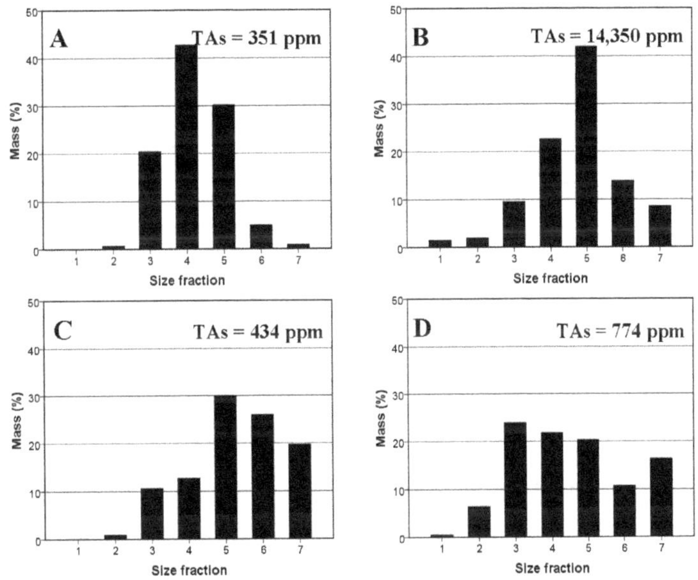

While most mining operations generate coarse dust, high temperature processes, such as smelting and coal combustion, are typically associated with fine particulates, accumulation-mode particulates, and vapors [10]. Coarse particles (≥2.5 μm diameter) are produced by mechanical processes such as the crushing and grinding of ore, and may be resuspended via wind erosion and mechanical disturbance [10,23]. Fine (≤2.5 μm) and accumulation mode particles (0.1–2.5 μm) are produced during smelting and combustion through the condensation of high temperature vapors, diffusion and coagulation [10,23].

Coarse and fine particulates have widely varying atmospheric residence times, and as a result, widely varying distributions. Arsenic associated with the fine fraction may remain in the atmosphere between seven [24] and up to 10 days (reviewed in Matschullat [3]), and can travel long distances [25].

Coarse particulates have a much shorter atmospheric residence time, typically minutes to hours due to a larger settling velocity [10]. Particle segregation of mine waste can occur during airborne transport, thereby reducing the size of the individual particles deposited [17]. In addition to mining operation type, atmospheric contaminant concentrations are also influenced by the distance and position of a sampling site in relation to the source, the height of the source (e.g., chimney or tailings pile), the type of dust suppression or flue gas cleaning, the exit velocity of the flue gas, and the prevailing wind speed [26] as well as changes in industrial technologies [27].

2.2. Origin, Production and Release of Particulate Arsenic

It is widely accepted that global atmospheric arsenic fluxes are dominated by mining-related industries involving high temperature processing [3]. An estimated 60% of global anthropogenically-generated atmospheric arsenic is attributed to copper smelting and coal combustion, with annual outputs of 12,080 and 6240 t respectively [3]. While it is well-documented that mine tailings represent major sources of arsenic-contaminated dust throughout the world [10,19,28,29], the contribution by these sources to total global atmospheric arsenic fluxes is yet to be assessed [3]. The occurrence of arsenic-bearing phases in unprocessed ore and the generation of particulate arsenic by different types of mining processes will be reviewed in the following sub-sections.

2.2.1. Smelting Operations

Gold, copper, lead and zinc ores typically contain arsenic-bearing minerals such as pyrite (FeS_2), galena (PbS), chalcopyrite ($CuFeS_2$) and the dominant arsenic-bearing mineral, arsenopyrite ($FeAsS$), which contains approximately 46% arsenic by weight [2]. The high temperature purification of arsenic-bearing ores during smelting and roasting volatilizes arsenic [30,31], and the resultant vapors may contain up to 95% arsenic [32]. Arsenic in close proximity to smelters and roasters is typically arsenic trioxide in particulate form [33,34], and depending on the feed material and extraction process, flue dusts can contain up to 30% arsenic trioxide [35,36]. Fugitive emissions of particulate arsenic may occur at various stages of high temperature processing, as well as during the transport and storage of ores, concentrates and waste heaps [37].

Although high efficiency control devices are often employed in smelters to reduce emissions, the quantity of total arsenic emitted from a single smelting operation can be substantially high. For example, around 300 t of arsenic are emitted annually from the Copper Smelter Complex Bor, in eastern Serbia [38]. Furthermore, uncontained smelter flue dusts represent an important potential source of airborne arsenic, compared with other secondary smelter by-products [39]. Over a period of 20 years, a copper smelter in Japan produced an estimated 9000 t of arsenic-rich flue dust (19.5 wt % of As) which is currently stockpiled at an undisclosed location in Japan [32]. Stockpiled by-products of the smelting process with high arsenic content present ongoing sources for redistribution.

2.2.2. Coal Combustion

Coal is a complex mixture of organic and inorganic compounds formed over millions of years from successive layers of fallen vegetation. Coal contains detectable levels of the vast majority of elements in the periodic table, including arsenic and other potentially toxic and environmentally sensitive elements [40,41]. Although much of the arsenic in coal is associated with the inorganic or mineral fraction (such as pyrite and other sulphide minerals), a significant portion is associated with organic matter [42,43]. Arsenic concentrations in coal typically range between 1–10 and 1500 mg·kg^{-1}, but concentrations as high as 32,000 mg·kg^{-1} have been reported in some super-enriched coal samples (reviewed in Kang *et al.* [42]). Arsenic in coal occurs in three non-exclusive distinct forms: arsenical pyrite, arsenopyrite and arsenate species [44,45].

During coal combustion, arsenic readily oxidizes to form arsenic oxide vapor [44] which combines with calcium oxide and condenses on the surface of fly ash particles in the form of calcium arsenate [46–48]. The inverse correlation between arsenic concentration and particle size which has been observed demonstrates that volatilized arsenic preferentially adsorbs or condenses on the finer particles [31]. Furthermore, higher combustion temperatures result in higher concentrations of particulate arsenic. For example, an increase in total arsenic concentration in PM_1 (particulate matter <1 μm) from 0.07 to 0.25 mg·m^{-3} at respective temperatures of 1100 and 1400 °C was reported in one study [48].

Solid by-products of the combustion process, including fly ash and bottom ash, are major sinks for arsenic. An estimated 90% to 100% of arsenic is captured in coal combustion by-products [49], with a preferential enrichment (up to 80%) for the fly ash component (reviewed in Yudovich and Ketris [50]). Removal efficiencies of arsenic by particulate control systems such as cyclones, electrostatic precipitators, wet scrubbers and fabric filters range between 43% and 99%, depending on the control device used [51]. An early study by Ondov *et al.* [52] reported that arsenic penetration through electrostatic precipitators (ESP) and wet scrubbers may be as high as 8.8% and 7.5%, respectively. Despite the widespread use of ESPs in Europe, a reported 575 t of arsenic were emitted from the combustion of coal during 1990 [35]. Similarly, in China around 550 t of arsenic were emitted from coal-fired power plants during 2007 [51]. Arsenic emissions arising from coal burning industries are an ongoing issue of global significance.

2.2.3. Mine Tailings

Fugitive dust emissions from mine wastes and mechanical processes associated with the hard rock mining industry such as crushing of sulphide ore and concentrates, and mechanical disturbance and wind erosion of uncontained mine tailings [10,53] are also associated with elevated levels of arsenic [17–19,54]. This is not surprising given that mine wastes and tailings are often characterized by extremely high arsenic concentrations. Concentrations in tailings ranging between 2250 and 21,400 mg·kg^{-1} have been detected in the Zimapan mining district in Mexico [55], and in some historical gold mine waste disposal areas in Victoria, Australia, concentrations of up to 15,000 mg·kg^{-1} have been recorded [56]. The preferential enrichment of arsenic in the finer size fraction in mine tailings [21,57] suggests that re-suspended dusts are characterized by higher arsenic content than the material from which it is suspended.

2.3. A Global Issue

The magnitude of the problems associated with arsenic contamination from mining operations is a serious ongoing issue in many localities throughout the world, and there are no indications of abatement. If the projected increase in global copper production over the next 20 years is correct [58], it could be reasonably expected that smelter emissions, and the generation of flue dust and other associated waste products, will also increase [39]. Furthermore, despite an overall increase in the number of coal plant retirements in some localities [59], the global demand for coal is predicted to rise at a rate of 1.3% per year, from 147 quadrillion Btu in 2010 to 180 quadrillion Btu in 2020 and 220 quadrillion Btu in 2040 [60]. Expansion of coal consumption reflects substantial increases in China and India [60]. In India, arsenic-contaminated fly ash from coal combustion processes occupies more than 65,000 acres, rendering the surrounding land unsuitable for agriculture [61].

Although not increasing substantially, the number of abandoned mines worldwide runs into millions [62], and their impact is likely to increase due to population growth and urban expansion. In the United States of America, 80% of an estimated 46,000 known abandoned mine sites require further investigation and/or remediation [63]. In Australia, there are more than 50,000 registered abandoned mines ranging from isolated minor surface works to more extensive and complex sites [64,65] In Mexico, the area affected by mining activities is estimated to be over 21.7 million hectares [66]. Each year in China the mining industry produces wastes that occupy an additional 2000 ha [67], and around 4000 Mt of tailings are stockpiled on land that is urgently needed for other purposes [68].

Given the widespread geographical distribution of arsenic-rich mine wastes and the global reliance on smelting and coal combustion for various products and services, the systematic characterization and ongoing monitoring of particulate arsenic generated by mining operations are becoming increasingly important for reliably determining the impacts on human health and the environment [45].

3. Monitoring and Assessment

A number of monitoring and assessment studies have been undertaken for different purposes: (i) to identify the dominant emissions sources of arsenic; (ii) to predict the potential contribution of an identified arsenic emission source to the atmosphere; and (iii) to identify the airborne arsenic species (Table 1). For monitoring and reporting purposes, atmospheric total arsenic concentrations are often compared with the annual mean target value of 6 $ng \cdot m^{-3}$, as set by current European Union air quality standards [69]. According to the World Health Organization (WHO) [70], the excess lifetime risk of contracting lung cancer if continuously exposed to 6.6 $ng \cdot m^{-3}$ is 1:100,000.

The different methodologies used to collect PM from mining operations are reflected in the contrasting size fractions and reporting units listed in Table 1. Air monitoring programs use various types of sampling equipment to collect PM, and the arsenic content of the PM is typically reported in terms of $ng \cdot m^{-3}$. Measurement of total suspended particulates (TSP) was the United States of America standard for atmospheric aerosol until the discovery of the relationship between particle size and lung deposition of inhaled particles [71].

The smaller the particle, the deeper it will travel into the respiratory tract (RT) and PM_{10} (particulate matter ≤ 10 μm) represents the upper limit for tracheobronchial and alveolar deposition in the human lung [72]. To meet the new PM_{10} health-based standard (adopted by the USA, Europe and elsewhere during the mid to late 1980s), collection devices such as the cascade impactor and multiple orifice uniform deposit impactor (MOUDI) have been used in various atmospheric monitoring studies [10,18,54]. These sampling systems are designed to collect a pre-selected suite of aerodynamically-fractionated samples which enables a systematic investigation into the arsenic content of particulates of interest to health. The relationship between particle size and human exposure will be reviewed in detail in Section 4.

Particulate arsenic may also be measured in size-fractionated mine waste samples generated through dry sieving bulk samples [21,57]. Similar to the cascade impactor mentioned above, this method facilitates a systematic characterization of collected mine waste samples but reports the concentrations in terms of $\mu g \cdot g^{-1}$. While this technique cannot provide a quantitative assessment of atmospheric arsenic at a particular location, the data may be useful for predicting potential particulate arsenic emissions from the source.

Atmospheric arsenic concentrations vary between localities and the type of emission source (Table 1). The following sub-sections examine the contribution of each emission source to atmospheric arsenic levels in various localities throughout the world.

3.1. Smelting

Much of the atmospheric arsenic research and monitoring published to date has focused on emissions from smelting operations. This reflects the dominant contribution by smelter emissions to global anthropogenic atmospheric arsenic inputs. As reviewed in Matschulatt [3], copper and zinc smelting activities contribute of 12,800 and 2210 t of arsenic respectively into the atmosphere per year, whereas steel production contributes a comparatively lower annual quantity of 60 t per annum. It should also be noted that in some industrial localities, smelting and other processes associated with the manufacturing of ceramic materials represent important sources of arsenic in the atmosphere [27]. Smelting operations produce the greatest localized air and soil arsenic concentrations while coal combustion distributes arsenic to the air in substantially lower concentrations over a wider area [73].

In the vast majority of case studies summarized in Table 1, concentrations exceeded, and in some cases, greatly exceeded, the annual WHO-prescribed target value [70]. In one extreme case, an average concentration of 330 $ng \cdot m^{-3}$ was reported in TSP collected approximately 1 km from a complex lead-copper smelter in Belgium [4]. Similarly, a maximum arsenic concentration of 572.3 $ng \cdot m^{-3}$ (mean, 93.9 $ng \cdot m^{-3}$) was recorded in TSP collected in the vicinity of a smelter in Walsall, UK, during an air monitoring program conducted between 1972 and 1989 [26]. Interestingly, a declining trend in atmospheric arsenic levels was reported at all of the UK monitoring locations, except the Walsall smelter site [26]. The authors postulated that widespread industrial switching from coal combustion to oil and gas as a domestic energy source for space heating was the probable cause for the overall decline in atmospheric arsenic in the UK [26]. Similar results were recorded in an industrial area in Spain, whereby reductions in atmospheric arsenic concentrations were significantly associated with decreases in industrial activities, specifically the production of ceramic materials [27].

Although the quantification of arsenic in TSP provides one measurement of arsenic contamination in the atmosphere, this measurement may underestimate the respiratory health risks to nearby communities due to the inverse relationship between particle size and arsenic content. After the introduction of particle size-selective criteria, various studies have measured and compared arsenic content in the PM_{10} and $PM_{2.5}$ fractions collected in the vicinity of smelting operations (Table 1). Data from these studies suggest a general trend for preferential enrichment in $PM_{2.5}$ [74–76]. For example, an air monitoring study conducted approximately 3.5 km from the Huelva copper smelter in southwestern Spain found that 85% of the total arsenic concentration in the PM_{10} size fraction was concentrated in $PM_{2.5}$ [77]. Similar studies conducted in the same locality yielded comparable results [74,75]. In contrast to these findings, one study reported that $PM_{2.5}$ collected in the vicinity of a copper smelter in Tacoma, WA, USA, contained only 37% of the total arsenic in the PM_{10} fraction (calculated from Polissar *et al.* [78]). These results highlight the importance of site-specific investigations during health-based risk assessments.

The greatest atmospheric arsenic levels generated by smelting operations occur in close proximity to the smelter, and decrease with increasing distance from the source [4,76,77]. Multiple reports suggest that the maximum concentrations are typically found within 1 km of the smelter site [4,78–81]. Furthermore, declines in concentrations have been observed over a relatively short distances. For example, atmospheric arsenic levels at a distance of 1 and 2.5 km from a complex copper-lead smelter in Belgium were 330 and 75 $ng{\cdot}m^{-3}$, respectively [4]. These results were supported by a complementary soil-based study that documented an exponential decline in soil arsenic and heavy metal concentrations within 1 km of a lead smelter in the Czech Republic, followed by a less-steep decrease between 1 and 6 km [37].

Meteorological variables, particularly surface wind circulation, play a critical role in determining the transport and spatial distribution of the pollution plume from smelting operations [82]. Contrary to the general trend between concentration and distance from the emission source, Serbula *et al.* [81] reported average arsenic levels of 131.4, 51.3 and 93.7 $ng{\cdot}m^{-3}$ at respective increasing distances of 0.8 (town park), 1.9 (institute) and 2.5 km (Jugopetrol) from a copper smelter in Bor, eastern Serbia. Compared with the mid-distance sampling location (institute), the farthest sampling location (Jugopetrol, which is downwind from the pollution source) experienced high-frequency exposure to the emissions as a result of dominant WNW and NW winds. To further highlight the impact of prevailing wind direction, the maximum concentration reported at Jugopetrol was equal to the maximum recorded at the sampling location closest to the smelter (Table 1). Similar relationships between atmospheric arsenic (and other metals), and surface wind characteristics in the vicinity of copper smelters have been documented [74,83]. In addition to wind direction, wind speed plays an important role in determining particulate arsenic distribution from smelting operations. The greatest concentrations of arsenic (and other metallic elements) emitted from the copper smelter in Bor occurred during calm conditions (wind speed less than 0.5 m/s) [38]. Low wind speeds inhibit the dispersal of local pollution away from the emission source and can therefore lead to very high localized concentrations of atmospheric pollutants [38].

3.2. Coal Combustion

Global coal combustion contributes an estimated 6240 t of arsenic to the atmosphere each year, equating to approximately half the contribution from copper smelting [3]. Atmospheric arsenic concentrations in coal combustion emissions are generally lower and typically distributed over a wider area. As a possible result of these two factors, coal combustion as a source of atmospheric arsenic has received less attention in the literature compared with copper/zinc/lead smelting.

Much of the research into coal combustion as a source of atmospheric arsenic has been undertaken in China (Table 1), and a recent review article listed this source as one of the key contributors to atmospheric arsenic in this country [84]. The mean atmospheric arsenic concentration for 32 localities across China was 51 ± 67 $ng{\cdot}m^{-3}$ (range, 0.03–200 $ng{\cdot}m^{-3}$). However, in heavily industrialized areas such as around Beijing, concentrations may be substantially greater [9].

Given that high temperature processes are typically associated with fine and accumulation-mode particles, arsenic levels in PM_{10} and $PM_{2.5}$ are frequently reported [85–88]. Comparable average PM_{10} arsenic concentrations were recorded in Beijing (58.3 ng·m^{-3}) and nearby Taiyuan (43.36 ng·m^{-3}) whereas the average $PM_{2.5}$ concentration in Ji'nan (40 ng·m^{-3}) was almost double that of Beijing (23.08 ng·m^{-3} Table 1). These values greatly exceed the recommended target value of 6 ng·m^{-3}.

Wind conditions appear to play an important role in the dispersal of atmospheric arsenic emitted by coal combustion sources [9]. Consistent with the trend found in the vicinity of smelting operations, one study [9] reported a statistically significant negative correlation between atmospheric arsenic concentration and wind speed in Beijing, China ($R = -0.31, p < 0.01$; Figure 2).

Figure 2. Relationship between total atmospheric arsenic concentration and wind speed in Beijing, China, for the period February 2009 to March 2011. Reprinted from Yang *et al.* [9] with permission from Elsevier.

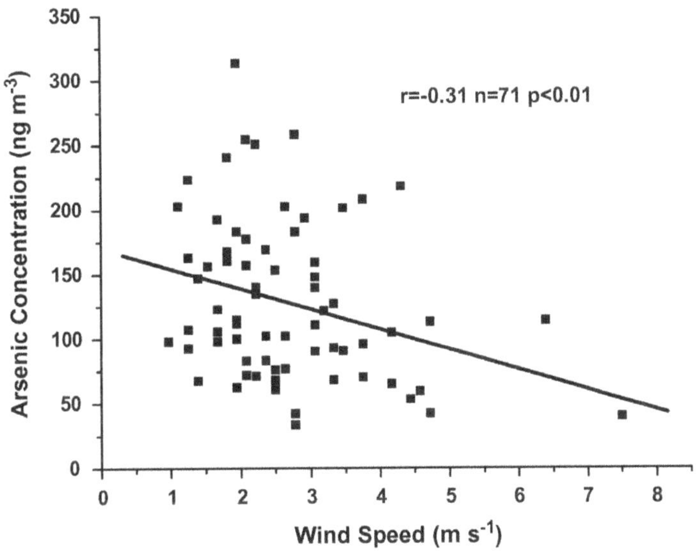

3.3. Mine Tailings

Research into mine tailings as a source of atmospheric arsenic has gained momentum in the last decade. Mine tailings have the potential to generate high levels of dust with extremely high atmospheric arsenic concentrations, particularly in arid and semi-arid environments [10]. The Rosh Pinah lead and zinc mine and ore processing plant in Namibia reported a maximum arsenic concentration of 9140 ng·m^{-3} (median, 4970 ng·m^{-3}) in wind-blown dust from tailings that cover more than 60 ha and are more than 20 m high [89]. Comparable with the trend observed around smelting operations, the impact of mine tailings on atmospheric arsenic levels are typically greatest at the source [11,17,18,54]. At the Rosh Pinah mine and ore processing plant atmospheric arsenic levels decreased from 4970 ng·m^{-3} at the tailings dam to 60 ng·m^{-3} at a distance of 2.5 km from the mine [89]. This relationship is most likely a result of the short atmospheric residence time of coarse particles (≥2.5 μm) typically found in mine tailings [10].

Arsenic enrichment in the finer fractions of size-fractionated mine tailings has been reported [19,21,57]. Although these findings are not reflective of actual atmospheric arsenic emissions from a particular source, the finer size fractions are more susceptible to wind-borne transport and are most likely to be re-suspended by wind or mechanical disturbance. Kim *et al.* [21] examined the distribution of arsenic concentration as a function of particle size in mine tailings samples collected from two different localities in the Randsburg historic mining district in south-central California, USA. Although there were distinct differences in the arsenic distributions amongst the wastes, there were obvious inverse relationships between grain size and arsenic concentration. The high arsenic content recorded in the dust size fraction of each sample (range, 356–8210 ppm) illustrates the potential of their corresponding sources to generate potentially hazardous emissions [21].

The effects of seasonality on particulate arsenic emissions from mine tailings have also been investigated. Meteorological factors associated with different seasons, especially rainfall and temperature, have been shown to have a dramatic impact on arsenic mobility through the air [54,90]. During the dry summer months in the City of Lavrion, Greece, concentrations of arsenic in PM_{10} increased dramatically (more than 6 times) compared with concentrations during late winter [54,90]. Similarly, a study in Aznalcazar, southwest Spain, found that sporadic rainfall and low convective atmospheric dynamics during the late winter were associated with relatively low re-suspension of PM from heavy metal mining wastes [54]. During summer, the combination of intensive convective circulation and low rainfall facilitates surface drying leading to enhanced re-suspension of PM. Low rainfall and decreased humidity lead to increased atmospheric particulates, and therefore, increased atmospheric arsenic concentration [90].

3.4. Arsenic Speciation in Particulate Matter

Environmental arsenic exists in four oxidation states including As(V), As(III), As(0) and As(-III) [91,92]. The most common forms of arsenic in the environment include the trivalent (arsenite) and pentavalent (arsenate) species [93], and they are often found occurring together [94,95]. Under oxidizing conditions, such as in surface soils and water, arsenic typically occurs in the pentavalent form [92], whereas in sufficiently reducing environments, or in the presence of a reducing agent, arsenite is the dominant form [94,96]. It is widely recognized that arsenite species have greater mobility in the environment [97] and are reported to be 25 to 60 times more toxic than the corresponding pentavalent forms [98]. Since the oxidation state of arsenic in soil, water, and other environmental matrices is one of the key factors governing toxicity, speciation analysis is of interest in human exposure studies.

Speciation analysis has been used widely for the identification and quantification of arsenic species in bulk samples of surface soils and mine wastes [94,95,99,100]. However, comparatively less work has been conducted in relation to arsenic speciation in atmospheric PM generated by mining operations [9,18,44,74–76,83]. Research conducted to date indicates that both arsenate and arsenite may co-exist in smelter, coal combustion and gold roaster emissions [9,44,45,74–76,83,94] although reported levels for the trivalent species are generally much lower than those for the arsenates (Table 1). For example, arsenate and arsenite concentrations in coal combustion emissions in China were 67 and 4.7 $ng \cdot m^{-3}$, respectively [9]. Similarly, Oliveira *et al.* [83] reported respective arsenate and arsenite concentrations of 10.4 and 1.2 $ng \cdot m^{-3}$ in copper smelter emissions in Spain. The presence of arsenite in smelter emissions may result from the reduction of arsenate by aerosol sulphur dioxide S(IV) complexes during transport of the emission plume [101].

Airborne monitoring programs combined with speciation analysis demonstrate clearly that airborne arsenic is a serious and ongoing issue in mining communities and heavily industrialized areas throughout the world.

Table 1. Summary of the average, minimum and maximum total arsenic (TAs) concentrations recorded in particulate matter (PM) from various mining operations, including smelting, coal combustion and mine waste. Values for TAs are expressed as nanogram per cubic meter ($ng \cdot m^{-3}$) unless otherwise specified. Where applicable, all units of distance measurement have been converted to metric system.

Pb-Cu smelter	Belgium	TSP (May–September 1978)	<1	330			[4]
			2.5	75			
Cu smelter	Tacoma, WA, USA	$PM_{2.5-10}$ (January 1985–Febrary 1986)	0.8	153.9 ± 269.4			[78]
		$PM_{2.5}$ (January 1985–Febrary 1986)		90.2 ± 170.7			
		$PM_{2.5-10}$ (January 1985–Febrary 1986)	10	3.7 ± 9.6			
		$PM_{2.5}$ (January 1985–Febrary 1986)		4.4 ± 3.6			
Cu smelter	Walsall, UK	TSP	<1	93.9 ± 89.7 (10.6–572.3)			[26]
Cu smelter	Quillota, Central Chile	PM_{10} (December 1999–November 2000)	≤40	32.5 ± 33.7 (1.7–196)			[102]
Cu smelter	Huelva, southwest Spain	TSP (January–December 2000)	2	12.3 ± 1.6 (3.0–33.8)	1.2 ± 0.3 (0.3–1.8)	10.4 ± 1.8 (2.1–30.6)	[83]
Cu smelter	Huelva, southwest Spain	PM_{10} (2001)	2	7.7 (1.6–29.4)	1.2 (0.6–2.2)	6.5 (0.01–25.7)	[75]
		PM_{10} (2002)		9.9 (1.3–79.8)	2.1 (0.4–3.4)	7.8 (0.01–56.2)	
Cu smelter	Huelva, southwest Spain	$PM_{2.5}$ (2001)	2	6.4 (0.8–30.2)	0.9 (0.01–1.6)	5.0 (0.01–25.3)	[74]
		$PM_{2.5}$ (2002)		7.9 (1.0–56.6)	1.4 (0.1–2.7)	6.6 (0.01–56.2)	
Cu smelter	Huelva, southwest Spain	PM_{10} (2004)	3.5	4.67 (max: 22.4)			[77]
		$PM_{2.5}$ (2004)	3.5	3.04 (max: 19.0)			
		PM_{10} (2005)	3.5	10.6 (max: 62.1)			
		$PM_{2.5}$ (2005)	3.5	9.18 (max: 60.3)			
Cu mining and smelter complex	Bor, eastern Serbia	PM_{10} (15–year average; 1994–2008)	0.8	131.4 (<2–669)			[81]
			1.9	51.3 (<2–356)			
			2.5	93.7 (<2–670)			
Cu mining and smelter complex	Bor, eastern Serbia	PM_{10} (24 March–1 April 2009)	0.65	32.97 ± 53.63 (2.4–149)			[38]
Ferromanganese plant	Dunkirk, France	PM_{10} (January 2003–March 2005)	2	5.1 ± 5.4 (0.5–35.1)			[103]
Cu smelter	Huelva, southwest Spain	$PM_{2.5}$ (16–22 October 2009)	5	2.1 ± 4.2 (0–20)			[82]

Table 1. *Cont.*

Complex Cu smelter	Tsumeb, Namibia	PM_{10} (2010–2011)	Smelter boundary	310			[80]
			Low exposure site	190			
Coal combustion	Beijing, China	PM_{10} (2001 and 2006)	12 sites across city	58.3 ± 60			[86]
Coal combustion	Beijing, China	TSP (February 2009–March 2011)	n.a.	130 ± 60 (30–310)	4.7 ± 3.6 (0.73–20)	67 ± 35 (14–250)	[9]
Coal combustion	Beijing, China	$PM_{2.5}$ (December 2012–January 2013)	n.a.	23.08			[85]
Coal combustion	Taiyuan, China	PM_{10} (2–16 March 2004)	n.a.	43.36 ± 27.61 (11.98–82.55)			[87]
Coal combustion	Ji'nan, eastern China	$PM_{2.5}$ (17–28 September 2010)	5	40 ± 40			[88]
Coal mine (raw coal)	Southwest Virginia, USA	PM_{10} (7 August 2008)	0.3	0.958			[12]
			1.6	0.735			
Gold mine tailings	Rodalquilar, southeastern Spain	PM_{10}	n.a.	1581 ppm			[19]
		Mechanically re-suspended in lab, n=2		1368 ppm			
Pb-Zn mine	Rosh Pinah, Namibia	TSP	0	4970 (2800–9140)			[89]
		Tailings dam	0	280 (130–920)			
		Ore treatment plant	1.5	30 (30–70)			
			2.5	60 (20–80)			
Cu-Pb-Zn mine tailings	Aznalcazar, South Spain	TSP (20 May–27 December 1998)	0	221 (4.9–2681)			[54]
			0.5	69 (2–921)			
Historical Ag-Pb mine tailings	City of Lavrion, Greece	PM_{10} Overall average	1	520 (1–3031)			[90]
		Winter		115 (1–791)			
		Summer		909 (121–3031)			
Abandoned Au mine tailings	Nova Scotia, Canada	>16 μm (2004)	0	8200		Present but not quantified	[18]
		16–8 μm (2004)		2020			
		8–4 μm (2004)		631			
		4–2 μm (2004)		337			
		2–1 μm (2004)		58.3			
		1–0.5 μm (2004)		13.3			

Table 1. *Cont.*

Former Au mine tailings	Yellcwknife, Canada	TSP (July–September 2004)	<1	19 (1–76)			[104]
		PM_{10} (July–September 2004)		6 (1–15)			
Different mine waste types	Butte, Montana, USA	PM_{10} Mine waste type 1	n.a.	406 ppm			[57]
		PM_{10} Mine waste type 2		467 ppm			
		PM_{10} Mine waste type 3		469 ppm			
		PM_{10} Mine waste type 4		769 ppm			
Ag-Au mine tailings	Descarga mine tailings site, USA	>2830 µm	n.a.	203 ppm			[21]
		2830–1700 µm		452 ppm			
		1700–1000 µm		976 ppm			
		1000–500 µm		1870 ppm			
		500–250 µm		2650 ppm			
		250–125 µm		3790 ppm			
		125–75 µm		3650 ppm			
		75–45 µm		4720 ppm			
		45–32 µm		7060 ppm			
		32–20 µm		8210 ppm			
Pb-Zn mine waste	Oklahoma, USA	PM2.5 (July–September 2005)	<1	0.64 ± 0.48			[11]
			5	0.62 ± 0.32			
			18	0.56 ± 0.33			
Cu-Au-Ag mine waste	Rio Tinto mines, Spain	Total bulk deposition (March 2009–February 2010/March 2010–February 2011)	0	4.4/2.1 $mg \cdot m^{-2}$			[17]
			0.5	0.7/0.5 $mg \cdot m^{-2}$			
			1.5	0.7/1.0 $mg \cdot m^{-2}$			
Smelter & coal combustion	China (various localities)	Average of PM10, PM2.5 TSP and dust		51.0 ± 67			[84]
Smelter & other industries	Aspropyrgyros Greece	TSP (December 2004–June 2006)	n.a.	3.4 ± 0.3	<0.2	3.2 ± 0.4	[76]
		PM_{10}–$PM_{2.5}$ (December 2004–June 2006)		1.9 ± 0.3	<0.2	1.7 ± 0.4	
		$PM_{2.5}$ (December 2004–June 2006)		1.1 ± 0.3	<0.2	1.0 ± 0.4	

4. Human Exposure

Communities living in the vicinity of mining operations may be exposed to airborne arsenic-contaminated particulates and be at risk of health deterioration though absorption after dermal and eye contact, or by ingestion after inhalation [28]. However, arsenic absorption through the skin following dermal and eye contact is a minor contributor compared with ingestion and inhalation exposures [25] and will not be further discussed here. Furthermore, incidental ingestion of arsenic-contaminated particulates, usually as a result of contaminated food or water supplies, has been the most thoroughly investigated pathway, and its significant range of adverse effects have been well documented following acute, intermediate and chronic exposures [25], negating the need for further detailed review here.

For the general population, ingestion is typically considered the primary exposure pathway to arsenic, and inhalation of arsenic bearing PM has been considered to be a minor exposure route [2]. The relatively neglected topic of inhalation exposure with consequent issues linked to airborne PM containing arsenic species from proximate mining industries needs to be addressed. For example, exposure assessments of communities living in the vicinity of smelting and coal combustion operations suggest that inhalation may play a similar, if not more important role than ingestion, in the overall exposure to airborne particulate arsenic [4,105–107]. In addition, it has been shown that children are particularly susceptible to inhalation exposure due to: (i) their increased likelihood of coming into contact with dust [78]; and (ii) children inhale a greater volume of air than adults relative to their size [108].

Therefore, in the following sections we will consider some of the ways in which inhaled arsenic-contaminated particulates generated by mining operations may lead to systemic absorption, toxicity, and arsenic-related disease endpoints. In order to understand how arsenic becomes mobile (or bioavailable) and exerts its toxic effects in the human body, we will begin with a discussion on the fate of inhaled particles in the RT with particular emphasis on the role that particle size plays in determining the ultimate absorption or defense mechanisms.

4.1. Deposition Location and Particle Clearance from the Respiratory Tract (RT)

The location and manner in which PM is deposited in the RT are critical for understanding how the arsenic-bearing particles might react with different lung constituents. When PM is inhaled, a proportion of the particles are retained while the remainder are expelled via exhalation. Retained particles are deposited in different regions of the RT according to their size [109–111] and as a general rule, the smaller the particle the deeper it will penetrate into the RT and the longer it will be retained (Table 2; [72,112]). To protect the body against foreign materials, the human respiratory system has developed a range of physiological lines of defense [113,114]. We will review the deposition location of inhaled particles as a function of particle size, the methods of clearance from each location, and pathways for absorption. When referring to the different "deposition regions", we use the morphometric model described by the International Commission on Radiological Protection [115]. This model divides the human RT into three major anatomical regions: (i) the extra-thoracic; (ii) the tracheobronchial, and; (iii) the alveolar, which are modeled deposition locations for the inhalable, thoracic and respirable particulate size fractions, respectively [116].

Table 2. Deposition of PM_{10} in different regions of the human respiratory tract [115,116] as a function of particle size (data from Newman [72]), including the estimated retention time of the particle size in each deposition location (data from Bailey [112]).

Anatomical Region (Corresponding Particulate Size Fraction)	PM Size (μm)	Deposition Location	Retention Time
Extra-thoracic (Inhalable)	7–10	Nasal passage	1 day; small fraction may be retained for longer
	5–7	Pharynx	Few minutes
Tracheobronchial (Thoracic)	3–5	Trachea	Few minutes
	2–3	Bronchi	Hours to weeks
	1.0–2.5	Terminal bronchioles	Hours to weeks
Alveolar (Respirable)	0.5–1.0	Alveoli	50 to 7000 days

4.1.1. Extra-Thoracic Region (Inhalable Particulate Fraction)

The inhalable particulate fraction (particles up to 10 μm in size) consists of particles that can be deposited into the extra-thoracic region and become trapped in the nasal cavity [109], mouth [116] and pharynx [117]. The vast majority of particles deposited in the extra-thoracic region are removed via a combination of nose-blowing, sneezing and mucociliary transport to the gastrointestinal (GI) tract [117]. Nose-blowing clears from 0.5% to 50% of particles from the front of the nose, while the remainder is slowly cleared into the GI tract [117]. Particles in the pharynx may reach the GI tract within one hour following deposition [117], and a very small proportion (around 0.05%) may be absorbed directly via the pharynx epithelium and cleared into the blood or lymphatic system [117]. Ingestion is therefore the dominant exposure pathway to particles deposited in the extra-thoracic region.

4.1.2. Tracheobronchial Region (Thoracic Particulate Fraction)

The thoracic particulate fraction is comprised of particles (1–5 μm in size) that penetrate the extra-thoracic region [116] and deposit in the tracheobronchial region. This region consists of the trachea, bronchi and terminal bronchioles [115]. Particles deposited here are of particular importance because lung carcinomas occur preferentially in the bronchial airways [110]. Particles trapped in the mucous produced by the bronchial epithelial cells are typically cleared by mucociliary transport into the throat, and then expectorated or swallowed [28,114,118]. While it is generally accepted that mucociliary transport is the principal clearance mechanism in the first 24 h [118], the rate of clearance depends upon on the clearance velocity of the mucous, particle shape, charge and surface geochemistry [119]. Furthermore, the ciliary movement is ineffective if the mucous is not of the correct viscosity due to illness or pharmacological action [109]. Other clearance mechanisms from the tracheobronchial region include coughing, absorption through airway epithelium into the blood or lymphatic system, and phagocytosis [113,118], and depending on the method of clearance, particles can be retained in the RT for weeks (Table 2; [112]). As described in sub-Section 4.2, the solubility of the particle plays an important role in determining which clearance mechanism is employed and the duration of the retention.

4.1.3. Alveolar Region (Respirable Particulate Fraction)

Airborne particles ≤1 μm can be deeply inhaled into the unciliated airways of the lung (the alveolar region) and absorbed directly into the pulmonary circulation system [113]. Alternatively, these particles may be phagocytosed and cleared by alveolar macrophages, and then either absorbed into regional lymph nodes via lymphatic vessels [120] or transported into the ciliated airways and cleared via mucociliary transport [121]. This latter process may take weeks to months to complete [122]. Alveolar macrophages are important cells of the immune system, exhibiting major phagocytic abilities and in response to inflammatory reactions, release reactive oxygen species (ROS). Under normal exposure conditions, the components of the inflammatory reaction interact synergistically with ROS to eliminate foreign material from the respiratory system [123].

4.2. Effects of Exposure Duration and Solubility

Variation in the solubility of different arsenic compounds is important for exposure and risk assessment studies [57]. In the case of short-term inhalation exposure (minutes to hours), the number of particles in the RT decreases over time until all particles have been cleared via phagocytosis and/or mucociliary transport [124]. Deposited particles containing soluble arsenic compounds may expose nearby cells to a high concentration of arsenic [125], which rapidly declines as the dissolved arsenic is removed from the lungs [126] via absorptive mechanisms through the airway epithelium [127]. Lantz *et al.* [128] proposed that this exposure regime would reduce the time for interaction with pulmonary cells and tissue. Less soluble particles on the other hand that are retained in the lung expose the target tissue to arsenic for a longer period of time (up to weeks), as observed in rodents after intratracheal instillation of inorganic arsenic compounds of varying solubility [125,126,129,130].

In the case of long-term exposure (days to years), a steady state between deposition and clearance will be reached and the retained fraction will remain in the lungs for most of the exposure period [110]. Consequently, retention of particles containing soluble and slightly soluble arsenic compounds, especially those particles deposited in the alveolar region and sequestered in the lymph nodes, may expose cells to low doses of arsenic for a prolonged period of time. It is frequently reported that long-term, low-level exposures to arsenic may be predictive of toxic effects [126,131,132] and the pathogenesis of lung diseases, such as lung carcinoma [130].

Figure 3 illustrates that following inhalation, arsenic can follow different pathways leading to systemic absorption, and each pathway is highly dependent upon particle solubility and method of clearance. Systemic exposure to arsenic may occur as a result of ingestion following mucociliary clearance, by dissolution in the lung fluid, direct entry into lymph nodes, or by phagocytosis. Systemic exposure to arsenic following inhalation of arsenic-bearing particulates could therefore be considered as a multi-pathway process with differing durations and intensities of exposure.

Figure 3. Potential pathways leading to systemic absorption of inhaled arsenic, including clearance mechanisms and their associated durations and intensities of exposure. Adapted from Wang [120].

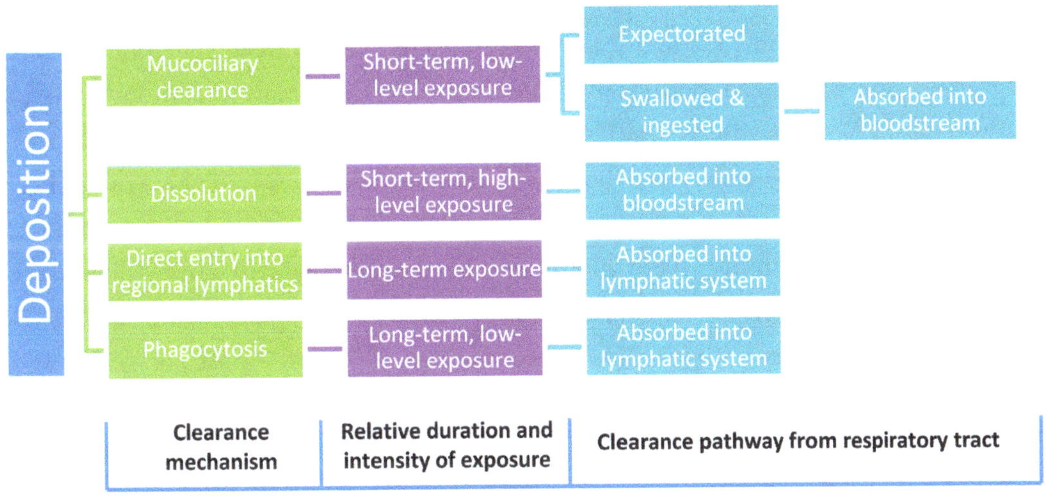

4.3. Pulmonary Bioavailability of Inhaled Arsenic

The bioavailable fraction of arsenic is considered to be an important determinant of toxicity and the associated disease response [133]. The term bioavailability may be interpreted in a number of different ways [134], however and for the purposes of this review paper, the terms bioavailability and bioaccessibility will be used in accordance with the definitions prescribed by Ng *et al.* [135]. Briefly, the portion of a contaminant that is absorbed into the body following exposure is referred to as the bioavailable fraction and is typically measured *in vivo* [135]. Bioaccessibility on the other hand refers to the soluble fraction of a compound following *in vitro* gastrointestinal or pulmonary extraction, and may be used as a surrogate for estimating the bioavailability of a contaminant [135].

In order to assess the relative risk of inhalation exposure to metal-laden particles of various origins, simulated lung fluids (SLF) such as Gamble's solution and artificial lysosomal fluids (ALF) have been used in various studies [136–139]. Gamble's solution is an electrolyte fluid similar in composition to that of interstitial fluid with a pH near 7.4, and aims to mimic the aqueous component of the lung [140]. ALF is analogous to the fluid produced by macrophages during phagocytosis [141] and has a pH of around 4.5 [137]. Biological fluid pH is an important parameter governing the solubility of arsenic and other metals. For example, arsenic solubility measured as a percentage of the total arsenic concentration of mine waste, was reported as 36.6% in simulated stomach fluid (pH 1.2) and 0.4% in SLF (pH 7.5) [57], suggesting that an acid medium is required for arsenic dissolution. When determining pulmonary arsenic bioaccessibility, it may therefore be prudent to also investigate the behavior of arsenic in the more acidic ALF solution.

A limited number of studies aimed at comparing the bioaccessibility of other metallic compounds in SLF and ALF solutions reported significantly higher dissolution rates of potentially toxic metals in ALF [137,139]. Conversely, Plumlee *et al.* [142] found that SLF (near-neutral pH) was effective in leaching arsenic from dust samples collected from a dry lake, and the oral and inhalation bioaccessible arsenic fractions found in these particular dust samples were comparable. While it is important to note that the contrasting results between these studies highlight the importance of site-specific bioaccessibility assessments, they also indicate that certain arsenic species are relatively mobile at near-neutral conditions. Furthermore, the differences may also be attributed to the contrasting dissolution times used in each study: the mine waste and the dry lake dust samples underwent dissolution times of around 2 h [57] and 24 h [142], respectively. Given that fine particles may be retained in the RT for prolonged periods of time (Table 2), incubation duration is a particularly important parameter in bioaccessibility studies.

Pulmonary bioaccessibility tests may be more reliable predictors of bioavailability than the widely-used aqueous solubility tests, since Rhoads and Sanders [125] reported that arsenic, and other metals with low aqueous solubility, were highly soluble in the lungs of rats. A more recent study observed that SLF was more effective than deionized water at leaching arsenic in the ≤20 μm size fraction of soil impacted by fire, with leachate concentrations of 19 and 2 μg/L, respectively [143].

4.4. Summary

A summary of some of the key factors governing bioavailability of inhaled arsenic-bearing particles is proposed (Figure 4). Particle size governs the deposition location of inhaled particulates in the RT. Knowledge of the location and solubility of deposited particles is important for predicting the methods of clearance from and retention time in the RT, and therefore the types of lung fluids with which the particles may interact. Contact with pulmonary fluids can then release arsenic from inhalable arsenic-bearing particulates. Since the retention of arsenic in the body is predictive of toxicity and the pathogenesis of disease [126,131,132], the long-term pulmonary bioavailability of arsenic represents important consideration in the health risk assessment of populations living in mining-affected regions.

Figure 4. Diagrammatic representation of the interactions between key factors governing the pulmonary bioavailability of arsenic.

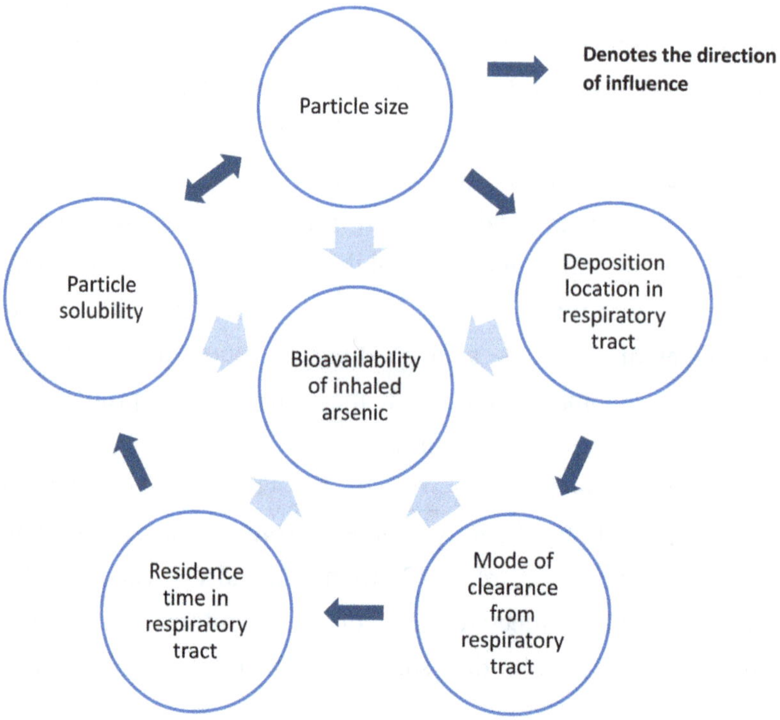

5. Importance of Metabolic Transformation in Arsenic Toxicity

5.1. Arsenic Biomethylation

The role of metabolism in arsenic toxicity has been the subject of several detailed reviews [144–149] therefore the following discussion will provide an overview of the key concepts only. Methylation is the major metabolic pathway for ingested inorganic arsenic in most mammals, and occurs via alternating reduction of pentavalent arsenic to the trivalent state, followed by oxidative addition of a methyl group [146,150–153]. Biotransformation of inorganic arsenicals occurs primarily in the liver with an estimated 70% [154] of metabolites readily excreted in urine [147,155–157]. The remaining portion deposits differentially in other target organs and tissues including the kidneys and the lungs, as well as keratinized tissues such as skin, nails, and hair [158–161].

In terms of clearly understanding arsenic biochemistry and toxicology, arsenic methylation presents a complex problem because the metabolic sequence (Figure 5) yields at least six distinct products, each with its own unique toxicology: arsenite, monomethylarsonic acid (MMA^{V}), monomethylarsonous acid (MMA^{III}), dimethylarsinic acid (DMA^{V}), dimethylarsinous acid (DMA^{III}) and dimethylthiolarsinic acid ($DMTA^{V}$) [146,162,163]. Various studies have demonstrated that the unstable trivalent intermediary products, MMA^{III} and DMA^{III}, are highly reactive and substantially more toxic than the inorganic and pentavalent compounds [149,152,162,164,165]. Arsenic methylation is therefore widely considered to be a bioactivation pathway rather than a detoxification process [144], with the resulting toxicity closely linked to the methylation status and valence state of the metabolites [166]. Therefore, understanding the arsenic biomethylation pathway is critical to elucidating its subsequent action as a toxin and carcinogen [167].

Figure 5. Metabolic pathway of inorganic arsenic. Reprinted from Chilakpati [168] with permission from Elsevier.

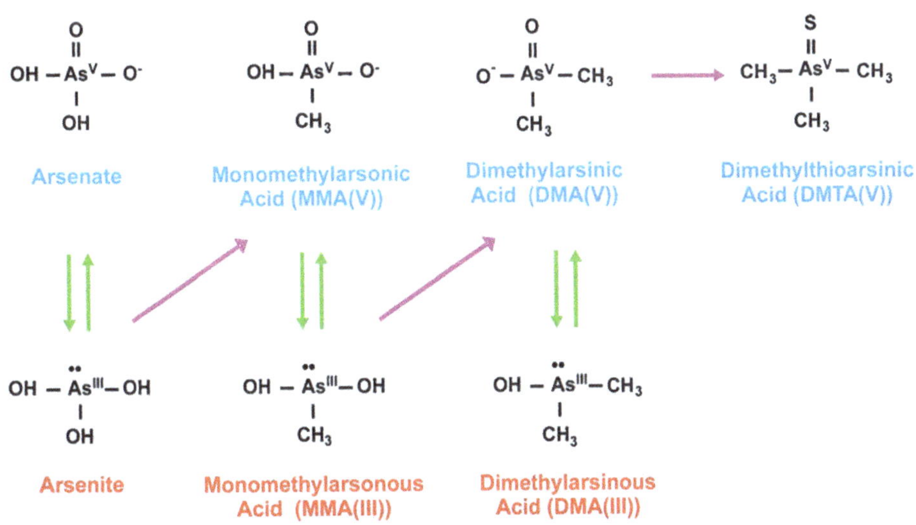

5.2. Oxidative Stress as a Mode of Action for Arsenic Carcinogenesis

Although several modes of action for arsenic carcinogenesis have been presented in the literature including oxidative stress, suppressed DNA repair, altered methylation patterns, genotoxicity and cell proliferation [144], the oxidative stress theory has been intensively investigated and is supported by a substantial mass evidence [168–171]. Oxidative stress refers to an imbalance between the production of reactive oxygen species (ROS), or free radicals, and antioxidant defense mechanisms [172]. Free radicals are characterized by the presence of unpaired electrons and the associated reactivity can lead to tissue injury [173].

The first oxidative stress theory for arsenic proposed that a minor metabolite of DMA^{V}, dimethylarsine (a trivalent arsenic compound), is produced via a process of reduction *in vivo* [170], possibly following a reaction between DMA^{III} and specific coenzymes important for cellular respiration [174]. Dimethylarsine is estimated to be around 100 times more toxic than DMA^{III} which is a potent genotoxin in its own right [174]. Dimethylarsine can react with molecular oxygen forming the dimethylarsenic ($(CH_3)_2As$) radical, and the superoxide anion O_2^- [175]. Through the addition of another molecule of oxygen, the dimethylarsenic radical forms the dimethylarsenic peroxyl ($(CH_3)_2AsOO$) radical. Finally, the hydroxyl radical ($HO^{\cdot}$) can be produced via reaction with cellular iron and other transition metals [170,175].

Although an excessive production of ROS, such as superoxide anion and hydroxyl radical, is commonly associated with impaired cellular functions, DNA damage and carcinogenesis [144,175,176], the dimethylarsenic and/or dimethylarsenic peroxyl radicals were found to play a crucial role in lung-specific DNA damage, tumorigenesis [169–171,174,177] and general arsenic-induced toxicity [178]. The generation of oxidative stress as a potential mode of action of arsenic for its disease endpoints is an ongoing area of research and the associated complexities have been comprehensively reviewed [145,158,175,179].

5.3. The Human Lung as a Target Organ for Arsenic Toxicity

Remarkably, arsenic is the only reported human lung carcinogen for which there is sufficient evidence of pulmonary carcinogenicity as a result of both inhalation and ingestion exposures [25,180]. Smith *et al.* [181] reported that the relative risk of lung cancer following inhalation and ingestion of arsenic was independent of the exposure pathway. Distinguishing between the different routes of exposure is complicated not only by the arsenic transformations that take place in the body, but also the common target organs following the different exposure pathways [163]. The high variability in pulmonary solubility observed for different arsenic compounds [126,129,130] also represents a confounding factor.

For systemically absorbed arsenic, via inhalation or ingestion, research suggests that the pulmonary system may function as a target tissue for toxicity based on the observation that dimethylarsine is excreted as a gas from the circulation via the lungs [170,177]. High partial pressures of molecular oxygen in the lungs may promote dimethylarsenic and dimethylarsenic peroxyl radical formation as dimethylarsine is excreted and passed through to the respiratory system [144,158,175].

Less soluble arsenic compounds can be retained in the lung as observed in humans [182] and rodents [126,129,130]. According to Styblo *et al.* [152], human lung epithelial cells have very low arsenic methylation capacity *in vitro*, which may translate to a lower capacity to convert inorganic arsenic methylate arsenicals *in vivo*. A reduced capacity to methylate arsenicals could be associated with an increased risk of toxicity due to prolonged retention of inorganic arsenic in the lung [183]. In support of these observations, various *in vivo* studies have reported that arsenic toxicity is closely linked with a prolonged retention of inorganic arsenic in the lungs of rodents [129,130]. Further studies to examine the direct effects of inorganic arsenic compounds on pulmonary cells in order to elucidate the carcinogenic mode of action of retained arsenic-bearing particulates are suggested.

5.4. Direct Effects of Arsenic on Pulmonary Cells

Some of the key effects of arsenic exposure on a range of different pulmonary cell lines are summarized in Table 3. Since the dose response of arsenic can be substantially different in animal models compared with *in vivo* human exposure [184], this section will primarily focus on studies involving pulmonary cell lines, specifically human bronchial epithelial (HBE) cells derived from human lung epithelium [168], alveolar macrophage (AM) cells, which are typically harvested from animals [185], and human pulmonary fibroblast (HPF) cells. HBE and AM cells represent the first lines of defense against foreign particles [185], while HPF cells are important for regeneration and repair of chemically or mechanically damaged tissues [186]. As discussed by Dodmane *et al.* [165], although the effects of *in vitro* arsenic exposure are likely to reflect the *in vivo* effects, a cautionary approach should be adopted when interpreting the data due to the variability of effects observed amongst experimental systems.

5.4.1. Pulmonary Cytotoxicity of Arsenic

Cytotoxicity assays, and the measurement of representative parameters associated with cell pathology, are widely used to quantitatively assess the *in vitro* potency of a toxicant in the whole animal. Clear dose-response relationships between arsenic concentration and cytoxicity have been established in HBE cells [165,168,187–189], HPF cells [189–191] and AM cells [185]. Figure 6 shows a notable decrease in HPF and HBE cell survival, in a time- and concentration-dependent manner, following 24 and 120 h treatments with sodium arsenite [189]. Relative cell survival rates indicate that sodium arsenite is more cytotoxic to HPF than HBE cells (Figure 6; [189]). A similar study found that arsenic trioxide was also toxic to HPF cells, however greater concentrations were required to produce similar effects [190]. The differential cytotoxicities observed between these two trivalent arsenic compounds can be attributed to the fact that arsenic trioxide has a lower solubility in the lung than sodium arsenite [126].

Consistent with other lines of evidence presented in previous sections, recent studies confirm that methylated arsenicals are more cytotoxic to pulmonary cells than the inorganic trivalent forms [165,168,188]. For example, the respective median lethal concentrations (LC50) of As^{III}, DMA^{III} and MMA^{III} in HBE cells were reported as 5.8, 1.4 and 1.0 μM, after a 72 h exposure period [165]. $DMTA^{V}$, exhibited a similar cytotoxicity potency to DMA^{III} [168]. While little is known about the pulmonary toxic effects of $DMTA^{V}$, gene expression analysis has shown that cells exposed to $DMTA^{V}$ and DMA^{III} share a relatively high number of differentially expressed genes (DEGs) following exposure to minimally cytotoxic arsenic concentrations, indicating the existence of associated similarities in the cellular mechanism of cytotoxicity of these two arsenicals at lower concentrations [168].

A systematic assessment of the cytotoxic effects and cellular uptake of As^{III}, MMA^{III}, DMA^{III}, MMA^{V}, DMA^{V} and thiodimethylarsinic acid (thio-DMA^{V}, $[(CH_3)_2As(S)OH]$) on human alveolar epithelial cells has been undertaken in complementary studies [187,188]. Thio-DMA^{V} is a human arsenic metabolite of inorganic arsenic and is formed immediately when DMTA^{V} is added to aqueous solution [187]. Cytotoxicity was quantified by measuring reductions in cell number, cell volume and colony formation following a 24 h exposure period [187,188]. In terms of these cytotoxicity endpoints, the cytotoxic order of extracellular arsenic concentrations was reported as DMA^{III} > MMA^{III} > thio-DMA^{V} ≥ As^{III} ≥ MMA^{V} ~ DMA^{V} [187]. Taking into consideration the bioavailability of each arsenic species, as measured by cellular uptake, the cytotoxic order was reported to change to thio-DMA^{V} ~ As^{III} ~ MMA^{III} > DMA^{III} ≥ MMA^{V} ~ DMA^{V} [187]. Cellular uptake of thio-DMA^{V} was strongly correlated with cytotoxicity endpoints, including cell number (correlation coefficient, −0.986) and colony forming ability (correlation coefficient, −0.998) [187].

Differences in arsenic-induced cytotoxicity endpoints reported in the literature may be attributed to variability in a number of experimental parameters: (i) the arsenic species or compound; (ii) the cell exposure duration; (ii) the cell systems used in each study; and (iii) the methods for assessing cytotoxicity endpoints.

Figure 6. Cytotoxicity of sodium arsenite in: (**A**) human lung fibroblast cells, and (**B**) human lung epithelial cells, following 24 and 12 h treatments. Reprinted from Xie *et al.* [189] with permission from Elsevier.

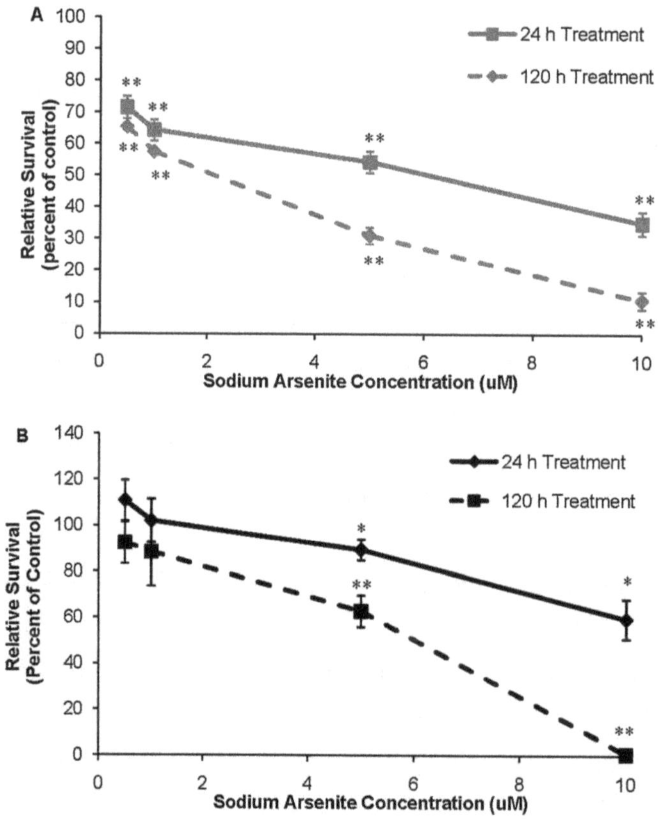

5.4.2. Effects of Arsenic-Induced Reactive Oxygen Species (ROS) Production on Human Bronchial Epithelial (HBE) Cells and Human Fibroblast (HF) Cells

Although ROS are widely recognized for their beneficial and growth-promoting effects on cells, overproduction can lead to toxic effects [192] including damage to cellular DNA and protein [144].

Studies show that HBE and HPF cells generate elevated ROS levels in a dose-dependent manner in the presence of arsenic [191,193]. Moreover, chronically exposed arsenic-transformed HBE cells constitutively generate cellular ROS (probably hydrogen peroxide) in the absence of further arsenic exposure [193]. Constitutive generation of ROS was found to be necessary for activating certain signaling pathways that regulate cell survival and cell proliferation [193].

Enhanced arsenic-induced ROS generation and accumulation have been associated with dose-dependent responses in rates of cell proliferation and colony formation in HBE cells [193–196] as well as anti-apoptotic signaling [195]. Increased cell proliferation is a distinguishing characteristic of cancer cells and is crucial for tumor formation, while apoptosis plays an important role in killing abnormal cells so that they cannot form tumors [193]. One study reported that increased cell proliferation of arsenic-exposed cells was mediated by anti-apoptotic-signaling induced by cyclooxygenase, COX-2 [197], an enzyme associated with inflammation and other pathogenesis [198]. Enhanced ROS levels play an important role in mediating COX-2 production in airway epithelial cells [199].

ROS production has also been linked with gene expression changes in HBE cells consistent with several of the proposed mechanisms for arsenic carcinogenesis [144] including oxidative stress, DNA damage and a weakened tumor-suppression response [165,168,195]. Suckle *et al.* [195] assessed the malignant potential of *in vitro* arsenic-transformed cells by injecting them into mice. The *in vivo* study identified phenotypic characteristics consistent with malignant lung epithelial cells [195], and whole genome expression profiling identified potential mitochondrial oxidative stress and increased metabolic energy output, which is indicative of increased mitochondrial energy production [195]. Importantly, chronic arsenic exposure may therefore target mitochondrial function leading to enhanced ROS generation and cancer-related gene signaling [195]. Antioxidants that target mitochondrial function could play a role in ameliorating some of the effects of arsenic in chronically-exposed populations [200].

Zhao *et al.* [201] recently discovered that long-term exposure to arsenic altered cellular energy metabolism through the induction of aerobic glycolysis (the Warburg effect), as observed in arsenite-treated HBE and other human cell lines cells. The Warburg effect is a metabolically supportive phenotype for the increased energy demands associated with the growth, proliferation and invasion of cancer cells (see the review by Vander Heiden *et al.* [202]). Unlike normal cells which produce lactate under anaerobic conditions only, the Warburg effect states that cancer cells generate large quantities of lactate regardless of oxygen availability [202]. This study was potentially the first to link an environmental toxicant with the induction of the Warburg effect, and thus this discovery may assist in identifying the role of arsenic toxicity in other diseases associated with disrupted energy metabolism, such as diabetes and atherosclerosis [201].

5.4.3. Arsenic-Induced Suppression of Alveolar Macrophage (AM) Function

Alveolar macrophages (AM) serve as the front line of cellular defence against foreign material by clearing the air spaces of any infectious, toxic or allergenic particles that have penetrated mechanical defences, such as the nasal passages and mucociliary transport system [203]. Under normal conditions, ROS are secreted by alveolar macrophages in response to phagocytosis or stimulation with specific agents, and play a key role in efficiently killing invading pathogens [204]. Various detrimental effects of arsenic on these important cell functions have been observed (Table 3). For example, Palmieri *et al.* [185] noted concentration-dependent reductions in AM viability and size following exposure to sodium arsenite concentrations of 2 and 2.5 μM, respectively, and a notable increase in apoptosis after 5 μM. In the presence of the lower sodium arsenite concentrations (<2 μM), AM cells maintained the ability to regulate cell homeostasis whereas higher doses (≥5 μM), reduced cell viability to 50% [185]. Increasing cell culture time generally played a key role in amplifying the observed adverse effects, particularly during exposure to the higher (5 and 10 μM) sodium arsenite concentrations [185].

Contrary to the commonly-observed response by arsenic-exposed HBE and HPF cells, AM cells typically exhibit a dose-dependent reduction in ROS production in the presence of arsenic [128,185,205–208]. Soluble trivalent arsenic was notably more potent at inhibiting ROS production than the corresponding pentavalent form, with superoxide inhibition occurring at respective concentrations of 0.1 and 1 μg/mL [208]. In contrast, the slightly soluble trivalent and pentavalent forms showed similar patterns in ROS production with inhibition occurring at a concentration of 10 μg/mL arsenic [128,207]. Gercken *et al.* [205] postulated that the depression of O_2^- (superoxide anion) production by arsenic-exposed AM may be linked with high concentrations of arsenic on the particle surface. Both the studies by Lantz *et al.* [128,208] observed that a 24 h period of arsenic exposure was required to suppress ROS production.

Suppression of ROS production, or a reduction in AM function as demonstrated by others [128,185,205,207,208], may therefore inhibit phagocytosis: an important clearance mechanism of foreign particles, such as dust and bacteria, from the lung. Suboptimal phagocytosis by AM cells has been associated with a decreased ability to clear dead or dying cells from the respiratory system thereby leading to pathological inflammation [209] as well as an increased susceptibility to pulmonary infection such as pneumonia, in respiratory health-compromised individuals [210].

5.4.4. Arsenic-Induced Inhibition of the Wound Healing Response in Human Bronchial Epithelial (HBE) Cells

As the respiratory epithelium is frequently injured by inhaled pollutants or micro-organisms, the epithelial wound repair response plays a critical role in the maintenance of epithelial barrier integrity [211]. Concentration-dependent arsenic-induced inhibition of wound healing in mechanically-wounded HBE cells has been demonstrated (Table 3). In the absence of arsenic, the wounded area of an epithelial monolayer of HBE cells was largely repaired (approximately 80%) by migrating cells after a period of 4 h [212]. In the presence of 30 and 60 ppb arsenic however, the amounts of wound closure were 48% and 24%, respectively [212]. The highest concentration (290 ppb) resulted in the expansion of the wound area in the first hour, followed by 16.5% healing at 4 h [212]. Further analyses indicated that overexpression of matrix metalloproteinase (MMP-9), an enzyme important for human respiratory healing and wound closure [213], leads to dysregulated wound repair in the presence of arsenic and reductions in cellular migration [212].

Regulation of MMP-9 and migration of airway epithelial cells are linked with ATP-dependent Ca^{2+} signalling [213]. Tightly coordinated Ca^{2+} transport and activity are vital during early wound healing processes; therefore Ca^{2+} is commonly used as an immediate damage indicator [214]. Furthermore, general interference with airway ATP signalling has been linked with chronic lung diseases, such as chronic obstructive pulmonary disease (COPD) [215]. To investigate whether arsenic disrupts Ca^{2+} signalling in mechanically-wounded HBE cells, Ca^{2+} concentrations were monitored following acute (24 h) and chronic (4–5 weeks) exposure with micromolar and nanomolar concentrations of sodium arsenite [216,217]. Significant and dose-dependent reductions in Ca^{2+} propagation in wounded cells compared to controls were observed (Figure 7; [216,217]). Arsenic-induced suppression of the wound healing response as a result of both acute and chronic exposures (well below levels typically associated with inhalation where arsenic has been linked with disease presentation) may ultimately result in a reduced ability of the lung epithelium to effectively and sufficiently close a barrier breach [212,216,217].

Figure 7. Wound healing assay of 16HBE14o- cells exposed chronically (4–5 weeks) to 0, 130, or 335 nM sodium-arsenite: (**A**) Representative images of initial wounding (left column), 30 min post-wounding (middle column), and 1 h post-wounding (right column). White scale bar represents 50 μM; (**B**) Quantification of percent wound closure over time at 30 and 60 min post-wounding. "*" indicates significant difference from untreated controls by a one-way ANOVA ($p < 0.05$). Reprinted with permission from Sherwood *et al.* [217].

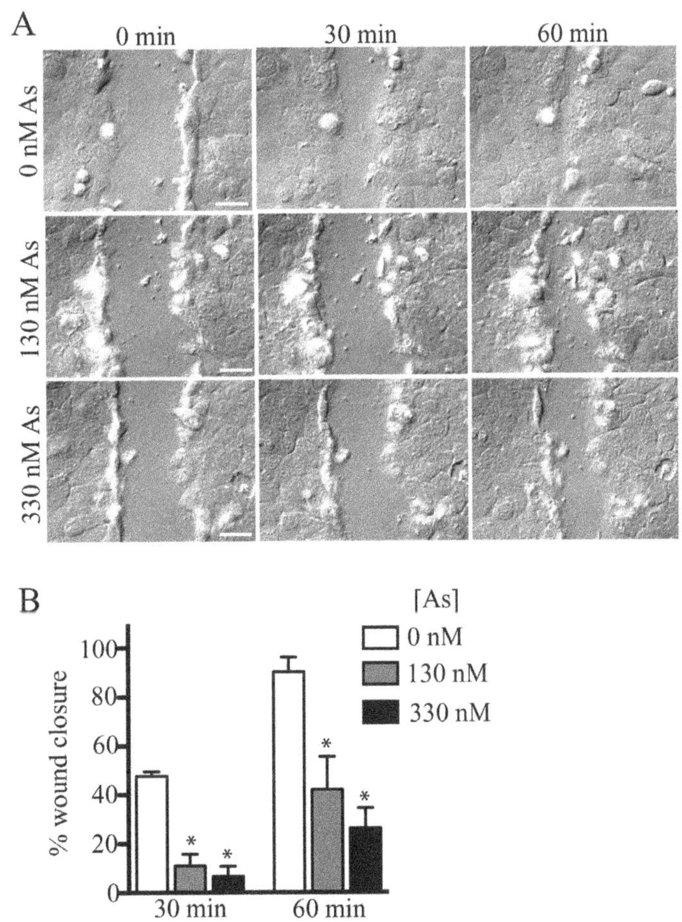

Table 3. Direct effects of arsenic exposure on human bronchial epithelial (HBE), cells, human pulmonary fibroblast (HPF) cells, and pulmonary alveolar macrophage (AM) cells. All experiments were conducted *in vitro*, unless otherwise specified. Specific cell lines are listed in accordance with the abbreviations used in each study.

pound		ne	gical Effects	al Human Effects	
bronchial (or alveolar epithelial) cells					
Na-arsenite	0.5–10 μM for 24 and 120 h	NHBE	Dose-dependent reduction in cell survival; chromosomal aberrations ive of DNA double strand breaks	Lung cancer	[189]
Na-arsenite, MMA^{III}, DMA^{III}	Variable for 3 days	HBE	MMA^{III} & DMA^{III} were more cytotoxic; dose-dependent alteration of inflammatory response at low concentrations; alterations in oxidative stress and DNA damage repair at increasing concentrations	Pulmonary diseases linked with inflammation and increased bronchial cell proliferation	[165]
Na-arsenite	0–4 μM for 2 weeks	HBEp	Concentration-dependent increase in cellular lactate production; lactate d via aerobic glycolysis (the Warburg effect)	Growth, proliferation and n of cancer cells	[201]
As-trioxide	2.5 μM for 6 months	2B *In vivo* (Nu/nu mice) *In silico* Signalling analysis	pendent cell proliferation; cells exhibited a cancer-like phenotype Tumour formation; time-dependent increase in tumour volume; cells exhibited a malignant and metastatic phenotype ROS generation; DNA damage; chronic inflammation; dysregulation of l anti-cancer gene signalling, anti-apoptosis and invasive signalling	Lung cancer	[195]
Na-arsenite	130 and 330 nM for 4–5 weeks and 3.9 for 24 h	16HBE14o-cells ed)	Dose-dependent reduction in the wound healing response (Ca^{2+} signalling), to inhibition of wound repair	Chronic lung disease, nchiectasis	[216,217]
Na-arsenite MMA^{III}, DMA^{III}, ^{V}, DMA^{V}, DMTA^{V}	Various (μM) for 24 h	A549	DMA^{III} and MMA^{III} showed pronounced cellular uptake; differential endpoints related to DNA repair	Arsenic-induced diseases	[187,188]
Na-arsenite	0.25–5 μM for 26 weeks	BEAS-2B	ROS-induced cell proliferation and colony formation; constitutive generation of ROS (probably H_2O_2); degree of effects were ration-dependent	Primary lung tumour formation	[193]
Na-arsenite	20 nM, 200 nM, 2 μM and for 12, 24 and 48 h	BEAS-2B	Enhanced cell growth and proliferation; up-regulation of protein, D1, is commonly over-expressed in cancer cells	Development/progression carcinogenesis	[196]
Arsenite, MMA^{III}, DMA^{III}, DMTA^{V}	Variable concentrations for 24 h	BEAS-2B	Arsenite was least cytotoxic; methylated forms shared similar cytotoxicities; dose-dependent increase in number of differentially expressed genes linked to carcinogenicity; minimally cytotoxic arsenic levels induced oxidative stress	Lung cancer	[168]

Table 3. *Cont.*

As Compound	Dose	Cell Line	Pathological Effects	Potential Human Effects	Ref.
Na-arsenite	30, 60, 290 ppb for 24 h	16HBE14o- (wounded)	Dose-dependent inhibition of the wound healing response	Compromised lung function	[212]
Na-arsenite	5–40 μM for 6–48 h	BEAS-2B	Overexpression of COX-2; apoptotic disruption; cell proliferation	Accumulation of genetically damaged cells leading to malignancy	[197]
Human pulmonary fibroblast cells					
Na-arsenite	0.5–10 μM for 24 and 120 h	HPF	Dose-dependent reduction in cell survival; concentration-dependent increase in chromosome damage such as DNA double strand breaks.	Lung cancer	[189]
As-trioxide	1–50 μM for 24 h	HPF	Dose-dependent reduction in cell survival between 10 and 50 μM As-trioxide		[190]
As-trioxide	1–50 μM for 0–180 h	NHBF	Dose-dependent increase in ROS (O_2^-) levels; cell growth inhibition and cell death		[191]
Alveolar macrophage cells (harvested from animals)					
Na-arsenite	1.25–10 μM for 24–96 h	Mouse AM	Dose-dependent reduction in macrophage viability and volume; time-dependent increase in apoptotic cell at higher arsenic concentrations; decrease in ROS (O_2^-) generation at low concentrations	Immunological disorders; decreased capacity to respond to toxicants	[185]
As-trioxide & Ca-arsenate (slightly soluble)	0.1–300 μg/mL for 24 h	Rat AM	Dose-dependent reduction of ROS (O_2^-) after 24 h; similar pattern for both arsenicals (around 10 μg/mL)	Alteration in AM function; compromised host defence	[128]
Na-arsenite & Na-arsenate (soluble forms)	0.1–300 μg/mL for 24 h	Rat AM	Dose-dependent reduction of ROS (O_2^-) after 24 h; As^{III} more potent than As^{V}; differential immune response between the two species	Compromised defence against infection and altered immune surveillance	[208]
Arsenic (fly ash)	50–230 ppm for 24 h	Rabbit AM	Concentration-dependent inhibition of ROS (H_2O_2 and O_2^-) production	Suppression of AM function	[206]
As-trioxide	0.1–1000 μM for 24 h	Rabbit AM	Concentration-dependent inhibition of ROS (H_2O_2 and O_2^-) production	Increased susceptibility to bacterial infections	[207]
As-trioxide (fly ash)	Industrially-relevant levels for 24 h	Rabbit AM	Suppressed ROS (O_2^-) production	Suppression of AM function	[205]

6. Epidemiological and Exposure Monitoring

Epidemiological studies provide an important link between health effects and air pollution exposure, because they provide an accurate representation of the health records and environmental conditions pertaining to a well-defined population [218]. In this regard epidemiological studies of industrially-exposed cohorts conducted during the mid-1900s have provided strong evidence of a causative role for airborne arsenic in respiratory cancer mortality. This has resulted in a diverse but important body of historical epidemiological evidence accrued on the health risks and disease outcomes associated with known, high level occupational inhalation exposures [219–221].

However, with increasing concerns regarding the effects of peripheral exposure to potential carcinogens, there is increasing attention directed at the health of communities living in the vicinity of smelting and mining operations and uncontained mine wastes and tailings. Notwithstanding the common source of the concerns, it has been observed that there are important differences between the situations of occupationally- and environmentally-exposed cohorts. Occupational studies usually differ methodologically from the environmental investigations in that there is a contained area of contamination and a restricted population who are exposed to high levels of airborne material. Whereas studies of environmental exposure in communities living in arsenic-affected areas usually start at birth, and the exposure itself may not be recognized for many years and may be intermittent, thereby rendering epidemiological studies more difficult to design and interpret, particularly since they are observational only. For these reasons, we report separately on the findings for each exposure type, since they will address different aspects of the effects of airborne particulate matter on health.

6.1. Known Occupational Exposures

An industrial hygiene study conducted between 1943 and 1965 at the Anaconda copper smelter in Montana, USA, recorded extremely high levels of airborne arsenic ($\geq 5000\ \mu g \cdot m^{-3}$), particularly in and around the ore roasting furnace, materials crushing plant and the arsenic refinery departments [222]. Similar conditions were reported at the Ronnskar smelter in Sweden [220]. Airborne arsenic concentrations in excess of 20,000 $\mu g \cdot m^{-3}$ were not uncommon at these two smelting operations [220,222]. Lower values for airborne arsenic were typically found in areas such as the administration departments, electrical and machine workshops, outdoor environment, building department and general office area [220,222]. Significantly, airborne arsenic concentrations reported at the latter two locations are 8- and 2000-fold greater than the current target value of 6 $ng \cdot m^{-3}$ proposed by EU regulations.

Symptoms of severe arsenic exposure among smelter workers observed during the 1920s included a notable rise in the rate of sick days due to various acute and chronic respiratory disorders [223]. Arsenic trioxide-laden dust (generated as a by-product of the copper smelting process) deposited in the nose and respiratory airways forms arsenous acid on contact with moisture, resulting in necrosis of the mucous membranes [223]. Diseases reported among smelter workers during the early 1930s were bronchitis, tracheitis, ulcers, laryngitis, rhinitis, perforation of the nasal septum, atrophy of the mucus membranes in the respiratory passages and occupational arsenical dermatitis (unpublished works by Inghe and Bursell [224], translated in Gerhardsson *et al.* [225]). Emphysema and ischemic heart disease were also noted [219]. Despite the prevalence of these non-malignant respiratory disorders, meta-analysis of the available epidemiological data did not detect any statistically significant excesses in mortality among smelter workers compared to the control cases [219,221].

The first cases of lung cancer that were traced to the work environment occurred at a Swedish smelter in the 1960s whereby a five-fold increase in lung cancer mortality compared with controls was observed [226]. Occupational health investigations at other smelting operations, as well as comprehensive reassessments and meta-analyses of previously reported data, demonstrated strong links between airborne arsenic exposure and respiratory cancer [220–222,227,228]. Lubin *et al.* [221] reported a statistically significant trend between the excess relative risk of respiratory cancer and cumulative exposure to airborne arsenic amongst a cohort of 8014 copper smelter workers in Montana, United States. Over a 50 year period, 446 deaths due to respiratory cancers were observed, comprising 428 lung cancers and 14 cancers of the larynx. No other cause of death was found to be associated with arsenic exposure, with the possible exception of COPD [221].

In addition to smelting, other studies have demonstrated a link between lung cancer and arsenic exposure at hard rock mining operations [228]. One of the most comprehensively investigated cases relates to four tin mines and three associated smelting operations in southern China, where underground miners were exposed to respirable concentrations of arsenic ranging between 0.1 and 38.3 $\mu g \cdot m^{-3}$ [229]. Chen and Chen [229] reported that the rates of lung cancer were strongly associated with cumulative dust exposure, arsenic exposure and duration of exposure. While the magnitude of risk from mining (odds ratio (OR), 8.8) was only slightly less than for smelting (OR, 12.3), exposure to both mining and smelting increased the risk to 22.0 [228]. The potential additive carcinogenic effects of inhaled crystalline silica, cigarette smoking and exposure to radon could not be ruled out [228].

To examine the distribution of arsenic in the body following long-term exposure, researchers collected and analysed tissues from deceased workers from the Ronnskar smelter in Sweden, and from various controls, and correlated these with the cause of death [225]. Post-mortem investigations discovered elevated levels of arsenic and seven other metals of concern in the lung, liver and kidneys of the deceased workers [182,225]. Median arsenic concentrations of 35 and 50 $\mu g \cdot kg^{-1}$ reported in lung tissue of the deceased smelter workers were six to seven times greater than the control cases [182,225], providing some evidence of a causative role for arsenic in respiratory cancer mortality among the exposed population [182]. Although the arsenic content diminished in liver tissue, a longer biological half-life of arsenic was observed in the lung [182]. Similar findings have been reported in animal studies [126]. An extended biological half-life and retention of arsenic in lung tissue may have implications for the development of respiratory disease. Lung cancer risk in a cohort of 107 Chinese tin miners was more dependent on the duration of arsenic exposure than then intensity [228]. Conversely, exposure intensity was more important in determining the lung cancer risk than duration in smelter workers [220,222], indicating a need for comparative studies with consistent exposure and outcome criteria.

Due to the use of exposure reduction measures by mining and mining-related industries, the number of published studies relating to rates of lung cancer and mortality in mining and mining-related industries has declined in recent years. However, occupational inhalation exposure to airborne arsenic remains a serious health issue in some localities. A recent study reported that copper smelter workers in northeastern China were exposed to airborne arsenic values that were up to 57% above the short-term exposure threshold limit value of 20 $\mu g \cdot m^{-3}$ [230]. Seven of the 38 copper smelter workers selected for investigation had arsenic-related skin disorders including hyperkeratosis and/or hyper-pigmentation, as well as elevated urinary arsenic levels [230]. Urinary arsenic speciation analysis revealed that higher occupational exposures and skin damage cases were associated with a decreased capacity for arsenic methylation [230]. Similar results have been reported elsewhere [231]. These findings support the premise that suppressed methylation capacity results in an increased risk of arsenic toxicity due to the retention of arsenic in the body [183].

6.2. Inadvertent Environmental Exposures

It has been found that a number of populations around the world live in the vicinity of active or abandoned mining operations [28], and there exists overwhelming epidemiological evidence suggesting that there is an increased risk of arsenic exposure for these communities [4–9,78,107,232]. These studies show that children are particularly susceptible to inhalation exposure since they respire a greater relative volume of air with respect to their size, and may therefore be exposed to correspondingly higher levels of airborne contaminants than adults. Children also have an increased likelihood of coming into contact with soil and dust through playing in dirt contaminated with arsenic residues [78,233,234]. As a consequence, many human exposure monitoring studies have focussed on measuring arsenic exposure in child populations [4,7,107,233,235,236].

Measurement of arsenic in human nails, hair, urine and blood concentrations are commonly used for determining arsenic uptake in humans [78,105,232,235,236]. Blood and urine arsenic levels provide a reliable short-term measure of arsenic exposure because arsenic is readily excreted from the bloodstream via the kidneys [25]. Analysis of arsenic deposited in the toenails and hair provides useful indicators when the measurement of long-term, low-level arsenic exposure is required [234–238]. It has also been shown that analysis of the arsenic content of particles that have adhered to the hands of children can also be used as an indicator of potential exposure [4].

It is important to note that although such biological markers of arsenic exposure as those reported above are useful for predicting the degree of risk, elucidating the exact pathway to environmental uptake of arsenic in localities where multiple exposure pathways exist is not straightforward [233]. As previously mentioned in this review, airborne arsenic-contaminated particulates generated by mining operations often may be small enough to be inhaled, and have the potential to directly reach the tracheobronchial and/or alveolar regions of the RT of populations living within the reach of the industrial plume or raised dust material [19,54]. However, particles that have been deposited on the ground or other surfaces may be either ingested due to physical contact, or resuspended as dust, and then inhaled [19,105]. Many studies therefore report the existence of multiple possible pathways for human exposure to arsenic-bearing particulates in the vicinity of mining operations which contributes to the complexity of epidemiological studies of this issue [4,7,105,233,238] A recent study reported that the ingestion and inhalation exposure pathways contributed equally to the arsenic-associated carcinogenic and non-carcinogenic risks in such populations [105].

From the work reported in the above investigations, it is clear that human arsenic exposure is governed by a number of variables. There are important inverse relationships which have been frequently reported between the concentration of airborne arsenic levels and the distance from the source, and between biological arsenic levels and the distance of the home, playground or school environment from metal smelters and other mining operations [4,7,107,233]. Buchet *et al.* [4] reported airborne arsenic concentrations of 330 and 75 $ng{\cdot}m^{-3}$, and dust concentrations of 1710 and 66 $\mu g{\cdot}g^{-1}$ at distances of 1 and 2.5 km from a lead smelter in Belgium, which are consistent with this inverse relationship. Correspondingly, the average arsenic concentration on the hands of children living within the 1 km zone was ten times greater than those children living further away [4]. Similarly, Hwang *et al.* [233] found that the urine arsenic content of children living near an extensively contaminated former copper smelter in Montana were significantly inversely correlated with distance from the smelter site.

As cautioned by Frost *et al.* [6], the assumption of a simple inverse relationship between arsenic uptake and distance from the emission source may oversimplify this phenomenon, since seasonality and wind direction are also important variables influencing exposure [9,107,231]. Milham and Strong [107] demonstrated that fluctuations in urine arsenic levels among children living near a copper smelter were closely associated with changes in prevailing wind direction. In this study, the urine arsenic concentrations of children living downwind of the smelter decreased simultaneously with shifts in wind direction [107]. Another study of children living near a former copper smelter site reported elevated biological arsenic levels during the summer, a time when seasonal factors enhance the mobilisation of dust from uncontained mine wastes, such as tailings and flue dust [233].

Carcinogenic and non-carcinogenic risks associated with inhalation exposure to atmospheric arsenic emitted by coal combustion have recently been estimated in exposed Chinese populations [9,105]. Because it has been observed that the average effective diameter of arsenic-containing aerosols from combustion processes is 1 μm [3], there exists a high potential for deposition in the terminal bronchioles and alveoli of exposed populations. Consequently, it has been estimated that more than two million residents in Beijing have an increased risk of developing cancer as a result of probable exposure to atmospheric arsenic, generated principally from coal combustion [9]. Recent measures of daily total inorganic arsenic inhalation exposure values for Beijing residents (0.3–0.8 $\mu g{\cdot}day^{-1}$) showed that they were 10 times greater than those in the United States (40–90 $ng{\cdot}day^{-1}$). These studies indicated that daily intakes of arsenite and arsenate in Beijing were 0.01–0.03 and 0.16–0.44 $\mu g{\cdot}day^{-1}$ by inhalation, respectively. Based on these exposures and the known effects of both arsenite and arsenate as carcinogens, an estimated excess cancer risk of $(4.2 \pm 2.0) \times 10^{-4}$ was predicted for the city's population [9]. In a similar study, Cao *et al.* [105] reported a median carcinogenic risk posed by arsenic inhalation of 2.91×10^{-3} in a community living near the largest coal refinery plant in a town of Shanxi Province, China.

6.3. Impacts of Climate Change

The effects of climate change are predicted to have an impact on mine waste chemistry and mobility. The predicted rise in global temperature is expected to increase the rate of mine waste weathering by a factor of approximately 1.3 by the year 2100 [239]. Prolonged weathering of mine waste materials will lead to the formation of a greater abundance of soluble salts [67]. Moreover, the anticipated increase in extreme weather conditions are likely to lead to a greater frequency and intensity of dust storms, as already observed in localities such as Asia, Africa, and Australia [240,241] which in combination with the weathering, is likely to result in an increase in the occurrence and bioavailability of airborne arsenic.

7. Conclusions and Research Priorities

The potential health effects of exposure to airborne arsenic-bearing particulates generated by current and/or past mining operations are widely recognized as a growing issue of significant global importance. Investigations surveyed in this review, taken from disparate but complimentary lines of inquiry, strongly support a causative role for inhalation exposure of inorganic arsenic species in the aetiology of lung cancer and other respiratory health disorders, suggesting that a strong focus on this exposure modality is crucial for the long-term health of affected populations.

This review has highlighted the need to conclusively elucidate the exact mechanisms of arsenic-induced toxicity from exposure to PM in order to facilitate the prediction and diagnosis of adverse health consequences, and thereby enable adequate risk assessments to be undertaken.

Recent developments in various complimentary areas of research within the overarching field of medical geology including geochemistry, biomedicine, toxicology and epidemiology, have identified a number of factors that play a key role in understanding these varied phenomena. These include: (i) the effects of differing environmental variables leading to exposure; (ii) the influence of particulate characteristics on the initial deposition location in the RT; (iii) the differing toxicity levels of particulate-borne arsenicals, their species and their metabolites, and (iv) the complex pathogenesis of arsenic-induced lung disease.

While it is clear that absorbed arsenic exerts cytotoxic and genotoxic effects on pulmonary cells following both acute and chronic exposures, important species- and dose-dependent differences in toxicities between the two exposure regimes have been observed. It is also clear that particle size plays a major role in governing the deposition location, solubility, methods of clearance and retention time of arsenic-bearing species in the RT, and hence has a direct effect on the range of arsenic metabolites released to the body. Current research indicates that the exposure to arsenic and of these metabolites is predictive of the pathogenesis of lung disease, which leads to the conclusion that the long-term pulmonary bioavailability of arsenic in PM requires serious consideration in health risk assessments. Development of a series of standardized lung bioavailability assays that assess both short- and long-term exposures would be beneficial, particularly when drawing comparisons between studies.

The potential for human exposure to airborne arsenic will inevitably increase in the future due to several key factors. Increases in global copper production and coal use, with which arsenic species are intimately related, are indicators of increasing global wealth and population. With increasing wealth and population, consequent increases in urbanization will inevitably lead to encroachment on and disturbance of existing contaminated sites. In addition, it is predicted that climate change will have a considerable impact on mine waste chemistry and mobility, effectively amplifying every other risk factor, and increasing the urgency in gaining a greater understanding of all aspects of arsenic in our environment.

It is strongly recommended that future research prioritizes identifying human populations and sensitive sub-populations at risk of exposure, as well as developing long-term, cost-effective methods to adequately contain or reduce airborne emissions from known sources.

Acknowledgments

Rachael Martin is supported by an Australian Postgraduate Award Scholarship. Open access publication of this article was funded by the Collaborative Research Network (CRN), Federation University Australia. The views of the authors do not necessarily represent those of the CRN. The authors would like to thank AINSE Ltd for providing financial assistance (Award-PGRA) to enable work on the original research component of this paper.

Author Contributions

All authors contributed substantially to the work presented in this manuscript. As principal researcher, Rachael Martin made a substantial contribution to this work which was undertaken in association with her PhD program. Kim Dowling provided critical analyses and commentary during the development of this manuscript, ensuring that the reviewed literature was accurately interpreted. Dora Pearce provided extensive commentary on the epidemiology and other health-related sections of this manuscript, ensuring that all findings related to health outcomes were accurately represented. With an extensive background in the field of chemistry, James Sillitoe has made substantial contributions to this paper, particularly regarding the technical aspects. Singarayer Florentine assisted with the development of the underpinning theory and conceptual framework for this manuscript, as well as assisting with major re-drafting and editing.

References

1. Mandal, B.K.; Suzuki, K.T. Arsenic round the world: A review. *Talanta* **2002**, *58*, 201–235.
2. International Agency for Research on Cancer (IARC). *IARC Monographs on the Evaluation of the Carcinogenic Risks to Humans, Vol 100 C, Arsenic, Metals, Fibers and Dusts*; IARC: Lyon, France, 2012.
3. Matschullat, J. Arsenic in the geosphere—A review. *Sci. Total Environ.* **2000**, *249*, 297–312.
4. Buchet, J.P.; Roels, H.; Lauwerys, R.; Braux, P.; Claeys-Thoreau, F.; Lafontaine, A.; Verduyn, G. Repeated surveillance of exposure to cadmium, manganese, and arsenic in school-age children living in rural, urban, and nonferrous smelter areas in Belgium. *Environ. Res.* **1980**, *22*, 95–108.
5. Carrizales, L.; Razo, I.; Tellez-Hernandez, J.I.; Torres-Nerio, R.; Torres, A.; Batres, L.E.; Cubillas, A.; Diaz-Barriga, F. Exposure to arsenic and lead of children living near a copper-smelter in San Luis Potosi, Mexico: Importance of soil contamination for exposure of children. *Environ. Res.* **2006**, *101*, 1–10.
6. Frost, F.; Harter, L.; Milham, S.; Royce, R.; Smith, A.H.; Hartley, J.; Enterline, P. Lung cancer among women residing close to an arsenic emitting copper smelter. *Arch. Environ. Health* **1987**, *42*, 148–153.
7. Landrigan, P.J.; Baker, E.L. Exposure of children to heavy metals from smelters: Epidemiology and toxic consequences. *Environ. Res.* **1981**, *25*, 204–224.

8. Newhook, R.; Hirtle, H.; Byrne, K.; Meek, M.E. Releases from copper smelters and refineries and zinc plants in Canada: Human health exposure and risk characterization. *Sci. Total Environ.* **2003**, *301*, 23–41.
9. Yang, G.; Ma, L.; Xu, D.; Li, J.; He, T.; Liu, L.; Jia, H.; Zhang, Y.; Chen, Y.; Chai, Z. Levels and speciation of arsenic in the atmosphere in Beijing, China. *Chemosphere* **2012**, *87*, 845–850.
10. Csavina, J.; Field, J.; Taylor, M.P.; Gao, S.; Landazuri, A.; Betterton, E.A.; Saez, A.E. A review on the importance of metals and metalloids in atmospheric dust and aerosol from mining operations. *Sci. Total Environ.* **2012**, *433*, 58–73.
11. Zota, A.R.; Willis, R.; Jim, R.; Norris, G.A.; Shine, J.P.; Duvall, R.M.; Schaider, L.A.; Spengler, J.D. Impact of mine waste on airborne respirable particulates in northeastern Oklahoma, United States. *J. Air Waste Manag. Assoc.* **2009**, *59*, 1347–1357.
12. Aneja, V.P.; Isherwood, A.; Morgan, P. Characterisation of particulate matter (PM_{10}) related to surface coal mining operations in Appalachia. *Atmos. Environ.* **2012**, *54*, 496–501.
13. Ghose, M.K.; Majee, S.R. Characteristics of hazardous airborne dust around an Indian surface coal mining area. *Environ. Monit. Assess.* **2007**, *130*, 17–25.
14. Soukup, J.M.; Becker, S. Human alveolar macrophage responses to air pollution particulates are associated with insoluble components of coarse material, including particulate endotoxin. *Toxicol. Appl. Pharmacol.* **2001**, *171*, 20–26.
15. Thompson, R.J.; Visser, A.T. Mine Haul Fugitive Dust Emission and Exposure Characterisation. In Proceedings of the 2nd International Conference on the Impact of Environmental Factors on Health, Catania, Sicily, Italy, 17–19 September 2003; pp. 117–141.
16. Ghose, M.K.; Majee, S.R. Assessment of dust generation due to opencast coal mining—An Indian case study. *Environ. Monit. Assess.* **2000**, *61*, 255–263.
17. Castillo, S.; de la Rosa, J.D.; de la Campa, A.M.S.; Gonzalez-Castanedo, Y.; Fernandez-Caliani, J.C.; Gonzalez, I.; Romero, A. Contribution of mine wastes to atmospheric metal deposition in the surrounding area of an abandoned heavily polluted mining district (Rio Tinto mines, Spain). *Sci. Total Environ.* **2013**, *449*, 363–372.
18. Corriveau, M.C.; Jamieson, H.E.; Parsons, M.B.; Campbell, J.L.; Lanzirotti, A. Direct characterization of airborne particles associated with arsenic-rich mine tailings: Particle size, mineralogy and texture. *Appl. Geochem.* **2011**, *26*, 1639–1648.
19. Moreno, T.; Oldroyd, A.; McDonald, I.; Gibbons, W. Preferential fractionation of trace metals-metalloids into PM_{10} resuspended from contaminated gold mine tailings at Rodalquilar, Spain. *Water Air Soil Pollut.* **2007**, *179*, 93–105.
20. Meza-Figueroa, D.; Maier, R.M.; de la O-Villanueva, M.; Gomez-Alvarez, A.; Moreno-Zazueta, A.; Rivera, J.; Campillo, A.; Grandlic, C.J.; Anaya, R.; Palafox-Reyes, J. The impact of unconfined mine tailings in residential areas from a mining town in a semi-arid environment: Nacozari, Sonora, Mexico. *Chemosphere* **2009**, *77*, 140–147.
21. Kim, C.S.; Wilson, K.M.; Rytuba, J.J. Particle-size dependence on metal(loid) distributions in mine wastes: Implications for water contamination and human exposure. *Appl. Geochem.* **2011**, *26*, 484–495.
22. Ragaini, R.C.; Ralston, H.R.; Roberts, N. Environmental trace metal contamination in Kellogg, Idaho, near a lead smelting complex. *Environ. Sci. Technol.* **1977**, *11*, 773–781.

23. Seinfeld, J.H.; Pandis, S.N. *Atmospheric Chemistry and Physics: From Air Pollution to Climate Change*; Wiley: New York, NY, USA, 2006.
24. Rahn, K.A. *The Chemical Composition of the Atmospheric Aerosol*; Technical Report; University of Rhode Island: Kingston, RI, USA, 1976.
25. Agency for Toxic Substances and Disease Registry (ATSDR). Toxicological Profile for Arsenic. Available online: http://www.atsdr.cdc.gov/ToxProfiles/tp.asp?id=22&tid=3 (accessed on 5 July 2013).
26. Lee, D.S.; Garland, J.A.; Fox, A.A. Atmospheric concentrations of trace elements in urban areas of the United Kingdom. *Atmos. Environ.* **1994**, *28*, 2691–2713.
27. Garcia-Aleix, J.R.; Delgado-Saborit, J.M.; Verdu-Martin, G.; Amigo-Descarrega, J.M.; Esteve-Cano, V. Trends in arsenic levels in PM_{10} and $PM_{2.5}$ aerosol fractions in an industrialized area. *Environ. Sci. Pollut. Res.* **2014**, *21*, 695–703.
28. Plumlee, G.S.; Morman, S.A. Mine wastes and human health. *Elements* **2011**, *7*, 399–404.
29. Schaider, L.A.; Senn, D.B.; Brabander, D.J.; McCarthy, K.D.; Shine, J.P. Characterization of zinc, lead, and cadmium in mine waste: Implications for transport, exposure, and bioavailability. *Environ. Sci. Technol.* **2007**, *41*, 4164–4171.
30. Andrade, C.F.; Jamieson, H.E.; Kyser, T.K.; Praharaj, T.; Fortin, D. Biogeochemical redox cycling of arsenic in mine-impacted lake sediments and co-existing pore waters near Giant Mine, Yellowknife Bay, Canada. *Appl. Geochem.* **2010**, *25*, 199–211.
31. Helsen, L. Sampling technologies and air pollution control devices for gaseous and particulate arsenic: A review. *Environ. Pollut.* **2005**, *137*, 305–315.
32. Shibayama, A.; Takasaki, Y.; William, T.; Yamatodani, A.; Higuchi, Y.; Sunagawa, S.; Ono, E. Treatment of smelting residue for arsenic removal and recovery of copper using pyro-hydrometallurgical process. *J. Hazard. Mater.* **2010**, *181*, 1016–1023.
33. Cullen, W.R.; Reimer, K.J. Arsenic speciation in the environment. *Chem. Rev.* **1989**, *89*, 713–764.
34. Wang, S.; Mulligan, C.N. Occurrence of arsenic contamination in Canada: Sources, behavior and distribution. *Sci. Total Environ.* **2006**, *366*, 701–721.
35. Maggs, R. A Review of Arsenic in Ambient Air in the UK. Available online: http://uk-air.defra.gov.uk/reports/empire/arsenic00/arsenic_97v.pdf (accessed on 12 November 2013).
36. Twidwell, L.G.; Mehta, A.K. Disposal of arsenic bearing copper smelter flue dust. *Nucl. Chem. Waste Manag.* **1985**, *5*, 297–303.
37. Rieuwerts, J.; Farago, M. Heavy metal pollution in the vicinity of a secondary lead smelter in the Czech Republic. *Appl. Geochem.* **1996**, *11*, 17–23.
38. Kovacevic, R.; Jovasevic-Stojanovic, M.; Tasic, V.; Milosevic, N.; Petrovic, N.; Stankovic, S.; Matic-Besarabic, S. Preliminary analysis of levels of arsenic and other metallic elements in PM_{10} sampled near copper smelter Bor, (Serbia). *Chem. Ind. Chem. Eng. Q.* **2010**, *16*, 269–279.
39. Montenegro, V.; Sano, H.; Fujisawa, T. Recirculation of high arsenic content copper smelting dust to smelting and converting processes. *Miner. Eng.* **2013**, *49*, 184–189.
40. Finkelman, R.B. Trace elements in coal: Environmental and health significance. *Biol. Trace Elem. Res.* **1999**, *67*, 197–204.
41. Finkelman, R.B.; Gross, P.M.K. The types of data needed for assessing the environmental and human health impacts of coal. *Int. J. Coal Geol.* **1999**, *40*, 91–101.

42. Kang, Y.; Liu, G.; Chou, C.; Wong, M.H.; Zheng, L.; Ding, R. Arsenic in Chinese coals: Distribution, modes of occurrence, and environmental effects. *Sci. Total Environ.* **2011**, *412–413*, 1–13.
43. Sia, S.; Abdullah, W.H. Enrichment of arsenic, lead, and antimony in Balingian coal from Sarawak, Malaysia: Modes of occurrence, origin, and partitioning behaviour during coal combustion. *Int. J. Coal Geol.* **2012**, *101*, 1–14.
44. Huggins, F.E.; Helble, J.J.; Shah, N.; Zhao, J.; Srinivasachar, S.; Morency, J.R.; Lu, F.; Huffman, G.P. Forms of occurrence of arsenic in coal and their behavior during coal combustion. *Abstr. Pap. Am. Chem. Soc.* **1993**, *38*, 265–271.
45. Nelson, P.F.; Shah, P.; Strezov, V.; Halliburton, B.; Carras, J.N. Environmental impacts of coal combustion: A risk approach to assessment of emissions. *Fuel* **2010**, *89*, 810–816.
46. Bolanz, R.M.; Majzlan, J.; Jurkovic, L.; Gottlicher, J. Mineralogy, geochemistry, and arsenic speciation in coal combustion waste from Novaky, Slovakia. *Fuel* **2012**, *94*, 125–136.
47. Furimsky, E. Characterization of trace element emissions from coal combustion by equilibrium calculations. *Fuel Process. Technol.* **2000**, *63*, 29–44.
48. Zhao, Y.; Zhang, J.; Huang, W.; Wang, Z.; Li, Y.; Song, D.; Zhao, F.; Zheng, C. Arsenic emission during combustion of high arsenic coals from Southwestern Guizhou, China. *Energy Convers. Manag.* **2008**, *49*, 615–624.
49. Brownfield, M.E.; Affolter, R.H.; Cathcart, J.D.; O'Connor, J.T.; Brownfield, I.K. Characterization of feed coal and coal combustion products from power plants in Indiana and Kentucky. In Proceedings of the 24th International Technical Conference on Coal Utilization and Fuel Systems, Clearwater, Florida, FL, USA, 8–11 March 1999; pp. 989–1000.
50. Yudovich, Y.E.; Ketris, M.P. Arsenic in coal: A review. *Int. J. Coal Geol.* **2005**, *61*, 141–196.
51. Tian, H.; Wang, Y.; Xue, Z.; Qu, Y.; Chai, F.; Hao, J. Atmospheric emissions estimation of Hg, As, and Se from coal-fired power plants in China, 2007. *Sci. Total Environ.* **2011**, *409*, 3078–3081.
52. Ondov, J.M.; Ragaini, R.C.; Bierman, A.H. Elemental emissions from a coal-fired power plant. Comparison of a venturi wet scrubber system with a cold-side electrostatic precipitator. *Environ. Sci. Technol.* **1979**, *13*, 588–601.
53. Hamilton, E.I. Environmental variables in a holistic evaluation of land contaminated by historic mine wastes: A study of multi-element mine wastes in West Devon, England using arsenic as an element of potential concern to human health. *Sci. Total Environ.* **2000**, *249*, 171–221.
54. Querol, X.; Alastuey, A.; Lopez-Soler, A.; Plana, F. Levels and chemistry of atmospheric particulates induced by a spill of heavy metal mining wastes in the Donana area, Southwest Spain. *Atmos. Environ.* **2000**, *34*, 239–253.
55. Mendez, M.; Armienta, M.A. Arsenic phase distribution in Zimapan mine tailings, Mexico. *Geofis. Int.* **2003**, *42*, 131–140.
56. Smith, E.; Smith, J.; Smith, L.; Biswas, T.; Correll, R.; Naidu, R. Arsenic in Australian environment: An overview. *J. Environ. Sci. Health Part. A* **2003**, *A38*, 223–239.
57. Mullins, M.J.P.; Norman, J.B. Solubility of metals in windblown dust from mine waste dump sites. *Appl. Occup. Environ. Hyg.* **1994**, *9*, 218–223.

58. Northey, S.; Mohr, S.; Mudd, G.M.; Weng, Z.; Giurco, D. Modelling future copper ore grade decline based on a detailed assessment of copper resources and mining. *Resour. Conserv. Recycl.* **2014**, *83*, 190–201.
59. U.S. Energy Information Administration (EIA). *Annual Energy Outlook 2014 with Projections to 2040*; U.S. EIA: Washington, DC, USA, 2014.
60. U.S. Energy Information Administration (EIA). International Energy Outlook 2013. Available online: http://www.eia.gov/forecasts/ieo/more_highlights.cfm (accessed on 18 August 2013)
61. Pandey, V.C.; Singh, J.S.; Singh, R.P.; Singh, N.; Yunus, M. Arsenic hazards in coal fly ash and its fate in Indian scenario. *Resour. Conserv. Recycl.* **2011**, *55*, 819–835.
62. European Commission. Abandoned Mines Can Be Used as Geothermal Energy Source. Available online: http://ec.europa.eu/environment/integration/research/newsalert/pdf/230na6.pdf (accessed on 18 December 2013).
63. Bureau of Land Management, U.S. Department of the Interior. Abandoned Mine Lands. Available online: http://www.blm.gov/wo/st/en/prog/more/Abandoned_Mine_Lands.html (accessed on 17 May 2013).
64. Ministerial Council on Mineral and Petroleum Resources/Minerals Council of Australia. Strategic Framework for Managing Abandoned Mines in the Minerals Industry. Available online: http://www.industry.gov.au/resource/Mining/Documents/StrategicFrameworkforManagingAbandonedMines.pdf (accessed on 2 February 2014).
65. Unger, C.; Lechner, A.; Glenn, V.; Edraki, M.; Mulligan, D.R. Mapping and prioritising rehabilitation of abandoned mines in Australia. In Proceedings of the 2012 Life-of-Mine Conference, Brisbane, Australia, 10–12 July 2012.
66. Gonzalez, R.C.; Gonzalez-Chavez, M.C.A. Metal accumulation in wild plants surrounding mining wastes. *Environ. Pollut.* **2006**, *144*, 84–92.
67. Lottermoser, B.G. *Mine Wastes: Characterisation, Treatment and Environmental Impacts*; Springer: New York, NY, USA, 2010.
68. Liao, B.; Huang, L.N.; Ye, Z.H.; Lan, C.Y.; Shu, W.S. Cut-off net acid generation pH in predicting acid-forming potential in mine spoils. *J. Environ. Qual.* **2007**, *36*, 887–891.
69. European Commission. Air Quality Standards. Available online: http://ec.europa.eu/environment/air/quality/ standards.htm (accessed on 3 June 2014).
70. World Health Organisation. *Air Quality Guidelines for Europe*, 2nd ed.; WHO Regional Publications: Geneva, Switzerland, 2000.
71. Vincent, J.H. *Aerosol Sampling: Science, Standards, Instrumentations and Applications*; Wiley: Chichester, UK, 2007.
72. Newman, L.S. Clinical pulmonary toxicology. In *Clinical Environmental Health and Exposures*, 2nd ed.; Sullivan, J.B., Krieger, G., Eds.; Lippincott Wiliams and Wilkins: Philadelphia, PA, USA, 2001; pp. 206–233.
73. United States Environmental Protection Agency. Locating and Estimating Air (L&E) Documents, EPA Document Number 454/r-98–013. Available online: http://www.epa.gov/ttnchie1/le/ (accessed on 10 November 2013).

74. De la Campa, A.M.S.; de la Rosa, J.D.; Sanchez-Rodas, D.; Oliveira, V.; Alastuey, A.; Querol, X.; Gomez-Ariza, J.L. Arsenic speciation study of PM2.5 in an urban area near a copper smelter. *Atmos. Environ.* **2008**, *42*, 6487–6495.
75. Sanchez-Rodas, D.; Sanchez de la Campa, A.M.; de la Rosa, J.D.; Oliveira, V.; Gomez-Ariza, J.L.; Querol, X.; Alastuey, A. Arsenic speciation of atmospheric particulate matter (PM10) in an industrialised urban site in southwestern Spain. *Chemosphere* **2007**, *66*, 1485–1493.
76. Tsopelas, F.; Tsakanika, L.; Ochsenkuhn-Petropoulou, M. Extraction of arsenic species from airborne particulate filters-application to an industrial area of Greece. *Microchem. J.* **2008**, *89*, 165–170.
77. Fernandez-Camacho, R.; de la Rosa, J.; de la Campa, A.M.S.; Gonzalez-Castanedo, Y.; Alastuey, A.; Querol, X.; Rodriguez, S. Geochemical characterization of Cu-smelter emission plumes with impact in an urban area of SW Spain. *Atmos. Res.* **2010**, *96*, 590–601.
78. Polissar, L.; Lowry-Coble, K.; Kalman, D.A.; Hughes, J.P.; van Belle, G.; Covert, D.S.; Burbacher, T.M.; Bolgiano, D.; Mottet, N.K. Pathways of human exposure to arsenic in a community surrounding a copper smelter. *Environ. Res.* **1990**, *53*, 29–47.
79. European Commission (EC). Ambient Air Pollution by As, Cd and Ni Compounds. Position Paper. Available online: http://www.itm.su.se/reflabmatningar/dokument/as_cd_ni_position_paper.pdf (accessed on 10 July 2013).
80. Johnson, B.D.; Myers, J.E. Preliminary validation of modelled environmental PM_{10} Arsenic Trioxide (As2O3) dust fallout from a copper smelter in Namibia. In Proceedings of the 4th International Congress on Arsenic in the Environment, Cairns, Australia, 22–27 July 2012; pp. 431–432.
81. Serbula, S.M.; Antonijevic, M.M.; Milosevic, N.M.; Milic, S.M.; Ilic, A.A. Concentrations of particulate matter and arsenic in Bor (Serbia). *J. Hazard. Mater.* **2010**, *181*, 43–51.
82. Chen, B.; Stein, A.F.; Castell, N.; de la Rosa, J.D.; de la Campa, A.M.S.; Gonzalez-Castanedo, Y.; Draxler, R.R. Modeling and surface observations of arsenic dispersion from a large Cu-smelter in southwestern Europe. *Atmos. Environ.* **2012**, *49*, 114–122.
83. Oliveira, V.; Gomez-Ariza, J.L.; Sanchez-Rodas, D. Extraction procedures for chemical speciation of arsenic in atmospheric total suspended particles. *Anal. Bioanal. Chem.* **2005**, *382*, 335–340.
84. Duan, J.; Tan, J. Atmospheric heavy metals and arsenic in China: Situation, sources and control policies. *Atmos. Environ.* **2013**, *74*, 93–101.
85. Greenpeace. Detecting the Heavy Metal Concentration of PM2.5 in Beijing. Available online: http://www.greenpeace.org/eastasia/Global/eastasia/publications (accessed on 3 March 2014).
86. Okuda, T.; Katsuno, M.; Naoi, D.; Nakao, S.; Shigeru, T.; He, K.; Ma, Y.; Lei, Y.; Jia, Y. Trends in hazardous trace metal concentrations in aerosols collected in Beijing, China from 2001 to 2006. *Chemosphere* **2008**, *72*, 917–924.
87. Xie, R.; Seip, H.M.; Wibetoe, G.; Nori, S.; McLeod, C.W. Heavy coal combustion as the dominant source of particulate pollution in Taiyuan, China, corroborated by high concentrations of arsenic and selenium in PM10. *Sci. Total Environ.* **2006**, *370*, 409–415.

88. Zhou, S.; Yuan, Q.; Li, W.; Lu, Y.; Zhang, Y.; Wang, W. Trace metals in atmospheric fine particles in one industrial urban city: Spatial variations, sources, and health implications. *J. Environ. Sci.* **2014**, *26*, 205–213.
89. Kribek, B.; Majer, V.; Pasava, J.; Kamona, F.; Mapani, B.; Keder, J.; Ettler, V. Contamination of soils with dust fallout from the tailings dam at the Rosh Pinah area, Namibia: Regional assessment, dust dispersion modeling and environmental consequences. *J. Geochem. Explor.* **2014**, doi:10.1016/j.gexplo.2014.01.010.
90. Protonotarios, V.; Petsas, N.; Moutsatsou, A. Levels and composition of atmospheric particulates (PM10) in a mining-industrial site in the city of Lavrion, Greece. *J. Air Waste Manag. Assoc.* **2002**, *52*, 1263–1273.
91. Jain, C.K.; Ali, I. Arsenic: Occurrence, toxicity and speciation techniques. *Water Res.* **2000**, *34*, 4304–4312.
92. Ferguson, J.F.; Gavis, J. A review of the arsenic cycle in natural waters. *Water Res.* **1972**, *6*, 1259–1274.
93. Akter, K.; Naidu, R. Arsenic speciation in the environment. In *Managing Arsenic in the Environment: From Soil to Human Health*; Naidu, R., Smith, E., Owens, G., Bhattacharya, P., Nadebaum, P., Eds.; CSIRO Publishing: Collingwood, VT, Australia, 2006; pp. 61–74.
94. Jamieson, H.E.; Walker, S.R.; Andrade, C.F.; Wrye, L.A.; Rasmussen, P.E.; Lanzirotti, A.; Parsons, M.B. Identification and characterization of arsenic and metal compounds in contaminated soil, mine tailings, and house dust using synchrotron-based microanalysis. *Hum. Ecol. Risk Assess.* **2011**, *17*, 1292–1309.
95. Walker, S.R.; Jamieson, H.E. The speciation of arsenic in iron oxides in mine wastes from the giant gold mine, N.W.T. Applications of synchrotron micro-XRD and micro-XANES at the grain scale. *Can. Mineral.* **2005**, *43*, 1205–1224.
96. Cherry, J.A.; Shaikh, A.U.; Tallman, D.E.; Nicholson, R.V. Arsenic species as an indicator of redox conditions in groundwater. *J. Hydrol.* **1979**, *43*, 373–392.
97. Meharg, A. Arsenic in rice—Understanding a new disaster for southeast Asia. *Trends Plant Sci.* **2004**, *9*, 415–417.
98. Korte, N.E.; Fernando, Q. A review of arsenic (III) in groundwater. *Crit. Rev. Environ. Control* **1991**, *21*, 1–39.
99. Garcia-Manyes, S.; Jimenez, G.; Padro, A.; Rubio, R.; Rauret, G. Arsenic speciation in contaminated soils. *Talanta* **2002**, *58*, 97–109.
100. Shuvaeva, O.V.; Bortnikova, S.B.; Korda, T.M.; Lazareva, E.V. Arsenic speciation in a contaminated gold processing tailings dam. *Geostand. Newsl.* **2000**, *24*, 247–252.
101. Eatough, D.J.; Christensen, J.J.; Eatough, N.L.; Hill, M.W.; Major, T.D.; Mangelson, N.F.; Post, M.E.; Ryder, J.F.; Hansen, L.D.; Meisenheimer, R.G.; *et al.* Sulfur chemistry in a copper smelter plume. *Atmos. Environ.* **1982**, *16*, 1001–1015.
102. Hedberg, E.; Gidhagen, L.; Johansson, C. Source contributions to PM10 and arsenic concentrations in Central Chile using positive matrix factorization. *Atmos. Environ.* **2005**, *39*, 549–561.

103. Alleman, L.Y.; Lamaison, L.; Perdrix, E.; Robache, A.; Galloo, J. PM10 metal concentrations and source identification using positive matrix factorization and wind sectoring in a French industrial zone. *Atmos. Res.* **2010**, *96*, 612–625.
104. Hrebenyk, B.W.; Iravani, A. *Air Quality Monitoring at Giant Mine Site—Yellowknife, A Baseline Study*; Report for the Indian and Northern Affairs Canada, Giant Mine Remediation Project; SENES Consultants Ltd: Ontario, USA, 2007.
105. Cao, S.; Duan, X.; Zhao, X.; Ma, J.; Dong, T.; Huang, N.; Sun, C.; He, B.; Wei, F. Health risks from the exposure of children to As, Se, Pb and other heavy metals near the largest coking plant in China. *Sci. Total Environ.* **2014**, *472*, 1001–1009.
106. Huang, M.; Chen, X.; Shao, D.; Zhao, Y.; Wang, W.; Wong, M.H. Risk assessment of arsenic and other metals via atmospheric particles, and effects of atmospheric exposure and other demographic factors on their accumulations in human scalp hair in urban area of Guangzhou, China. *Ecotoxicol. Environ. Saf.* **2014**, *102*, 84–92.
107. Milham, S.; Strong, T. Human arsenic exposure in relation to a copper smelter. *Environ. Res.* **1974**, *7*, 176–182.
108. United States Environmental Protection Agency. Questions About Your Community: Indoor Air. Available online: http://www.epa.gov/region1/communities/indoorair.html (accessed on 5 January 2014).
109. Davies, C.N. Inhalation risk and particle size in dust and mist. *Brit. J. Ind. Med.* **1949**, *6*, 245–253.
110. Hofmann, W. Modelling inhaled particle deposition in the human lung-A review. *J. Aerosol Sci.* **2011**, *42*, 693–724.
111. Lippman, M.; Yeates, D.B.; Albert, R.E. Deposition, retention, and clearance of inhaled particles. *Br. J. Ind. Med.* **1980**, *37*, 337–362.
112. Bailey, M.R. The new ICRP model for the respiratory tract. *Radiat. Prot. Dosim.* **1994**, *53*, 107–114.
113. Labiris, N.R.; Dolovich, M.B. Pulmonary drug delivery. Part I: Physiological factors affecting therapeutic effectiveness of aerosolized medications. *J. Clin. Pharmacol.* **2003**, *56*, 588–599.
114. Nicod, L.P. Lung defences: An overview. *Eur. Respir. J.* **2005**, *14*, 45–50.
115. Taylor, D.M. Human respiratory tract model for radiological protection. *J. Radiol. Prot.* **1996**, *16*, doi:10.1088/0952-4746/16/1/013.
116. World Health Organization (WHO). *Hazard Prevention and Control in the Work Environment: Airborne Dust*; Occupatonal and Environmental Health Department of Protection of the Human Environment, WHO: Geneva, Switzerland, 1999.
117. Smith, J.R.H.; Etherington, G.; Shutt, A.L.; Youngman, M.J. A study of aerosol deposition and clearance from the human nasal passage. *Ann. Occup. Hyg.* **2002**, *46*, 309–313.
118. Asgharian, B.; Hofmann, W.; Miller, F.J. Mucociliary clearance of insoluble particles from the tracheobronchial airways of the human lung. *Aerosol Sci.* **2001**, *32*, 817–832.
119. Kirch, J.; Guenther, M.; Doshi, N.; Schaefer, U.F.; Schneider, M.; Mitragotri, S.; Lehr, C.M. Mucociliary clearance of micro- and nanoparticles is independent of size, shape and charge—An *ex vivo* and in silico approach. *J. Controll. Release* **2012**, *159*, 128–134.
120. Wang, C. *Inhaled particles*; Elsevier Academic Press: New York, NY, USA, 2005.
121. Folkesson, H.G.; Matthay, M.A.; Westrom, B.R.; Kim, K.J.; Karlsson, B.W.; Hastings, R.H. Alveolar epithelial clearance of protein. *J. Appl. Physiol.* **1996**, *80*, 1431–1445.

122. Martonen, T.B. Mathematical model for the selective deposition of inhaled pharmaceuticals. *J. Pharm. Sci.* **1993**, *82*, 1191–1199.
123. Hakim, J. Reactive oxygen species and inflammation. *C R Seances Soc. Biol. Fil* **1993**, *187*, 286–295.
124. Hofmann, W.; Asgharian, B. The effect of lung structure on mucociliary clearance and particle retention in human and rat lungs. *Toxicol. Sci.* **2003**, *73*, 448–456.
125. Rhoads, K.; Sanders, C.L. Lung clearance, translocation, and acute toxicity of arsenic, beryllium, cadmium, cobalt, lead, selenium, vanadium, and ytterbium oxides following deposition in rat lung. *Environ. Res.* **1985**, *36*, 359–378.
126. Marafante, E.; Vahter, M. Solubility, retention, and metabolism of intratracheally and orally administered inorganic arsenic compounds in the hamster. *Environ. Res.* **1987**, *42*, 72–82.
127. Edsbacker, S.; Wollmer, P.; Selroos, O.; Borgstrom, L.; Olsson, B.; Ingelf, J. Do airway clearance mechanisms influence the local and systemic effects of inhaled corticosteroids? *Pulm. Pharmacol. Ther.* **2008**, *21*, 247–258.
128. Lantz, R.C.; Parliman, G.; Chen, G.J.; Barber, B.; Winski, S.; Carter, D.E. Effect of arsenic exposure on alveolar macrophage function. II. Effect of slightly soluble forms of As(III) and As(V). *Environ. Res.* **1995**, *68*, 59–67.
129. Pershagen, G.; Lind, B.; Bjorklund, N. Lung retention and toxicity of some inorganic arsenic compounds. *Environ. Res.* **1982**, *29*, 425–434.
130. Takeo, I.; Akira, H.; Noburu, I. Comparison of arsenic trioxide and calcium arsenate retention in the rat lung after intratracheal instillation. *Toxicol. Lett.* **1982**, *12*, 1–5.
131. O'Bryant, S.E.; Edwards, M.; Menon, C.V.; Gong, G.; Barber, R. Long-term low-level arsenic exposure is associated with poorer neuropsychological functioning: A project FRONTIER study. *Int. J. Environ. Res. Public Health* **2011**, *8*, 861–874.
132. Zhang, C.; Mao, G.; He, S.; Yang, Z.; Yang, W.; Zhang, X.; Qiu, W.; Ta, N.; Cao, L.; Yang, H.; *et al.* Relationship between long-term exposure to low-level arsenic in drinking water and the prevalence of abnormal blood pressure. *J. Hazard. Mater.* **2013**, *262*, 1154–1158.
133. Caussy, D. Case studies of the impact of understanding bioavailability: Arsenic. *Ecotoxicol. Environ. Saf.* **2003**, *56*, 164–173.
134. Naidu, R.; Bolan, N.S.; Megharaj, M.; Juhasz, A.L.; Gupta, S.; Clothier, B.; Schulin, R. Bioavailability, definition, assessment and implications for risk assessment. In *Chemical Bioavailability in Terrestrial Environment*; Elsevier: Amsterdam, The Netherland, 2008; pp. 1–8.
135. Ng, J.C.; Juhasz, A.L.; Smith, E.; Naidu, R. *Contaminant Bioavailability and Bioaccessibility. Part. 2: Guidance for Industry*; Report for the Cooperative Research Centre for Contamination Assessment and Remediation of the Environment (CRC CARE), Technical Report series no. 14; CRC CARE: Salisbury South, Australia, 2009.
136. Broadway, A.; Cave, M.R.; Wragg, J.; Fordyce, F.M.; Bewley, R.J.F.; Graham, M.C.; Ngwenya, B.T.; Farmer, J.G. Determination of the bioaccessibility of chromium in Glasgow soil and the implications for human health risk assessment. *Sci. Total Environ.* **2010**, *409*, 267–277.
137. Colombo, C.; Monhemius, A.J.; Plant, J.A. Platinum, palladium and rhodium release from vehicle exhaust catalysts and road dust exposed to simulated lung fluids. *Ecotoxicol. Environ. Saf.* **2008**, *71*, 722–730.

138. Hedberg, Y.; Gustafsson, J.; Karlsson, H.L.; Moller, L.; Wallinder, I.O. Bioaccessibility, bioavailability and toxicity of commercially relevant iron- and chromium-based particles: *In vitro* studies with an inhalation perspective. *Part. Fibre Toxicol.* **2010**, *7*, 1–14.
139. Herting, G.; Wallinder, I.O.; Leygraf, C. Metal release from various grades of stainless steel exposed to synthetic body fluids. *Corros. Sci.* **2007**, *49*, 103–111.
140. Plumlee, G.S.; Ziegler, T.L. The medical geochemistry of dusts, soils and other earth materials. In *Environmental Geochemistry: Treatise of Geochemistry*; Lollar, B.S., Holland, H.D., Turekian, K.K., Eds.; Elsevier Ltd: Oxford, UK, 2003; Volume 9, pp. 263–310.
141. Marques, M.R.C.; Loebenberg, R.; Almukainzi, M. Simulated biological fluids with possible application in dissolution testing. *Dissolution Technol.* **2011**, *18*, 15–28.
142. Plumlee, G.S.; Morman, S.A.; Ziegler, T.L. The toxocological geochemistry of earth materials: An overview of processes and the interdisciplinary methods used to understsand them. *Rev. Mineral. Geochem.* **2006**, *64*, 5–57.
143. Wolf, R.E.; Morman, S.A.; Hageman, P.L.; Hoefen, T.M.; Plumlee, G.S. Simultaneous speciation of arsenic, selenium, and chromium: Species stability, sample preservation, and analysis of ash and soil leachates. *Anal. Bioanal. Chem.* **2011**, *401*, 2733–2745.
144. Kitchin, K.T. Recent advances in arsenic carcinogenesis: Modes of action, animal model systems, and methylated arsenic metabolites. *Toxicol. Appl. Pharmacol.* **2001**, *172*, 249–261.
145. Vahter, M.; Concha, G. Role of metabolism in arsenic toxicity. *Pharmacol. Toxicol.* **2001**, *89*, 1–5.
146. Vahter, M. Mechanisms of arsenic biotransformation. *Toxicology* **2002**, *181–182*, 211–217.
147. Roy, P.; Saha, A. Metabolism and toxicity of arsenic: A human carcinogen. *Curr. Sci.* **2002**, *82*, 38–45.
148. Thomas, D.J. Molecular processes in cellular arsenic metabolism. *Toxicol. Appl. Pharmacol.* **2007**, *222*, 365–373.
149. Styblo, M.; Drobna, Z.; Jaspers, I.L.S.; Thomas, D.J. The role of biomethylation in toxicity and carcinogenicity of arsenic: A research update. *Environ. Health Perspect.* **2002**, *110*, 767–771.
150. Brima, E.I.; Haris, P.I.; Jenkins, R.O.; Polya, D.A.; Gault, A.G.; Harrington, C.F. Understanding arsenic metabolism through a comparative study of arsenic levels in the urine, hair and fingernails of healthy volunteers from three unexposed ethnic groups in the United Kingdom. *Toxicol. Appl. Pharmacol.* **2006**, *216*, 122–130.
151. Gebel, T.W. Arsenic methylation is a process of detoxification through accelerated excretion. *Int. J. Hyg. Environ. Health* **2002**, *205*, 505–508.
152. Styblo, M.; Del Razo, L.M.; Vega, L.; Germolec, D.R.; LeCluyse, E.L.; Hamilton, G.A.; Reed, W.; Wang, C.; Cullen, W.R.; Thomas, D.J. Comparative toxicity of trivalent and pentavalent inorganic and methylated arsenicals in rat and human cells. *Arch. Toxicol.* **2000**, *74*, 289–299.
153. Thomas, D.J.; Waters, S.B.; Styblo, M. Elucidating the pathway for arsenic methylation. *Toxicol. Appl. Pharmacol.* **2004**, *198*, 319–326.
154. Rossman, T. Arsenic. In *Environmental and Occupational Medicine*; Rom, W., Markowitz, S., Eds.; Lippincott Williams and Wilkins: Hagerstown, MD, USA, 2007; pp. 1006–1017.

155. Aposhian, H.V.; Zheng, B.; Aposhian, M.M.; Le, X.C.; Cebrian, M.E.; Cullen, W.; Zakharyan, R.A.; Ma, M.; Dart, R.C.; Cheng, Z.; *et al.* DMPS-Arsenic challenge test. II. Modulation of arsenic species, including monomethylarsonous acid (MMAIII), excreted in human urine. *Toxicol. Appl. Pharmacol.* **2000**, *165*, 74–83.
156. Buchet, J.P.; Lauwerys, R.; Roels, H. Comparison of the urinary excretion of arsenic metabolites after a single oral dose of sodium arsenite, monomethylarsonate, or dimethylarsinate in man. *Int. Arch. Occup. Environ. Health* **1981**, *48*, 71–79.
157. Raml, R.; Rumpler, A.; Goessler, W.; Vahter, M.; Li, L.; Ochi, T.; Francesconi, K.A. Thio-dimethylarsinate is a common metabolite in urine samples from arsenic-exposed women in Bangladesh. *Toxicol. Appl. Pharmacol.* **2007**, *222*, 374–380.
158. Flora, S.J.S. Arsenic-induced oxidative stress and its reversibility. *Free Radic. Biol. Med.* **2011**, *51*, 257–281.
159. Kenyon, E.M.; Del Razo, L.M.; Hughes, M.F. Tissue distribution and urinary excretion of inorganic arsenic and its methylated metabolites in mice following acute oral administration of arsenate. *Toxicol. Sci.* **2005**, *85*, 468–475.
160. Naranmandura, H.; Bu, N.; Suzuki, K.T.; Lou, Y.; Ogra, Y. Distribution and speciation of arsenic after intravenous administration of monomethylmonothioarsonic acid in rats. *Chemosphere* **2010**, *81*, 206–213.
161. Ratnaike, R.N. Acute and chronic arsenic toxicity. *Postgrad. Med. J.* **2003**, *79*, 391–396.
162. Aposhian, H.V.; Zakharyan, R.A.; Avram, M.D.; Sampayo-Reyes, A.; Wollenberg, M.L. A review of the enzymology of arsenic metabolism and a new potential role of hydrogen peroxide in the detoxication of the trivalent arsenic species. *Toxicol. Appl. Pharmacol.* **2004**, *198*, 327–335.
163. Carter, D.E.; Peraza, M.A.; Ayala-Fierro, F.; Casarez, E.; Barber, D.S.; Winski, S.L. Arsenic metabolism after pulmonary exposure. In Proceedings of the Third International Conference on Arsenic Exposure and Health Effects, San Diego, CA, USA, 12–15 July 1998; pp. 299–309.
164. Cohen, S.M.; Arnold, L.L.; Eldan, M.; Lewis, A.S.; Beck, B.D. Methylated arsenicals: The implications of metabolism and carcinogenicity studies in rodents to human risk assessment. *Crit. Rev. Toxicol.* **2006**, *36*, 99–133.
165. Dodmane, P.R.; Arnold, L.L.; Kakiuchi-Kiyota, S.; Qiu, F.; Liu, X.; Rennard, S.I.; Cohen, S.M. Cytotoxicity and gene expression changes induced by inorganic and organic trivalent arsenicals in human cells. *Toxicology* **2013**, *312*, 18–29.
166. Tseng, C. A review on environmental factors regulating arsenic methylation in humans. *Toxicol. Appl. Pharmacol.* **2009**, *235*, 338–350.
167. Abernathy, C.O.; Thomas, D.J.; Calderon, R.L. Health effects and risk assessment of arsenic. *J. Nutr.* **2003**, 1536–1538.
168. Chilakapati, J.; Wallace, K.; Ren, H.; Fricke, M.; Bailey, K.; Ward, W.; Creed, J.; Kitchin, K. Genome-wide analysis of BEAS-2B cells exposed to trivalent arsenicals and dimethylthioarsinic acid. *Toxicology* **2010**, *268*, 31–39.
169. An, Y.; Kato, K.; Nakano, M.; Otsu, H.; Okada, S.; Yamanaka, K. Specific induction of oxidative stress in terminal bronchiolar Clara cells during dimethylarsenic-induced lung tumor promoting process in mice. *Cancer Lett.* **2005**, *230*, 57–64.

170. Yamanaka, K.; Okada, S. Induction of lung-specific DNA damage by metabolically methylated arsenics via the production of free radicals. *Environ. Health Perspect.* **1994**, *102*, 37–40.
171. Yamanaka, K.; Kato, K.; Mizoi, M.; An, Y.; Nakanao, M.; Hoshino, M.; Okada, S. Dimethylarsine likely acts as a mouse-pulmonary tumor initiator via the production of dimethylarsine radical and/or its peroxy radical. *Life Sci.* **2009**, *84*, 627–633.
172. Halliwell, B. Biochemistry of oxidative stress. *Biochem. Soc. Trans.* **2007**, *35*, 1147–1150.
173. Betteridge, D.J. What is oxidative stress. *Metabolism* **2000**, *49*, 3–8.
174. Andrewes, P.; Kitchin, K.T.; Wallace, K. Dimethylarsine and trimethylarsine are potent genotoxins *in vitro*. *Chem. Res. Toxicol.* **2003**, *16*, 994–1003.
175. Kitchin, K.T.; Ahmad, S. Oxidative stress as a possible mode of action for arsenic carcinogenesis. *Toxicol. Lett.* **2003**, *137*, 3–13.
176. Burdon, R.H. Superoxide and hydrogen peroxide in relation to mammalian cell proliferation. *Free Radic. Biol. Med.* **1995**, *18*, 775–794.
177. Yamanaka, K.; Kato, K.; Mizoi, M.; An, Y.; Takabayashi, F.; Nakano, M.; Hoshino, M.; Okada, S. The role of active arsenic species produced by metabolic reduction of dimethylarsinic acid in genotoxicity and tumorigenesis. *Toxicol. Appl. Pharmacol.* **2004**, *198*, 385–393.
178. Dopp, E.; von Recklinghausen, U.; Diaz-Bone, R.; Hirner, A.V.; Rettenmeier, A.W. Cellular uptake, subcellular distribution and toxicity of arsenic compounds in methylating and non-methylating cells. *Environ. Res.* **2010**, *110*, 435–442.
179. Flora, S.J.S. Arsenic induced oxidative stress and the role of antioxidant supplementation during chelation: A review. *J. Environ. Biol.* **2007**, *28*, 333–347.
180. Tchounwou, P.B.; Centeno, J.A.; Patlolla, A.K. Arsenic toxicity, mutagenesis, and carcinogenesis—A health risk assessment and management approach. *Mol. Cell Biochem.* **2004**, *255*, 47–55.
181. Smith, A.H.; Ercumen, A.; Yuan, Y.; Steinmaus, C.M. Increased lung cancer risks are similar whether arsenic is ingested or inhaled. *J. Exposure Sci. Environ. Epidemiol.* **2009**, *19*, 343–348.
182. Wester, P.O.; Brune, D.; Nordberg, G. Arsenic and selenium in lung, liver, and kidney tissue from dead smelter workers. *Br. J. Ind. Med.* **1981**, *38*, 179–184.
183. Hall, M.N.; Gamble, M.V. Nutritional manipulation of one-carbon metabolisms: Effects on arsenic methylation and toxicity. *J. Toxicol.* **2012**, *2012*, 1–11.
184. Bhattacharjee, P.; Chatterjee, D.; Singh, K.K.; Giri, A. Systems biology approaches to evaluate arsenic toxicity and carcinogenicity: An overview. *Int. J. Hyg. Environ. Health* **2013**, *216*, 574–586.
185. Palmieri, M.A.; Tasat, D.R.; Molinari, B.L. Oxidative metabolism of lung macrophages exposed to sodium arsenite. *Toxicol. In Vitro* **2007**, *21*, 1603–1609.
186. Sappino, A.P.; Schurch, W.; Gabbiani, G. Differentiation repertoire of fibroblastic cells: Expression of cytoskeletal proteins as marker of phenotypic modulations. *Lab. Invest.* **1990**, *63*, 144–161.
187. Bartel, M.; Ebert, F.; Leffers, L.; Karst, U.; Schwerdtle, T. Toxicological characterization of the inorganic and organic arsenic metabolite thio-DMAV in cultured human lung cells. *J. Toxicol.* **2011**, *2011*, 1–9.

188. Ebert, F.; Weiss, A.; Bultemeyer, M.; Hamann, I.; Hartwig, A.; Schwerdtle, T. Arsenicals affect base excision repair by several mechanisms. *Mutat. Res. Fundam. Mol. Mech. Mutagen.* **2011**, *715*, 32–41.
189. Xie, H.; Huang, S.; Martin, S.; Wise, J.P., Sr. Arsenic is cytotoxic and genotoxic to primary human lung cells. *Mutat. Res. Genet. Toxicol. Environ. Mutagen.* **2014**, *760*, 33–41.
190. Park, W.H.; Kim, S.H. Arsenic trioxide induces human pulmonary fibroblast cell death via the regulation of Bcl-2 family and caspase-8. *Mol. Biol. Rep.* **2012**, *39*, 4311–4318.
191. You, B.R.; Park, W.H. Arsenic trioxide induces human pulmonary fibroblast cell death via increasing ROS levels and GSH depletion. *Oncol. Rep.* **2012**, *28*, 749–757.
192. Acharya, A.; Das, I.; Chandhok, D.; Saha, T. Redox regulation in cancer: A double-edged sword with therapeutic potential. *Oxid. Med. Cell Longev.* **2010**, *3*, 23–34.
193. Carpenter, R.L.; Jiang, Y.; Jing, Y.; He, J.; Rojanasakul, Y.; Liu, L.; Jiang, B. Arsenite induces cell transformation by reactive oxygen species, AKT, ERK1/2, and P70s6K1. *Biochem. Biophys. Res. Commun.* **2011**, *414*, 533–538.
194. Chowdhury, R.; Chatterjee, R.; Giri, M.C.; Chaudhuri, K. Arsenic-induced cell proliferation is associated with enhanced ROS generation, Erk signaling and CyclinA expression. *Toxicol. Lett.* **2010**, *198*, 263–271.
195. Stueckle, T.A.; Lu, Y.; Davis, M.E.; Wang, L.; Jiang, B.; Holaskova, I.; Schafer, R.; Barnett, J.B.; Rojanasakul, Y. Chronic occupational exposure to arsenic induces carcinogenic gene signaling networks and neoplastic transformation in human lung epithelial cells. *Toxicol. Appl. Pharmacol.* **2012**, *261*, 204–216.
196. Wang, F.; Shi, Y.; Yadav, S.; Wang, H. p52–Bcl3 complex promotes cyclin D1 expression in BEAS-2B cells in response to low concentration arsenite. *Toxicology* **2010**, *273*, 12–18.
197. Ding, J.; Li, J.; Xue, C.; Wu, K.; Ouyang, W.; Zhang, D.; Yan, Y.; Huang, C. Cyclooxygenase-2 induction by arsenite is through a nuclear factor of activated T-cell-dependent pathway and plays an antiapoptotic role in Beas-2B cells. *J. Biol. Chem.* **2006**, *281*, 24405–24413.
198. Kuwano, T.; Nakao, S.; Yamamoto, H.; Tsuneyoshi, M.; Yamamoto, T.; Kuwano, M.; Ono, M. Cyclooxygenase 2 is a key enzyme for inflammatory cytokine-induced angiogenesis. *FASEB J.* **2004**, *18*, 300–310.
199. Zhao, Y.; Usatyuk, P.V.; Gorshkova, I.A.; He, D.; Wang, T.; Moreno-Vinasco, L.; Geyh, A.S.; Breysse, P.N.; Samet, J.M.; Spannhake, E.W.; *et al.* Regulation of COX-2 expression and IL-6 release by particulate matter in airway epithelial cells. *Am. J. Respir. Cell Mol. Biol.* **2009**, *40*, 19–30.
200. Frantz, M.; Wipf, P. Mitochondria as a target in treatment. *Environ. Mol. Mutagen.* **2010**, *51*, 462–475.
201. Zhao, F.; Severson, P.; Pacheco, S.; Futscher, B.W.; Klimecki, W.T. Arsenic exposure induces the Warburg effect in cultured human cells. *Toxicol. Appl. Pharmacol.* **2013**, *271*, 72–77.
202. Vander Heiden, M.G.; Cantley, L.C.; Thompson, C.B. Understanding the Warburg effect: The metabolic requirements of cell proliferation. *Science* **2009**, *324*, 1029–1033.
203. Rubins, J.B. Alveolar macrophages: Wielding the double-edged sword of inflammation. *Am. J. Respir. Crit. Care Med.* **2003**, *167*, 103–104.

204. Slauch, J.M. How does the oxidative burst of macrophages kill bacteria? Still an open question. *Mol. Microbiol.* **2011**, *80*, 580–583.

205. Gercken, G.; Labedzka, M.; Geertz, R.; Gulyas, H. Influence of heavy metals and mineral dusts on superoxide anion release by alveolar macrophages. *J. Aerosol Sci.* **1988**, *19*, 1133–1136.

206. Gulyas, H.; Labedzka, M.; Gercken, G. Depression of alveolar macrophage hydrogen peroxide and superoxide anion release by mineral dusts: Correlation with antimony, lead, and arsenic contents. *Environ. Res.* **1990**, *51*, 218–229.

207. Labedzka, M.; Gulyas, H.; Schmidt, N.; Gercken, G. Toxicity of metallic ions and oxides to rabbit alveolar macrophages. *Environ. Res.* **1989**, *48*, 255–274.

208. Lantz, R.C.; Parliman, G.; Chen, G.J.; Carter, D.E. Effect of arsenic exposure on alveolar macrophage function. *Environ. Res.* **1994**, *67*, 183–195.

209. Liang, Y.; Harris, F.L.; Brown, L.A.S. Alcohol induced mitochondrial oxidative stress and alveolar macrophage dysfunction. *BioMed Res. Int.* **2013**, *2014*, 1–13.

210. Cohen, A.B.; Cline, M.J. The human alveolar macrophage: Isolation, cultivation *in vitro*, and studies of morphologic and functional characteristics. *J. Clin. Invest.* **1971**, *50*, 1390–1398.

211. Zahm, J.; Kaplan, H.; Herard, A.; Doriot, F.; Pierrot, D.; Somelette, P.; Puchelle, E. Cell migration and proliferation during the *in vitro* wound repir of the respiratory epithelium. *Cell Motil. Cytoskeleton* **1997**, *37*, 33–43.

212. Olsen, C.E.; Liguori, A.E.; Zong, Y.; Lantz, R.C.; Burgess, J.L.; Boitano, S. Arsenic upregulates MMP-9 and inhibits wound repair in human airway epithelial cells. *Am. J. Physiol.* **2008**, *295*, 293–302.

213. Wesley, U.V.; Bove, P.F.; Hristova, M.; McCarthy, S.; van der Vllet, A. Airway epithelial cell migration and wound repair by ATP-mediated activation of dual oxidase 1. *J. Biol. Chem.* **2007**, *282*, 3213–3220.

214. Cordeiro, J.V.; Jacinto, A. The role of transcription-independent damage signals in the initiation of epithelial wound healing. *Nat. Rev. Mol. Cell Biol.* **2013**, *14*, 249–262.

215. Lommatzsch, M.; Cicko, S.; Muller, T.; Lucattelli, M.; Bratke, K.; Stoll, P.; Grimm, M.; Curk, T.; Zissel, G.; Ferrari, D.X. Extracellular adenosine triphosphate and chronic obstructive pulmonary disease. *Am. J. Respir. Crit. Care Med.* **2010**, *181*, 928–934.

216. Sherwood, C.L.; Lantz, R.C.; Burgess, J.L.; Boitano, S. Arsenic alters ATP-dependent Ca^{2+} signaling in human airway epithelial cell wound response. *Toxicol. Sci.* **2011**, *121*, 191–206.

217. Sherwood, C.L.; Lantz, R.C.; Boitano, S. Chronic arsenic exposure in nanomolar concentrations compromises wound response and intercellular signaling in airway epithelial cells. *Toxicol. Sci.* **2012**, *132*, 222–234.

218. Kelly, F.J.; Fussell, J.C. Size, source and chemical composition as determinants of toxicity attributable to ambient particulate matter. *Atmos. Environ.* **2012**, *60*, 504–526.

219. Enterline, P.E.; Day, R.; Marsh, G.M. Cancers related to exposure to arsenic at a copper smelter. *Occup. Envirn. Med.* **1995**, *52*, 28–32.

220. Jarup, L.; Pershagen, G.; Wall, S. Cumulative arsenic exposure and lung cancer in smelter workers: A dose-response study. *Am. J. Ind. Med.* **1989**, *15*, 31–41.

221. Lubin, J.H.; Pottern, L.M.; Stone, B.J.; Fraumeni, J.F. Respiratory cancer in a cohort of copper smelter workers: Results from more than 50 years of follow-up. *Am. J. Epidemiol.* **2000**, *151*, 554–565.
222. Welch, K.; Higgins, I.; Oh, M.; Burchfiel, C. Arsenic exposure, smoking, and respiratory cancer in copper smelter workers. *Arch. Environ. Health* **1982**, *37*, 325–335.
223. Dunlap, L.G. Perforatons of the nasal septum due to inhalation of arsenous oxid. *J. Am. Med. Assoc.* **1921**, *76*, 568–569.
224. Inghe, G.; Bursell, A. The Ronnskar study. Report of investigation. Stockholm, Sweden. Unpublished works, 1937.
225. Gerhardsson, L.; Brune, D.; Nordberg, G.F.; Wester, P.O. Multielemental assay of tissues of deceased smelter workers and controls. *Sci. Total Environ.* **1988**, *74*, 97–110.
226. Axelson, O.; Dahlgren, E.; Jansson, C.D.; Rehnlund, S.O. Arsenic exposure and mortality: A case-referent study from a Swedish copper smelter. *Br. J. Ind. Med.* **1978**, *35*, 8–15.
227. Englyst, V.; Lundstrom, N.; Gerhardsson, L.; Rylander, L.; Nordberg, G. Lung cancer risks among lead smelter workers also exposed to arsenic. *Sci. Total Environ.* **2011**, *273*, 77–82.
228. Taylor, P.R.; Qiao, Y.; Schatzkin, A.; Yao, S.; Lubin, J.; Mao, B.; Rao, J.; McAdams, M.; Xuan, X.; Li, J. Relations of arsenic exposure to lung cancer among tin miners in Yunnan Province, China. *Br. J. Ind. Med.* **1989**, *46*, 881–886.
229. Chen, W.; Chen, J. Nested case-control study of lung cancer in four Chinese tin mines. *Occup. Environ. Med.* **2002**, *59*, 113–118.
230. Xi, S.; Zheng, Q.; Zhang, Q.; Sun, G. Metabolic profile and assessment of occupational arsenic exposure in copper- and steel-smelting workers in China. *Int. Arch. Occup. Environ. Health* **2011**, *84*, 347–353.
231. Wen, J.; Wen, W.; Li, L.; Liu, H. Methylation capacity of arsenic and skin lesions in smelter plant workers. *Environ. Toxicol. Pharmacol.* **2012**, *34*, 624–630.
232. Wu, B.; Chen, T. Changes in hair arsenic concentration in a population exposed to heavy pollution: Follow-up investigation in Chenzhou city, Hunan province, southern China. *J. Environ. Sci.* **2010**, *22*, 283–289.
233. Hwang, Y.H.; Bornschein, R.L.; Grote, J.; Menrath, W.; Roda, S. Environmental arsenic exposure of children around a former copper smelter site. *Environ. Res.* **1997**, *72*, 72–81.
234. Wickre, J.B.; Folt, C.L.; Sturup, S.; Karagas, M.R. Environmental exposure and fingernail analysis of arsenic and mercury in children and adults in a Nicaraguan gold mining community. *Arch. Environ. Health* **2004**, *59*, 400–409.
235. Martin, R.; Dowling, K.; Pearce, D.; Bennett, J.; Stopic, A. Ongoing soil arsenic exposure of children living in an historical gold mining area in regional Victoria: Identifying risk factors associated with uptake. *J. Asian Earth Sci.* **2013**, *77*, 256–261.
236. Pearce, D.C.; Dowling, K.; Gerson, A.R.; Sim, M.R.; Sutton, S.R.; Newville, M.; Russell, R.; McOrist, G. Arsenic microdistribution and speciation in toenail clippings of children living in a historic gold mining area. *Sci. Total Environ.* **2010**, *408*, 2590–2599.
237. Button, M.; Jenkin, G.R.T.; Harrington, C.F.; Watts, M.J. Human toenails as a biomarker of exposure to elevated environmental arsenic. *J. Environ. Monit.* **2009**, *11*, 610–617.

238. Hinwood, A.L.; Sim, M.R.; Jolley, D.; de Klerk, N.; Bastone, E.B.; Gerostamoulos, J.; Drummer, O.H. Hair and toenail arsenic concentrations of residents living in areas with high environmental arsenic concentrations. *Environ. Health Perspect.* **2003**, *111*, 187–193.
239. Nordstrom, D.K. Acid rock drainage and climate change. *J. Geochem. Explor.* **2009**, *100*, 97–104.
240. Middleton, N.J. A geography of dust storms in south-west Asia. *J. Climatol.* **1986**, *6*, 183–196.
241. Zhang, X.Y.; Gong, S.L.; Zhao, T.L.; Arimoto, R.; Wang, Y.Q.; Zhou, Z.J. Sources of Asian dust and role of climate change *versus* desertification in Asian dust emission. *Geophys. Res. Lett.* **2003**, *30*, doi:10.1029/2003GL018206.

10

Exposure to Selected Geogenic Trace Elements (I, Li, and Sr) from Drinking Water in Denmark

Denitza Dimitrova Voutchkova [1,2,*], Jörg Schullehner [2,3,4], Nikoline Nygård Knudsen [5], Lisbeth Flindt Jørgensen [6], Annette Kjær Ersbøll [5], Søren Munch Kristiansen [1] and Birgitte Hansen [2]

1. Department of Geoscience, Aarhus University, Høegh-Guldbergs Gade 2, DK-8000 Aarhus C, Denmark; E-Mail: smk@geo.au.dk
2. Geological Survey of Denmark and Greenland (GEUS), Lyseng Allé 1, DK-8270 Højbjerg, Denmark; E-Mails: jsc@geus.dk (J.S); bgh@geus.dk (B.H.)
3. Department of Public Health, Aarhus University, Bartholins Allé 2, DK-8000 Aarhus C, Denmark
4. Centre for Integrated Register-Based Research at Aarhus University (CIRRAU), Fuglesangs Allé 4, DK-8210 Aarhus V, Denmark
5. National Institute of Public Health, University of Southern Denmark, Øster Farimagsgade 5A, 2nd floor, DK-1353, Copenhagen K, Denmark; E-Mails: nink@si-folkesundhed.dk (N.N.K.); ake@si-folkesundhed.dk (A.K.E.)
6. Geological Survey of Denmark and Greenland (GEUS), Øster Voldgade 10, DK-1350 Copenhagen K, Denmark; E-Mail: lfj@geus.dk

* Author to whom correspondence should be addressed: E-Mail: ddv@geo.au.dk;

Academic Editors: Jose A. Centeno, Robert B. Finkelman and Olle Selinus

---

Abstract: The naturally occurring geogenic elements iodine (I), lithium (Li), and strontium (Sr) have a beneficial effect on human health. Iodine has an essential role in human metabolism while Li and Sr are used, respectively, as a treatment for various mental disorders and for post-menopausal osteoporosis. The aim here is to evaluate the potential for future epidemiological investigations in Denmark of lifelong and chronic exposure to low doses of these compounds. The drinking water data represents approximately 45% of the annual Danish groundwater abstraction for drinking water purposes, which supplies approximately 2.5 million persons. The spatial patterns were studied using inverse distance weighted interpolation and cluster analysis. The exposed population was estimated based on two datasets: (1) population density in the smallest census unit, the parishes, and (2) geocoded addresses where at least one person is residing. We found significant spatial variation in the exposure for all three elements, related mainly to geochemical processes. This suggests a prospective opportunity for future epidemiological investigation of long-term effects of I, Li, and Sr, either alone or in combinations with other geogenic elements such as Ca, Mg or F.

Keywords: iodine; lithium; strontium; drinking water; treated groundwater; spatial trends; exposure; Denmark; epidemiology

---

1. Introduction

Although most chemical elements do not occur exclusively in drinking water (DW), exposures via DW, even at low concentrations, may have important consequences across the entire population [1].

The three trace elements which are in focus here (I, Li, and Sr) have in common that they are essential (I) or possibly essential (Li, Sr) for humans and are currently used as part of pharmaceuticals or dietary supplements. Also, their concentrations in DW can vary spatially, and lifelong exposure to different naturally occurring levels may have an impact on public health in various ways.

1.1. Sources of I, Li, and Sr in Ground- and Drinking Water

Iodine (I) is a trace element from the halogen group and occurs in oxidation states −1, 0, +1, +3, +4, +5, and +7 [2]. However, in the hydrogeochemical cycle, I is found in the stable inorganic forms iodide (I^-) and iodate (IO_3^-), as well as in various dissolved organic iodine compounds. The speciation data of I in Danish DW reported in [3] showed that there were six speciation combinations. Also, the complex spatial distribution of DW-I was attributed to differences in geological layers, hydrogeochemical reactions, and/or treatment procedures at the waterworks [3]. Iodine concentrations in Danish groundwater are characterised by both small-scale heterogeneity and large-scale spatial trends [4]. Voutchkova *et al.* [4] found that elevated groundwater-I concentrations originate from Palaeocene and Cretaceous limestone/chalk aquifers, and saw an association between I, Li, Ba, and Br. These elevated concentrations of I in Danish groundwater seemed to be caused by leaching from soil, the marine origin of the aquifers, and/or saline water influence; however, the processes governing the I concentrations were site and depth specific [5].

The lithium (Li) ion at +1 oxidation state is generally soluble and mobile in groundwater; however, sorption onto clay minerals and zeolite occurs [2]. Lithium in groundwater may have multiple geogenic sources. It occurs in the minerals spodumene ($LiAlSi_2O_6$) and lepidolite ($K_2Li_3Al_4Si_7O_{21}(OH,F)_3$), but also in many other minerals. Pegmatite and brines especially are strongly enriched in Li [6]. In a European study, a median value of 2.6 μg/L Li (min. <0.2 μg/L and max. 75 μg/L) in tap water was found based on 579 samples from all over Europe [2]. To our knowledge, there are no studies focusing on Li sources in Danish groundwater, except for a baseline study, where Hinsby *et al.* [7] concluded that Li in Miocene aquifers was of natural origin.

Strontium (Sr) occurs in nature in the +2 oxidation state and is the 15th most abundant element on Earth [2]. The size of the Sr^{2+} ion is intermediate between those of Ca^{2+} and K^{+}; thus, it substitutes them in many rock-forming minerals [2]. High concentrations of Sr in Danish groundwater were studied by Bonnesen *et al.* [8], who found that Sr concentrations increased with depth more than would be expected from diffusion of deep connate seawater alone. They concluded that dissolution of small amounts of Sr-rich aragonite ($Ca_{1-x}Sr_xCO_3$) or equilibrium with the Sr-rich minerals celestite ($SrSO_4$) and strontianite ($SrCO_3$) was the cause of elevated Sr in these chalk formations. Ramsay [9] found a correlation between Mg and Sr, and concluded that recrystallization of Sr-containing aragonite to pure calcite was the main cause of observed elevated Sr concentrations in the chalk aquifers in eastern Denmark. Strontium-enriched groundwater is hence an indicator of limited hydrogeological flushing with fresh water, as carbonate recrystallization takes place on a millennial time scale. Strontium (together with B, Br, Cs, Ge, Li and Rb) is especially enriched in hydrogeochemically mature groundwater [2].

1.2. Public Health and I, Li, and Sr in Drinking Water

Although there are no EU or U.S. standards for I, Li, or Sr, there are national standards for some European countries [2]. A DW standard (maximum values) for I exists in Russia (125 μg/L), for Li in both Russia and Ukraine (30 μg/L), and for Sr in Bosnia and Herzegovina (2 mg/L), Russia (7 mg/L), and Ukraine (7 mg/L) (see references in [2]). The Danish DW standard is 1 mg/L for Li, and 10 mg/L for Sr (provisional), while there is no standard for I [10].

1.2.1. Iodine

Iodine has an essential role in human metabolism [11]. Both insufficient and excessive dietary I intake can cause health problems. Worldwide, the focus is on iodine deficiency (ID), as it is "*the single most important preventable cause of brain damage*" [12]. Lower IQ, learning capacities, quality of life, and economic productivity are just a few of the adverse effects of severe ID [12]. Even mild ID can result in learning disabilities, poor growth and diffuse goitre in school children [13]. ID is not confined to developing countries [14]: Zimmermann and Andersson [15] estimated that 43.9% (n = 30.5 million) of 6–12-year-old children and 44.2% (n = 393.1 million) of the general population in the World Health Organization (WHO) European Region have insufficient I-intake. Denmark is amongst the 30 countries with ID status worldwide; however, subnational surveys are used for estimating the status in Denmark, as recent nationwide ones are lacking [16].

The recommended daily nutrient intake (RNI) for I is 150 μg for adults (250 μg at pregnancy and lactation), 120 μg for 6–12-year-old children, and 90 μg for babies 0–59 months old [11]. Iodine in the human body originates mainly from food and DW; however, most foods (except sea products) are naturally I low. Therefore, universal salt iodization (USI) programs have been established in many countries, as this is the strategy officially recommended by WHO and United Nations Children's Fund (UNICEF) for elimination of ID worldwide [11,12]. The sustainability of USI as an ID prevention measure depends on continuous monitoring [12], as well as its integration/coordination with the nationwide strategies for reduction of salt consumption [17]. In the context of the ongoing debate on how to address this issue [14,16,18,19], it is important to focus on regional (local) differences in other I-rich products [18] such as water, milk, *etc.*

Generally, DW is not considered a major dietary I source, providing only 10% [20]. After the mandatory USI was introduced in Denmark in 2001 [21], about 14% of the dietary I intake was derived from DW and other beverages (*w/o* juices and milk) [22]. Before the mandatory USI this percentage was 24%–25% [23,24]. It has been shown that local or regional geographical variation of I in DW exists and can be important for the I intake of the population, especially in areas where DW is of groundwater origin, as in Denmark [3,21,25] or China [26,27]. As part of our previous study, the DW contribution to dietary I intake in Denmark was estimated to vary in different parts of the country from 0% to above 100% (adults) or 50% (adolescents) of the RNI [3].

1.2.2. Lithium

Lithium has been used as a treatment for various mental disorders for more than 60 years. The therapeutic doses are much higher than naturally occurring Li levels in DW and typically within a clinical range of 300–1200 mg Li_2CO_3 per day [28,29]. A substantial amount of studies and meta-analyses investigating patients with mood disorders show that Li significantly reduces suicide mortality in both long-term and short-term treatment [30,31]. It has been hypothesised that if Li in therapeutic doses was effective in preventing suicide in people who already suffer from a mental illness, perhaps Li in small doses over the course of a lifetime could prevent suicide in the general population. This idea has been investigated in several ecological studies on aggregated data. A study from Texas, USA [32] found that counties with high Li levels in DW were associated with significantly lower suicide rates. More recent studies from Japan [33], the U.S. [34], and Austria [35,36]—the latter three also accounting for socioeconomic factors that are closely related to suicide—suggest that long-term intake of small doses of Li via DW may reduce the risk of suicide. Another study in the east of England found no correlation between Li levels in DW and suicide rates [37]. The biochemical mechanisms of action of Li are complex and not fully understood. Studies suggest that Li has a direct antisuicidal effect through a reduction of aggressivity and impulsivity, which are both associated with an increased risk of suicide [38].

1.2.3. Strontium

Osteoporosis is characterised by reduced bone mass and disruption of bone architecture, resulting in increased bone fracture and fragility, and thereby imposing a significant burden on both the individual and society [39]. Hernlund *et al.* [39] estimated, using a diagnostic criterion from WHO, that approximately 22 million women and 5.5 million men residing in the EU in 2010 had osteoporosis. Of these, approximately 0.28 million were from Denmark (female: 0.22 million, male: 0.06 million) [39,40]. The beneficial effects of stable Sr in the treatment of post-menopausal osteoporosis was reported as early as in the 1950–1960s; however, perhaps because of undue association of the stable naturally occurring isotope with the radioactive Sr isotope, those studies did not receive sufficient attention, and the clinical use of Sr nearly ceased in the 1980s [41]. Currently, therapy for osteoporosis includes dietary supplementation of Ca and Vitamin D, in addition to treatment with oestrogen, pharmaceutical products, or fluoride [42]. Strontium ranelate (Sr^{2+} and ranelic acid) was licenced and introduced to the European market for treatment of osteoporosis in 2004 [39].

The typical adult body burden of Sr is 0.3–0.4 g (99% in the skeleton), and the primary exposure sources are DW, grains, leafy vegetables, and dairy products [43]. Watts and Howe [43] estimated that the total daily intake of Sr in many parts of the world is up to 4 mg/day, with DW contributing 0.7–2 mg/day (based on 2 L daily consumption of DW with Sr concentrations of 0.34–1.1 mg/L). However, they noted that intakes may be higher in areas where DW concentrations are higher. Watts and Howe [43] and Agency for Toxic Substances and Disease Registry (ATSDR) [44] found that there was not enough evidence for Sr toxicity to humans and that human data were inadequate for setting a tolerable intake and a tolerable concentration of Sr.

The positive effects of Sr supplementation on bone have been examined in rats, monkeys, laying hens, and humans in various studies (a few examples are given in [41,42,45]). Very few studies of lifelong Sr exposure effects exist, as reviewed by ATSDR [44]. Dawson *et al.* [46] measured Sr in DW and urine ($n = 2187$) in families that had been residing within their respective communities for at least 10 years, and found a statistically significant product-moment correlation for decreased community mortality rate (in people over 45 years old) for hypertension with heart disease. Polyakova [47] proposed a classification dividing the Arkhangelsk region (Russia) into three zones with different probabilities of Kashin-Beck or similar bone disease manifestation based on the hypothesis that areas with DW characterised by Ca/Sr < 100 are coinciding with Kashin-Beck endemic regions. Curzon [48] found an association between caries prevalence and Sr in DW for lifelong residents in four Ohio cities, with minimum caries prevalence at DW concentrations around 5–6 mg Sr/L. There are few indications that Sr, likely in combination with other trace elements, such as F^- or Ba, could be beneficial to enhancing remineralisation of teeth, and hence protection against caries (for more references see [49]). To our best knowledge, there are no published reports on the potential public health effects (beneficial or adverse) of long-term exposure to different levels of naturally occurring Sr in DW in combination with Ca, F, or other DW constituents.

1.3. Study Objectives

The general objective of this study is to evaluate the potential for future epidemiological investigations of long-term (lifelong, chronic) exposure to low doses of three naturally occurring compounds (I, Li, and Sr) from DW. The specific study aims are accordingly (1) to characterise the nationwide spatial patterns of I, Li, and Sr concentrations in Danish DW and (2) to quantify the exposure to I, Li, and Sr from Danish DW.

2. Experimental Section

2.1. Danish Public Drinking Water Supply

Denmark is a relatively small country (approximately 43,000 km^2) with about 5.6 million inhabitants. The Danish DW supply is entirely of groundwater origin. The major part of the population is supplied by public waterworks. The reported groundwater abstraction for DW purposes for 2010 was 397 million m^3 (by 2585 public waterworks) [50]. Next to the public waterworks, there are single wells and small waterworks (supplying <10 households), which were estimated to supply about 0.4 million people (7%) [51].

The DW supply is highly decentralised. Sørensen and Møller [52] reported that about 72% of the active waterworks have annual abstractions of <0.1 million m^3, whereas only about 3% are abstracting >1 million m^3.

Bottled water consumption in Denmark was amongst the lowest in Europe in 2013 (22.8 L/cap or 0.127 million m^3 [53]) and below the global average (30 L/cap [54]). Thus, the major source of potable water in Denmark is delivered by public waterworks.

Generally, Danish groundwater requires simple treatment with aeration and sand filtration only. In the aeration step, naturally occurring gasses such as methane are removed and substituted by oxygen. During filtration, oxidised iron and manganese are removed. A few other components are detained in the sand filters in various magnitudes. Only 74 waterworks, producing about 50.47 million m^3, use some sort of more advanced water treatment [55]. However, neither chlorination nor ozone treatment was used in Denmark by 2012 [55].

The aquifers used for DW abstraction in Denmark are mainly unconsolidated Quaternary glacial sand, Tertiary marine and fluvial sand or Cretaceous limestone and chalk.

2.2. Water Chemistry Data (I, Li, and Sr)

The chemical data used here is from a DW sampling campaign conducted from April to June 2013 and reported in detail in [3,56]. The samples represent treated DW from groundwater origin, ready to be supplied to consumers (sampling point: exit waterworks). The treatment consists of aeration and sand filtration, except for 10.4% (n = 15) of the 144 waterworks, where a somewhat more advanced water treatment method is used [3].

Iodine data were collected for all of the waterworks included in the study (n = 144); however, where there were no total I measurements (n = 5), iodide (I^-) determined by Ion-exchange chromatography (IC) was used instead. Lithium and Sr data were obtained for 139 of the locations. The 144 waterworks abstract about 175 million m^3 annually, which accounts for 45% of the total groundwater abstraction by all public water supplies (excluding small waterworks or wells supplying fewer than 10 households) [3]. The samples were filtered in the lab (0.45 μm pore size Q-max syringe filter, Frisenette Aps, Ebeltoft, Denmark). Inductively coupled plasma mass spectrometry (ICP-MS) was used for determining I, Li, and Sr concentrations. A short summary of I, Li, and Sr data is presented in Table 1. Further details on the laboratory methods, sampling design and execution, hydrogeochemical characterisation, and water treatment are provided in [3,56].

2.3. Water Supply Areas

Schullehner and Hansen [57] recently compiled a map with the water supply areas of all 2852 public waterworks in Denmark but excluding a number of very small waterworks and wells supplying <10 households. For the purposes of our study, we have used only the areas supplied by the 144 included waterworks (Figure 1). It should be noted that: some of the selected areas are supplied by more than one waterworks (Figure 1) and it is possible that some of the residents in these areas are not connected to the public water supply but get their water from a privately owned well [57].

Table 1. Summary of the iodine, lithium, and strontium datasets (concentrations in drinking water) used in this study.

Title	Iodine (I)	Lithium (Li)	Strontium (Sr)
Unit	µg/L	µg/L	mg/L
Lab method	ICP-MS *	ICP-MS	ICP-MS
Count (*n*)	144 *	139	139
Detection limit (d.l.)	0.2	5	0.005
<d.l. (%)	6.25	18.7	0
Substitution (0.5*d.l.)	0.1	2.5	-
Min. concentration	0.1	2.5	0.07
Max. concentration	126	30.7	14.45
Mean concentration	13.97 *	11.04	1.31
Median concentration	11.25 *	10.30	0.59

Notes: * Here I^- was used where total iodine was not measured ($n = 5$); IC is the method for I^-; because these I^- measurements are included, the mean and median calculated here differ slightly from [3].

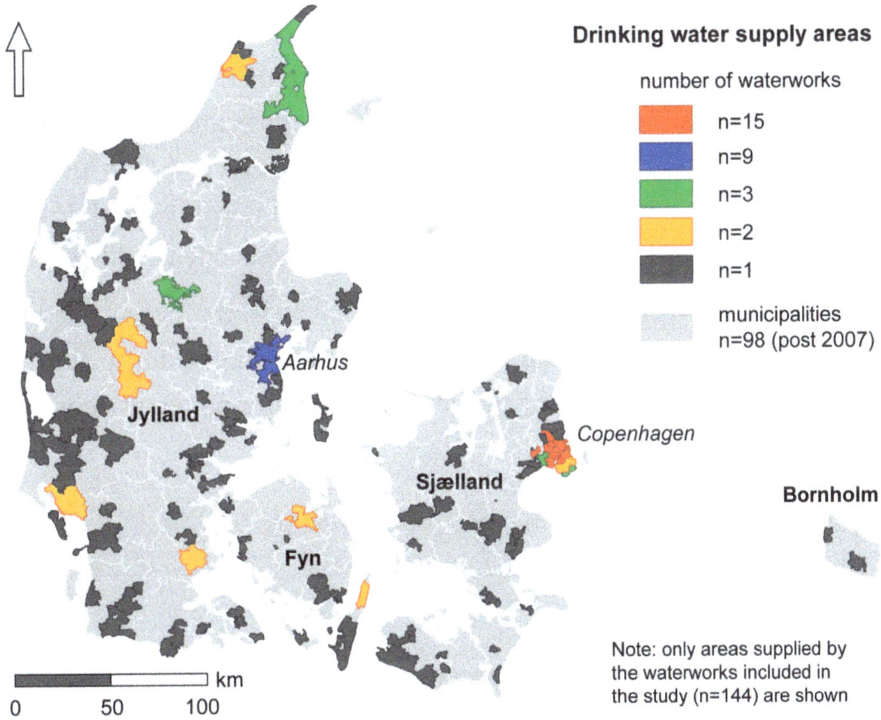

Figure 1. Water supply areas of the waterworks included in the study (n = 144); the areas in red, blue, green, and orange are supplied by more than one of the included waterworks (source: map on supply areas of 2852 Danish waterworks [57]).

All selected water supply areas were assigned the water quality measurements (I, Li, and Sr) of the waterworks by which they are supplied. The areas supplied by more than one waterworks were assigned the average concentrations measured at the waterworks supplying the specific area (Figure 1). The two largest cities, Copenhagen and Aarhus, are supplied with water treated by at least 15 and nine waterworks, respectively. An effort was made to pinpoint specific parts of the cities (neighbourhoods), which are preferentially supplied with water from one/some of these waterworks. Previously collected data from the water supply companies (as part of two studies [3,57]) was used for this purpose.

However, for parts of the cities (blue and red areas from Figure 1) this was not possible, as the water from all these waterworks is mixed together in the water distribution system. More precise estimations of I, Li, and Sr concentrations are possible only if water samples are obtained at carefully selected points in the distribution system, which was not feasible for this study.

2.4. Estimation of the Population Living in the Selected Water Supply Areas

Two datasets were used for estimating the population living in the selected areas:

1st dataset: a population density map based on the population counts in the smallest census unit (parishes) for 2008 (further details can be found in [57]). This method yields "number of residents" in the selected supply areas.

2nd dataset: a database including geocoded addresses with at least one registered resident from the Danish Civil Registration System (DCRS), provided by the Centre for Integrated Register-Based Research at Aarhus University (CIRRAU). This database contains one record for each specific address (municipality, road, house number, and, if relevant, door number) used as a residence in DCRS [58]. The DCRS was established in 1968 and has since recorded current and historical information not only on the place of residence, but also on vital status, gender, place and date of birth, parents, spouses, and siblings and twins for all persons living in Denmark [59]. This information is regarded as being of very high quality and yields an important and rare asset which can be used for epidemiological research [59]. A subset of this database has been used here. It consists of the geocoded addresses for 2012 only ($n = 2{,}092{,}090$), which are further referred to as "households".

The number of residents (1st dataset) and the number of household addresses (2nd dataset) within each water supply area were calculated using the geographical information system ArcMap 10.0 (Esri, Redlands, CA, USA).

2.5. Inverse Distance Weighted Interpolation and Cluster Analysis

2.5.1. Data Pretreatment

Due to skewed distributions of I and Sr concentrations, a square root transformation of I and a logarithmic transformation of Sr were applied prior to analysis. The transformations were selected by comparing the distribution of the transformed measurements with a normal distribution.

2.5.2. Inverse distance weighted interpolation

Inverse distance weighting (IDW) was used to estimate a density surface for each of the elements I, Li, and Sr. This method assigns a weighted average of the neighbouring values to each unmeasured grid cell on the map. The weight given to each observation is a function of the distance between that observation's location s_i and the grid point s_0 at which the interpolation is desired. Generally, the inverse distance interpolator is given as in Equation (1):

$$\hat{Z}(s_0) = \frac{\sum_{i=1}^{n} \omega(s_i) Z(s_i)}{\sum_{i=1}^{n} \omega(s_i)} \tag{1}$$

where $\hat{Z}(s_0)$ is the predicted value at the unsampled location s_0 and $Z(s_i)$ is the observed value at the ith location within a given maximum distance for $i = 1, \ldots, n$, with n being the number of locations in the study. The weights ω attributed to the observations were computed as in Equation (2):

$$\omega(s_i) = ||s_i - s_0||^{-p} \quad (2)$$

where $||s_i - s_0||$ is the Euclidian distance between locations s_0 and s_i and p is an inverse distance weighting power. The weighting power is selected in order to determine how fast the weights tend towards zero as the distance from the grid point increases [60–62].

Grid cells of 1 × 1 km, a power of $p = 2$, and a maximum distance of 75 km were applied. The density maps of I and Sr were derived using a square root and a logarithm transformation, respectively. Back-transformed interpolated values were calculated and mapped.

2.5.3. Cluster Analysis

A local cluster analysis was performed to investigate areas with significantly higher or lower levels of I, Li, or Sr in the DW. I and Sr were transformed prior to the analysis. The presence, significance, and approximate location of clusters were evaluated using spatial scan statistics implemented by Kulldorff [63] in the software SaTScan (v9.3.1, http://www.satscan.org/). The spatial scan statistic searches for clusters by using a search window of varying shape and size. For each location, a test is performed, evaluating whether the mean value is significantly higher (or lower) within the search window compared to outside. Given the continuous data, a normal distribution was used as the probability model in which the null hypothesis was that all observations come from the same distribution, whereas the alternative hypothesis was that there was one cluster location where the measurements have either a larger or smaller mean than outside that cluster. A central feature of this method is that the statistical inference is still valid, even if the true distribution is not normal [64].

The significance of identified clusters was tested using a likelihood ratio test with a p-value obtained using Monte Carlo simulations (999 permutations). The likelihood function is maximized over all window locations and sizes, and the one with the maximum likelihood constitutes the most likely cluster. An elliptic search window with a centre at the location of each waterworks was used, allowing no geographical overlap between clusters. The maximum percentage of the measurements to be included in a cluster was varied at 10%, 20%, 25%, 30%, and 50%, respectively. Changing the maximum percentage of the measurements included in a cluster did not change the location and number of clusters identified. A maximum percentage of 20% of the measurements included in a cluster was used.

2.6. Exposure Analysis

To estimate the exposure to I, Li, and Sr from DW the following data were used: (1) water chemistry data, which was assigned to each of the supply areas and (2) the 1st and 2nd datasets with the number of residents and the number of households in the selected supply areas, respectively. A schematic visualisation of the different datasets (and subsets) and the links between them is provided in Figure 2.

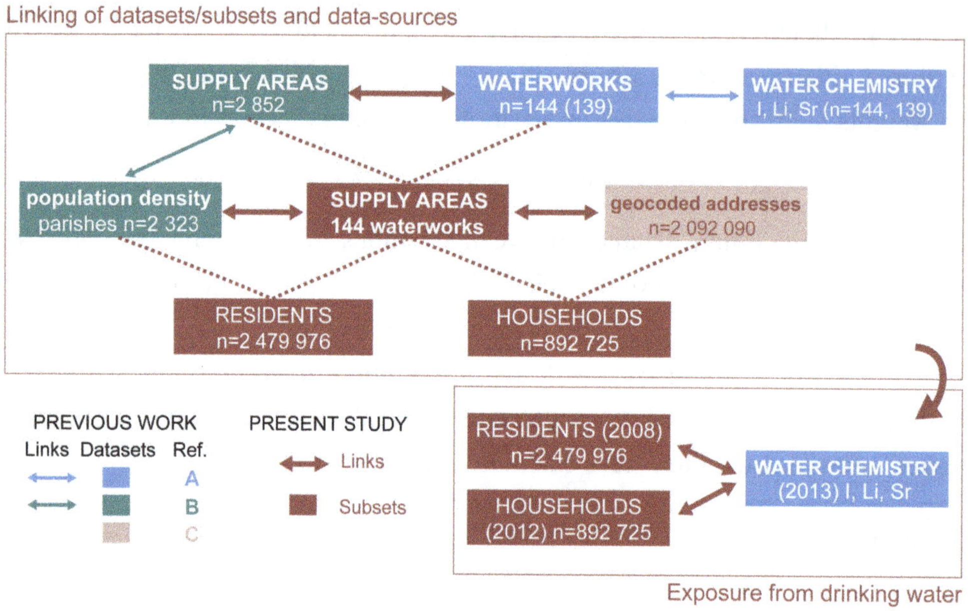

Figure 2. Scheme presenting the datasets, their subsets, and the links between them used in this study. Some of these datasets and links were prepared in previous studies (colour coded, references: A [3], B [57], and C [58]).

It was estimated that 2,479,976 residents (about 45.3% of all residents in 2008) and 892,725 households (42.7% of all households in 2012) are supplied with DW by the 144 waterworks analysed in this study. For the 139 waterworks where Li and Sr data are present, the number of residents is 2,442,705 (about 44.6%) and the number of households is 874,375 (41.8%). Thus, the exposure analysis covers close to half the population of Denmark (see Figure 1 for spatial reference).

The calculation of residents and households exposed to different levels of I, Li, and Sr are given as a percentage of the households and population included in this study, respectively.

3. Results and Discussion

3.1. Spatial Distribution of Drinking Water I, Li and Sr

The spatial distribution of I, Li, and Sr concentrations in treated DW of groundwater origin was examined using IDW interpolation and cluster analysis. The IDW interpolated maps are presented in Figure 3a,c,e. The cluster analysis identified areas with significantly high concentrations and significantly low concentrations of each of the elements I, Li, and Sr. The number of measurements (*i.e.*, waterworks) in a cluster, mean concentrations inside and outside the clusters, and *p*-values for the three elements are shown in Table 2. The ellipses of the significant hot and cold spots are presented overlaying the maps with the supply areas (see Figure 3b,d,f). However, it should be kept in mind that the cluster analyses are based on point data.

The lowest concentrations for all three elements are observed in the western part of Jylland, where the significant cold spots of I, Li, and Sr also are located. Another similarity in the spatial patterns is the general east-west trend: relatively higher concentrations are found in the eastern part and lower in the western part of the country. Despite that, the spatial distribution of I, Li, and Sr also show differences.

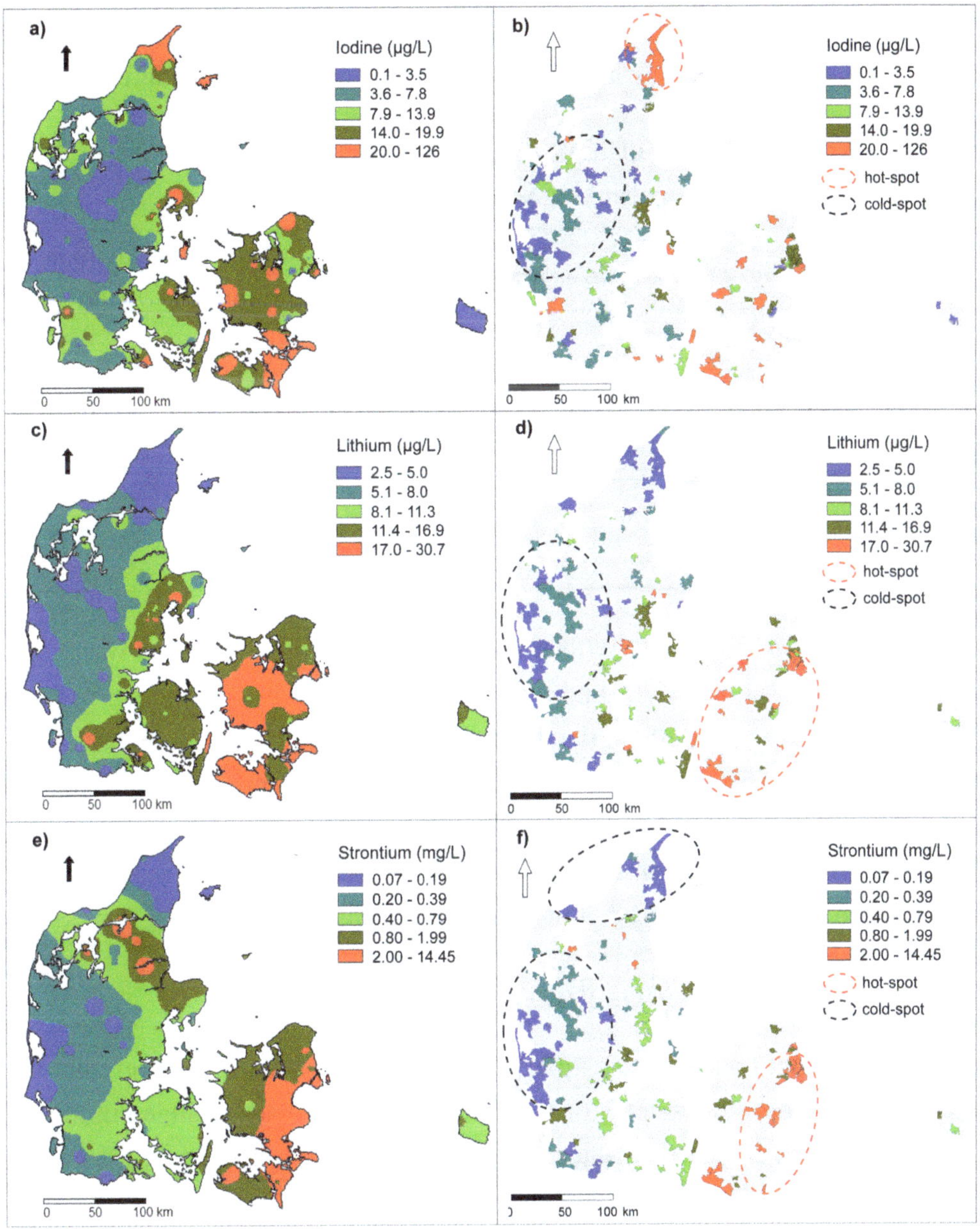

Figure 3. Iodine, lithium, and strontium in drinking water in Denmark; (**a**,**c**,**e**) IDW interpolation; (**b**,**d**,**f**) drinking water concentrations in the selected supply areas and hot and cold spot clusters. Note: each category represents ~20% of the observations; the cluster analysis is based on the point data. See Section 2 for details.

An east-west trend for I concentrations in DW was reported by [25,65] and is thereafter largely used by others. However, based on a cluster analysis of I data characterised by higher spatial sampling resolution, Voutchkova *et al.* [3] concluded that there is complex spatial variation and the east-west trend is an oversimplification. The same data as in [3] are used in the current study, while the different analyses employed here add to our previous work; e.g., the IDW interpolated maps (Figure 3a) visually confirm our statement about the complexity of the spatial variation. Northern Jylland is found to be a significant hot spot of DW-I by both the present and the previous analysis [3]. However, due to different data pretreatment (here: square root transformation *vs.* normal score transformation in [3]) and analytical method (here: spatial scan statistics *vs.* Local Moran's I in [3]), a second hot spot

(Sjælland according to [3]) was not found here. The governing factors for this complex spatial pattern have been attributed to both the geology and the groundwater treatment procedures [3].

Table 2. Geographical clusters of high (hot spot) and low concentrations (cold spot) of iodine, lithium, and strontium in drinking water.

Element	Type of Cluster	$N_{measurements}$ Inside Cluster	Mean Concentration		*p*-value
			Inside Cluster	**Outside Cluster**	
Iodine (μg/L)	Hot spot	4	77.09	9.92	0.001
	Cold spot	26	2.37	13.69	0.003
Lithium (μg/L)	Hot spot	27	19.08	9.10	0.001
	Cold spot	27	4.56	21.60	0.002
Strontium (mg/L)	Hot spot	27	2.66	0.45	0.001
	Cold spot	27	0.21	0.84	0.001
	Cold spot	10	0.15	0.72	0.049

Of all three elements, Li is the one with the most clearly manifested east-west trend: a smooth transition between the low (Li < 8 μg/L) and the high concentrations (Li > 17 μg/L) is characteristic. A significant hotspot is covers parts of Sjælland and the islands to the south (Figure 3c).

The highest Sr concentrations (>2 mg/L) are observed in the eastern part of Sjælland (covered by the significant hot spot, too), as well as in a few locations in Jylland. The hot spot for Sr is slightly smaller than the one for Li. Strontium is also the only element from the three which has a second significant cold spot, located on the raised Holocene seabed in northern Jylland.

3.2. Exposure to I, Li, and Sr via Drinking Water

The exposure to different concentrations of I, Li, and Sr from treated DW (groundwater origin) is given as percentage of exposed consumers or households from the ones included in this study, *i.e.*, the residents and households within each water supply area where I, Li, and Sr measurements were available (Figure 4; see Table 3 for absolute numbers).

The largest proportion of households (*h*) and residents (*r*) in this study are exposed to I concentrations in the range of 14–20 μg/L (*h*: 44%, *r*: 50%), Li concentrations in the highest range of 17–30.7 μg/L (*h*: 33%, *r*: 38%), and Sr concentrations in the range of 2–14 mg/L (*h*: 37%, *r*: 42%). However, only a small proportion of the population is exposed to the highest levels of the observed concentrations: 0.8% (*h*) or 0.4% (*r*) are exposed to Sr > 10 mg/L, which is the current provisional DW standard in Denmark; 1.7% (*h*) or 1.8% (*r*) are exposed to Li > 25 μg/L; and 0.5% (*h*) or 0.6% (*r*) are exposed to I > 50 μg/L. This exposure calculation takes into account the population density for 2008 (*r*) or all geocoded residential addresses in 2012 (*h*) in the areas supplied by the selected waterworks. Thus, it provides information on the differences in exposure based on the spatial variation of I, Li, and Sr in DW. The spatial distribution of DW supply areas exposed to different levels of I, Li, and Sr is provided in Figure 3b,d,f. From the results presented in Figure 4 (and Table 2), it can be concluded that there is a contrast in the exposure of the Danish population to I, Li, and Sr from DW. Possible health effects of these exposure contrasts could be studied by combining these results with data from the Danish health registers [66].

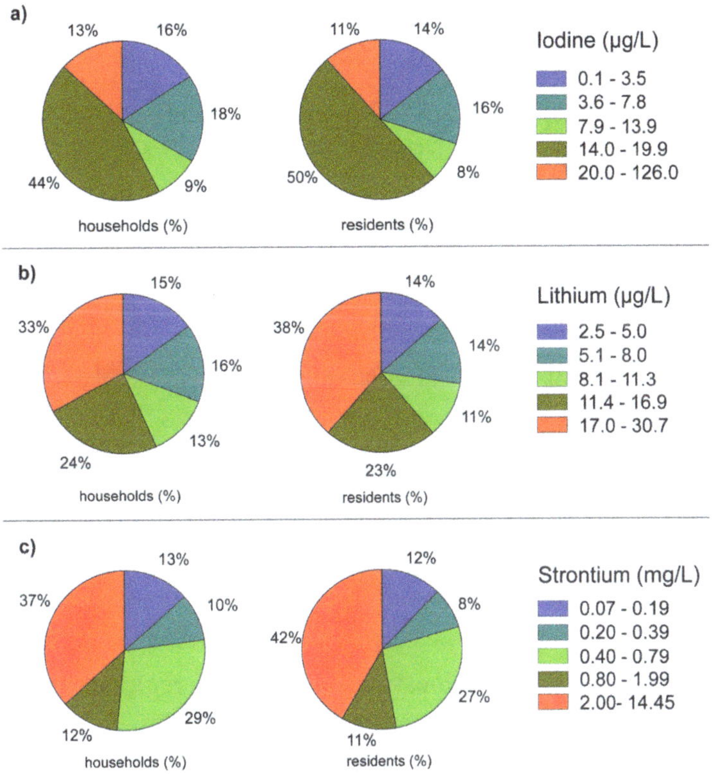

Figure 4. Proportion of households and residents exposed to different concentrations of (**a**) iodine, (**b**) lithium, and (**c**) strontium. Note: the number of households and number of residents are estimated using two different datasets (see Section 2); see Table 3 for absolute numbers.

Table 3. Households and residents exposed to different concentrations of iodine, lithium, and strontium in absolute numbers (*n*) and in percentages (%; see also Figure 4).

Element	Concentration	Households		Residents	
		n	%	*n*	%
Iodine	<3.6 µg/L	140,593	15.7	356,533	14.4
	3.6 to 7.8 µg/L	158,213	17.7	388,008	15.6
	7.9 to 13.9 µg/L	80,677	9.0	201,478	8.1
	14.0 to 19.9 µg/L	396,070	44.4	1,250,457	50.4
	20.0 to 126.0 µg/L	117,172	13.1	283,500	11.4
	Total	892,725	100	2,479,976	100
Lithium	<5.1 µg/L	130,954	15.0	332,613	13.6
	5.1 to 8.0 µg/L	138,441	15.8	335,875	13.8
	8.1 to 11.3 µg/L	109,879	12.6	277,078	11.3
	11.4 to 16.9 µg/L	207,907	23.8	556,759	22.8
	17.0 to 30.7 µg/L	287,194	32.8	940,380	38.5
	Total	874,375	100	2,442,705	100
Strontium	<0.2 mg/L	116,284	13.3	300,856	12.3
	0.20 to 0.39 mg/L	84,145	9.6	199,114	8.2
	0.40 to 0.79 mg/L	250,705	28.7	654,183	26.8
	0.80 to 1.99 mg/L	103,087	11.8	272,128	11.1
	2.00 to 14.45 mg/L	320,154	36.6	1,016,424	41.6
	Total	874,375	100	2,442,705	100

3.3. Discussion

The spatial variation of I concentrations in Danish groundwater is characterised both by a large-scale east-west trend [4] and by small-scale variation [4,5]. This is also clearly reflected in the geographical trend of the treated DW-I, which was shown here and in [3]. The elevated I concentrations in Danish DW and groundwater were found to be associated mainly with the Palaeocene to Cretaceous limestone or chalk and postglacial marine-sand aquifers [3–5].

There is limited information about the Li content in Quaternary and Tertiary deposits [7], and especially about the geochemical processes governing the release of Li to groundwater. Lithium is strongly enriched in ocean water compared to freshwater, and in brines. This may lead to the hypothesis that Danish aquifers of marine origin are Li enriched compared to those of glacial and fluvial origin. Moreover, an association between I and Li pointing at saline water influence was found based on Danish historical groundwater data [4].

Strontium concentrations in Danish DW seem to be similar to average concentrations in U.S. streams (between 0.5 and 1.5 mg/L) but higher than average Sr concentrations in U.S. groundwater (<0.5 mg/L) as reported by ATSDR [44]. The hot-spot location supports the regional findings by Ramsay [9] that local differences in the pre-Quaternary chalk and limestone aquifer geology and hydrogeology are responsible for elevated Sr concentrations in present-day groundwater. However, the lower Sr concentrations in DW (western part of Denmark) are most probably governed by the relatively constant contributions from the weathering of Sr-poor silicates in the soil, which is strongly dependent on texture and mineralogy, and from the dissolution of Sr-poor carbonates at the acidification front.

The significant spatial difference in the concentrations of I, Li, and Sr in Danish DW results in varying human exposure to these elements. Therefore, there is great potential for future epidemiological investigations of the long-term (lifelong, chronic) exposure to low doses of the three selected naturally occurring compounds from DW. In addition to exposure to a single element, there is a potential for studying the effects related to a combination of these and additional elements.

For example, in a project from Norway, nationwide data on municipal DW was combined with data on all registered treated hip fractures to study whether Ca and Mg have a protective function [67]. Corresponding studies based on Sr in a single exposure or in combination with Ca, Mg, or F^- in Danish DW, residential history and the various nationwide registers on health and social issues [66] can be conducted. The spatial distribution of Sr in Danish DW resembles somewhat the spatial distribution of F^- [68] and Ca and Mg [69]. Hence, this first prospective data analysis reveals a large potential for future nationwide public health studies, especially if Sr in DW is combined with Ca, Mg, and F. Findings relating Sr in DW to life-long health, as reported by Curzon [48] and Dawson *et al.* [46] on hypertension and caries, could most likely be improved considerably with such a multi-element approach, as Sr is closely related to Ca incorporation in human bones [42].

Similarly, an epidemiological investigation can elucidate whether the observed spatial differentiation in exposure to I from DW (see also [3]) influences the health status of the Danish population. The DCRS yields the unique possibility to connect past exposure of mothers (e.g., during pregnancy) to I from DW with the health status of their children in order to explore, whether the observed spatial differences in DW-I affect the children's performance (e.g., physical and mental development).

With respect to Li, there is currently an ongoing nationwide study conducted at the National Institute of Public Health (University of Southern Denmark, Copenhagen, Denmark) using geospatial methods to investigate whether long-term intake of naturally occurring low doses of Li in DW is protective against suicide, when accounting for socioeconomic as well as other factors.

The presented exposure analysis is based on water chemistry data from a single point in time. There is only limited data on the temporal variability of the studied geogenic elements in both treated DW and groundwater in Denmark. A comparison between the Li data used here and other, previously unreported Li measurements can be seen in Figure 5a, showing that the Li levels are similar even though the analytical methods (ICP-MS *vs.* Atomic absorption spectroscopy (AAS)) and the sampling dates differ (2013 *vs.* 2009–2010).

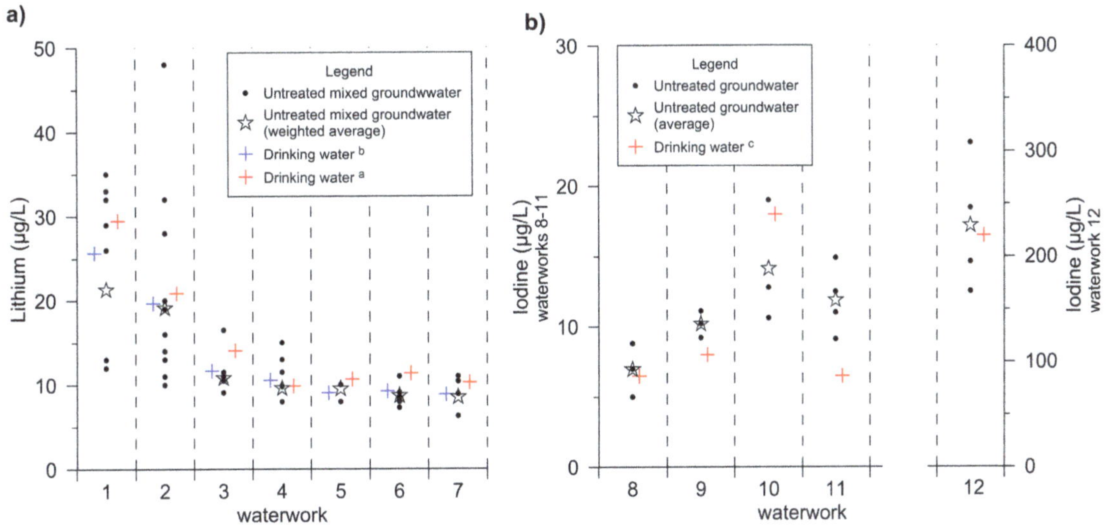

Figure 5. (**a**) Lithium concentrations in untreated mixed groundwater from well sites (black dots) at seven waterworks in the Copenhagen area and in treated drinking water (data from two studies are used: [a] the ICP-MS data reported here and in [3] (red +), [b] unreported AAS data provided by the waterworks (blue +; see Supplementary materials for further detail). (**b**) Comparison between I concentrations in drinking water (red +) and untreated groundwater from wells (black dots) of five waterworks located in Jylland ([c] data from 2012 reported in [70]).

These results imply that the Li concentration in DW at the given waterworks can be assumed to be stable over time. Another interesting aspect is that most of the large waterworks extract water from many wells, often grouped in well sites. As there are differences in I, Li, and Sr concentrations in the abstracted groundwater (Figure 5a, black dots), abstraction volumes and pumping strategies will govern the resulting concentrations in the treated DW. An illustration of the differences in Li concentrations in mixed groundwater at/between the well sites of seven waterworks in the Copenhagen area and the Li concentrations in treated DW at these waterworks is also presented in Figure 5a. Further, the results imply that there is no Li removal or enrichment during the treatment. A similar comparison between groundwater and treated DW is made for I at five waterworks located in Jylland (Figure 5b) based on the 2012 data reported in [70]. This comparison implies that at least at some waterworks, I can be partially removed by treatment (DW-I is lower than the groundwater-I concentrations). The issue of the effect of treatment and the temporal variation of the I concentrations in DW is further discussed in [3]. To our best knowledge, no such analysis exists on Sr in Danish DW or groundwater.

Another limitation of this exposure analysis (or future epidemiological studies based on these data) is that some misclassification could have occurred, as some of the households/residents included here may be supplied by private wells. There is also uncertainty associated with the concentrations in the supply areas where more than one waterworks distributes DW to the consumers (see Figure 1). Yet another issue is connected to the fact that we used I, Li, and Sr concentrations in DW at the exit of the waterworks but not much is known about whether these elements are involved in chemical processes in the distribution system before the DW reaches the consumer. Further investigations are needed in order to evaluate the effect of these misclassifications and/or uncertainties.

Last but not least, some limitations with respect to the exposure levels are due to the data on geographical location of the residency addresses. For the purposes of carrying out an epidemiological study on possible health effects, it is important to take the residential history of each studied individual into account. This is possible using the DCRS database. However, the exposure estimation will still be associated with uncertainty due to e.g., individuals commuting to areas with different exposure characteristics. Data from Statistics Denmark for 2013 shows that 470,950 people or about 31% of the employed Danish population commute less than 5 km, whereas about 7.6% commute more than 50 km (202,289 people).

4. Conclusions

This study revealed significant spatial variations in I, Li, and Sr concentrations in Danish DW representing approximately 45% of the annual groundwater abstraction for DW purposes. A general east-west trend of relatively high concentrations in the eastern part and lower ones in the western part of the country was observed. However, there are element-specific smaller-scale differences, so the general trend should be interpreted cautiously. The exposure to different I (Li, Sr) levels covers about 45.3% (44.6%) of all residents (2008) and 42.7% (41.8%) of all households (2012) that were supplied with DW by the investigated waterworks (I: 144; Sr and Li: 139). The spatial distribution of I, Li, and Sr in DW results in an exposure contrast of these elements. The largest part of the population (about 40%) is exposed to 14–20 μg I/L, 17–30.7 μg Li/L, and 2–14 mg Sr/L. The rest of the population covered here is exposed to both higher and lower I concentrations from DW. For Li and Sr, this range is at the upper end of the observed concentrations; thus the rest of the population is exposed only to lower Li and Sr concentrations in DW. The results presented here show that there is a great potential for future epidemiological studies on the long-term (lifelong, chronic) effects of exposure to I, Li, and Sr from DW as single elements. Additionally, it is also possible to include other relevant elements.

Acknowledgments

We would like to thank Malene Thygesen and the Centre for Integrated Register-Based Research at Aarhus University (CIRRAU) for the provision of the geocoded Danish addresses, and, Ann-Katrin Pedersen from HOFOR (The Greater Copenhagen Water Supply Company) for performing the AAS data analyses on lithium (Figure 5a and Supplementary materials), and providing these data for the present study. The rest of the water chemistry data as well as some of the data on supply areas was collected as part of a GEOCENTER (Denmark) project (2011–2014) funded by the Geological Survey of Denmark and Greenland (GEUS) and Aarhus University (Denmark). The authors express their sincere gratitude to the rest of the GEOCENTER project participants.

Author Contributions

The linking of the different data sources and the exposure analyses was done by D.D.V. and J.S. The IDW and the cluster analyses were performed by N.N.K. and A.K.E. The data for Figure 5 on Li in the groundwater and drinking water, as well as interpretation was provided by L.F.J. B.H. and S.M.K. provided background information and supervised the project. D.D.V compiled the initial version of this manuscript, with all authors contributing by writing different sections of it. All authors have equally participated in the revisions and the final editing of this text prior to its submission.

References

1. Villanueva, C.M.; Kogevinas, M.; Cordier, S.; Templeton, M.R.; Vermeulen, R.; Nuckols, J.R.; Nieuwenhuijsen, M.J.; Levallois, P. Assessing exposure and health consequences of chemicals in drinking water: Current state of knowledge and research needs. *Environ. Health Perspect.* **2014**, *122*, 213–221.
2. Reimann, C.; Birke, M. *Geochemistry of European Bottled Water*; Borntraeger Science Publishers: Stuttgart, Germany, 2010.
3. Voutchkova, D.D.; Ernstsen, V.; Hansen, B.; Sørensen, B.L.; Zhang, C.; Kristiansen, S.M. Assessment of spatial variation in drinking water iodine and its implications for dietary intake: A new conceptual model for Denmark. *Sci. Total Environ.* **2014**, *493*, 432–444.
4. Voutchkova, D.D.; Kristiansen, S.M.; Hansen, B.; Ernstsen, V.; Sørensen, B.L.; Esbensen, K.H. Iodine concentrations in Danish groundwater: Historical data assessment 1933–2011. *Environ. Geochem. Health* **2014**, *36*, 1151–1164.
5. Voutchkova, D.D.; Hansen, B.; Ernstsen, V.; Kristiansen, S.M. Hydro-geochemical characterisation of Danish groundwaters in relation to iodine. Paper III in PhD thesis [70].
6. Kesler, S.E.; Gruber, P.W.; Medina, P.A.; Keoleian, G.A.; Everson, M.P.; Wallington, T.J. Global lithium resources: Relative importance of pegmatite, brine and other deposits. *Ore Geol. Rev.* **2012**, *48*, 55–69.

7. Hinsby, K.; Rasmussen, E.S.; Henriksen, H.J. European Reference Aquifers: The Miocene Sand Aquifers of Western Denmark. In *Report for the EU Research Project ('BASELINE'): Natural Baseline Quality of European Groundwater: A basis for Aquifer Management*; Geological Survey of Denmark and Greenland (GEUS): Copenhagen, Denmark, 2003; pp. 1–18.
8. Bonnesen, E.P.; Larsen, F.; Sonnenborg, T.O.; Klitten, K.; Stemmerik, L. Deep saltwater in Chalk of North-West Europe: Origin, interface characteristics and development over geological time. *Hydrogeol. J.* **2009**, *17*, 1643–1663.
9. Ramsay, L. *Strontium i Grundvand & Drikkevand i Roskilde Amt*; Roskilde Amt: Roskilde, Denmark, 2005. (In Danish)
10. Danish Ministry of the Environment (DME). *Bekendtgørelse om Vandkvalitet og Tilsyn Med Vandforsyningsanlæg BEK nr 292 af 26/03/2014*; Miljøministeriet: Copenhagen, Denmark, 2014. (In Danish)
11. World Health Organization (WHO). *Iodine Deficiency in Europe: A Continuing Public Health Problem*; World Health Organization, United Nations Children's Fund: Geneva, Switzerland, 2007; pp. 1–86.
12. World Health Organization (WHO). *Assessment of Iodine Deficiency Disorders and Monitoring Their Elimination: A Guide for Programme Managers*, 3rd ed.; World Health Organization: Geneva, Switzerland, 2007; pp. 1–97.
13. Soldin, O.P. Iodine Status Reflected by Urinary Concentrations: Comparison with the USA and Other Countries. In *Comprehensive Handbook of Iodine: Nutritional, Biochemical, Pathological and Therapeutic Aspects*; Preedy, V.R., Burrow, G.N., Watson, R., Eds.; Elsevier: Amsterdam, The Netherlands, 2009; pp 1129–1137.
14. Zimmermann, M.B. Iodine deficiency in industrialized countries. *Clin. Endocrinol.* **2011**, *75*, 287–288.
15. Zimmermann, M.B.; Andersson, M. Update on iodine status worldwide. *Curr. Opin. Endocrinol. Diabetes Obes.* **2012**, *19*, 382–387.
16. Pearce, E.N.; Andersson, M.; Zimmermann, M.B. Global iodine nutrition: Where do we stand in 2013? *Thyroid* **2013**, *23*, 523–528.
17. World Health Organization (WHO). *Salt Reduction and Iodine Fortification Strategies in Public Health: Report of a Joint Technical Meeting*; World Health Organization: Geneva, Switzerland, 2014; pp. 1–34.
18. Speeckaert, M.M.; Speeckaert, R.; Wierckx, K.; Delanghe, J.R.; Kaufman, J.M. Value and pitfalls in iodine fortification and supplementation in the 21st century. *Br. J. Nutr.* **2011**, *106*, 964–973.
19. Campbell, N.; Dary, O.; Cappuccio, F.P.; Neufeld, L.M.; Harding, K.B.; Zimmermanne, M.B. Collaboration to optimize dietary intakes of salt and iodine: A critical but overlooked public health issue. *Bull. World Health Organ.* **2012**, *90*, 73–74.
20. Fuge, R. Soils and Iodine Deficiency. In *Essentials of Medical Geology: Impacts of the Natural Environment on Public Health*; Selinus, O., Alloway, B.J., Centeno, J.A., Finkelman, R.B., Fuge, R., Lindh, U., Smedley, P., Eds.; Elsevier: Amsterdam, The Netherlands, 2005; pp. 417–433.
21. Laurberg, P.; Jørgensen, T.; Perrild, H.; Ovesen, L.; Knudsen, N.; Pedersen, I.B.; Rasmussen, L.B.; Carlé, A.; Vejbjerg, P. The Danish investigation on iodine intake and thyroid disease, DanThyr: Status and perspectives. *Eur. J. Endocrinol.* **2006**, *155*, 219–228.

22. Pedersen, A.N.; Fagt, S.; Groth, M.V.; Christensen, T.; Biltoft-Jensen, A.; Matthiessen, J.; Andersen, N.L.; Kørup, K.; Hartkopp, H.; Ygil, K.H.; Hinsch, H.J.; Saxholt, E.; Trolle, E. *Danskernes Kostvaner 2003–2008*; National Food Institute, Technical University of Denmark (DTU Fødevareinstituttet): Kongens Lyngby, Denmark, 2010; pp. 1–200. (In Danish)
23. Rasmussen, L.B.; Larsen, E.H.; Ovesen, L. Iodine content in drinking water and other beverages in Denmark. *Eur. J. Clin. Nutr.* **2000**, *54*, 57–60.
24. Rasmussen, L.B.; Ovesen, L.; Bülow, I.; Jørgensen, T.; Knudsen, N.; Laurberg, P.; Perrild, H. Dietary iodine intake and urinary iodine excretion in a Danish population: Effect of geography, supplements and food choice. *Br. J. Nutr.* **2002**, *87*, 61–69.
25. Pedersen, K.M.; Laurberg, P.; Nøhr, S.; Jørgensen, A.; Andersen, S. Iodine in drinking water varies by more than 100-fold in Denmark. Importance for iodine content of infant formulas. *Eur. J. Endocrinol.* **1999**, *140*, 400–403.
26. Shen, H.M.; Liu, S.J.; Sun, D.J.; Zhang, S.B.; Su, X.H.; Shen, Y.F.; Han, H.P. Geographical distribution of drinking-water with high iodine level and association between high iodine level in drinking-water and goitre: A Chinese national investigation. *Br. J. Nutr.* **2011**, *106*, 243–247.
27. Lv, S.; Wang, Y.; Xu, D.; Rutherford, S.; Chong, Z.; Du, Y.; Jia, L.; Zhao, J. Drinking water contributes to excessive iodine intake among children in Hebei, China. *Eur. J. Clin. Nutr.* **2013**, *67*, 961–965.
28. Del Grande, C.; Muti, M.; Musetti, L.; Corsi, M.; Pergentini, I.; Turri, M.; Corsini, G.U.; Dell'Osso, L. Lithium and valproate in manic and mixed states: A naturalistic prospective study. *J. Psychopathol.* **2014**, *20*, 6–10.
29. Grunze, H.; Vieta, E.; Goodwin, G.M.; Bowden, C.; Licht, R.W.; Möller, H.J.; Kasper, S. The world federation of societies of biological psychiatry (WFSBP) guidelines for the biological treatment of bipolar disorders: Update 2012 on the long-term treatment of bipolar disorder. *World J. Biol. Psychiatry* **2013**, *14*, 154–219.
30. Cipriani, A.; Pretty, H.; Hawton, K.; Geddes, J.R. Lithium in the prevention of suicidal behavior and all-cause mortality in patients with mood disorders: A systematic review of randomized trials. *Am. J. Psychiatry* **2005**, *162*, 1805–1819.
31. Baldessarini, R.J.; Tondo, L.; Davis, P.; Pompili, M.; Goodwin, F.K.; Hennen, J. Decreased risk of suicides and attempts during long-term lithium treatment: A meta-analytic review. *Bipolar Disord.* **2006**, *8*, 625–639.
32. Schrauzer, G.N.; Shrestha, K.P. Lithium in drinking water and the incidences of crimes, suicides, and arrests related to drug addictions. *Biol. Trace Elem. Res.* **1990**, *25*, 105–113.
33. Ohgami, H.; Terao, T.; Shiotsuki, I.; Ishii, N.; Iwata, N. Lithium levels in drinking water and risk of suicide. *Br. J. Psychiatry* **2009**, *194*, 464–465.
34. Blüml, V.; Regier, M.D.; Hlavin, G.; Rockett, I.R.H.; König, F.; Vyssoki, B.; Bschor, T.; Kapusta, N.D. Lithium in the public water supply and suicide mortality in Texas. *J. Psychiatr. Res.* **2013**, *47*, 407–411.
35. Helbich, M.; Leitner, M.; Kapusta, N.D. Geospatial examination of lithium in drinking water and suicide mortality. *Int. J. Health Geogr.* **2012**, *11*, 1–8.

36. Kapusta, N.D.; Mossaheb, N.; Etzersdorfer, E.; Hlavin, G.; Thau, K.; Willeit, M.; Praschak-Rieder, N.; Sonneck, G.; Leithner-Dziubas, K. Lithium in drinking water and suicide mortality. *Br. J. Psychiatry* **2011**, *198*, 346–350.
37. Kabacs, N.; Memon, A.; Obinwa, T.; Stochl, J.; Perez, J. Lithium in drinking water and suicide rates across the East of England. *Br. J. Psychiatry* **2011**, *198*, 406–407.
38. Kovacsics, C.E.; Gottesman, I.I.; Gould, T.D. Lithium's Antisuicidal Efficacy: Elucidation of Neurobiological Targets Using Endophenotype Strategies. *Annu. Rev. Pharmacol. Toxicol.* **2009**, *49*, 175–198.
39. Hernlund, E.; Svedbom, A.; Ivergård, M.; Compston, J.; Cooper, C.; Stenmark, J.; McCloskey, E.V.; Jönsson, B.; Kanis, J.A. Osteoporosis in the European Union: Medical management, epidemiology and economic burden. A report prepared in collaboration with the International Osteoporosis Foundation (IOF) and the European Federation of Pharmaceutical Industry Associations (EFPIA). *Arch. Osteoporos.* **2013**, *8*, doi:10.1007/s11657-013-0136-1.
40. Svedbom, A.; Hernlund, E.; Ivergård, M.; Compston, J.; Cooper, C.; Stenmark, J.; McCloskey, E.V.; Jönsson, B.; Kanis, J.A. Osteoporosis in the European Union: A compendium of country-specific reports. *Arch. Osteoporos.* **2013**, *8*, doi:10.1007/s11657-013-0137-0.
41. Skoryna, S.C. Effects of oral supplementation with stable strontium. *Can. Med. Assoc. J.* **1981**, *125*, 703–712.
42. Dahl, S.G.; Allain, P.; Marie, P.J.; Mauras, Y.; Boivin, G.; Ammann, P.; Tsouderos, Y.; Delmas, P.D.; Christiansen, C. Incorporation and distribution of strontium in bone. *Bone* **2001**, *28*, 446–453.
43. Watts, P.; Howe, P. *Strontium and Strontium Compounds (Concise International Chemical Assessment Document, No 77)*; World Health Organization (WHO): Geneva, Switzerland, 2010; pp. 1–67.
44. Agency for Toxic Substances and Disease Registry (ATSDR). *Toxicological Profile for Strontium*; Agency for Toxic Substances and Disease Registry, Division of Toxicology/Toxicology Information Branch: Atlanta, GA, USA, 2004.
45. Shahnazari, M.; Sharkey, N.A.; Fosmire, G.J.; Leach, R.M. Effects of strontium on bone strength, density, volume, and microarchitecture in laying hens. *J. Bone Miner. Res.* **2006**, *21*, 1696–1703.
46. Dawson, E.B.; Frey, M.J.; Moore, T.D.; McGanity, W.J. Relationship of metal metabolism to vascular disease mortality rates in Texas. *Am. J. Clin. Nutr.* **1978**, *31*, 1188–1197.
47. Polyakova, E.V. Strontium in water-supply sources of arkhangelsk region and its impact on human health. *Hum. Ecol.* **2012**, *2*, 9–14.
48. Curzon, M.E. The relation between caries prevalence and strontium concentrations in drinking water, plaque, and surface enamel. *J. Dent. Res.* **1985**, *64*, 1386–1388.
49. Rygaard, M.; Albrechtsen, H.-J. *Redegørelse om Sundhedseffekter af Blødgøring i København Specielt Med Fokus på Caries*; Technical University of Denmark (DTU): Kongens Lyngby, Denmark, 2012. (In Danish)
50. Geological Survey of Denmark and Greenland (GEUS). JUPITER—Danmarks geologiske & hydrologiske database 2011. Available online: http://www.geus.dk/DK/data-maps/jupiter/Sider/default.aspx (accessed on 6 December 2012).

51. Danish Nature Agency (DNA). Kvaliteten af Det Danske Drikkevand for Perioden 2008–2010. Available online: http://naturstyrelsen.dk/media/nst/Attachments/Indberetningsrapportdrikkevand20082010.pdf (accessed on 17 February 2015).
52. Sørensen, B.L.; Møller, R.R. Evaluation of total groundwater abstraction from public waterworks in Denmark using principal component analysis. *Geol. Surv. Den. Greenl. Bull.* **2013**, *28*, 37–40.
53. Union of European Soft Drinks Associations (UNESDA). Sales Volume Statistics by Industry Analyst "Canadean". Available online: http://www.unesda.eu/products-ingredients/consumption/ (accessed on 17 February 2015).
54. Marcussen, H.; Holm, P.E.; Hansen, H.C.B. Composition, Flavor, Chemical Foodsafety, and Consumer Preferences of Bottled Water. *Compr. Rev. Food Sci. Food Saf.* **2013**, *12*, 333–352.
55. Danish Nature Agency (DNA). *Videregående Vandbehandling*; Danish Nature Agency (Naturstyrelsen), Ministry of the Environment (Miljøministeriet): Copenhagen, Denmark, 2012; pp. 1–65. (In Danish)
56. Voutchkova, D.D.; Hansen, B.; Ernstsen, V.; Kristiansen, S.M. Design of a nationwide drinking-water sampling campaign for assessment of dietary iodine intake and human health outcomes. Technical Note I in PhD thesis [70].
57. Schullehner, J.; Hansen, B. Nitrate exposure from drinking water in Denmark over the last 35 years. *Environ. Res. Lett.* **2014**, *9*, 095001.
58. Thygesen, M. Geocoding of All Danish Addresses from the Residence Database (Version 2). Available online: http://cirrau.au.dk/data-resources/data-documentation/ (accessed on 17 February 2015).
59. Pedersen, C.B. The Danish civil registration system. *Scand. J. Public Health* **2011**, *39*, 22–25.
60. Bivand, R.S.; Pebesma, E.J.; Gómez-Rubio, V. *Applied Spatial Data Analysis with R*; Springer: Berlin, Germany, 2008.
61. Waller, L.A.; Gotway, C.A. *Applied Spatial Statistics for Public Health Data*; John Wiley & Sons: Hoboken, NJ, USA, 2004.
62. Pfeiffer, D.; Robinson, T.; Stevenson, M.; Stevens, K.B.; Rogers, D.J.; Clements, A.C. *Spatial Analysis in Epidemiology*; Oxford University Press: Oxford, UK, 2008.
63. Kulldorff, M. A spatial scan statistic. *Commun. Stat. Theory Methods* **1997**, *26*, 1481–1496.
64. Kulldorff, M.; Huang, L.; Konty, K. A scan statistic for continuous data based on the normal probability model. *Int. J. Health Geogr.* **2009**, *8*, doi:10.1186/1476-072X-8-58.
65. Andersen, S.; Lauberg, P. The Nature of Iodine in Drinking Water. In *Comprehensive Handbook of Iodine Nutritional, Biochemical, Pathological and Therapeutic Aspects*; Preedy, V.R., Burrow, G.N., Watson, R., Eds.; Academic Press: London, UK, 2009; pp. 125–134.
66. Thygesen, L.C.; Daasnes, C.; Thaulow, I.; Brønnum-Hansen, H. Introduction to Danish (nationwide) registers on health and social issues: Structure, access, legislation, and archiving. *Scand. J. Public Health* **2011**, *39*, 12–16.
67. Dahl, C.; Søgaard, A.J.; Tell, G.S.; Flaten, T.P.; Hongve, D.; Omsland, T.K.; Holvik, K.; Meyer, H.E.; Aamodt, G. Nationwide data on municipal drinking water and hip fracture: Could calcium and magnesium be protective? A NOREPOS study. *Bone* **2013**, *57*, 84–91.

68. Kirkeskov, L.; Kristiansen, E.; Bøggild, H.; Von Platen-Hallermund, F.; Sckerl, H.; Carlsen, A.; Larsen, M.J.; Poulsen, S. The association between fluoride in drinking water and dental caries in Danish children. Linking data from health registers, environmental registers and administrative registers. *Community Dent. Oral Epidemiol.* **2010**, *38*, 206–212.
69. GEUS. Interactive Map on Water Hardness as an Average per Municipality. Available online: http://www.geus.dk/DK/data-maps/Sider/haardhedskort-dk.aspx (accessed on 17 February 2015).
70. Voutchkova, D.D. Iodine in Danish Groundwater and Drinking Water. Ph.D. Thesis, Aarhus University, Aarhus, Denmark, 2014.

11

Assessment of Geogenic Contaminants in Water Co-Produced with Coal Seam Gas Extraction in Queensland, Australia: Implications for Human Health Risk

William Stearman [1,*], Mauricio Taulis [1], James Smith [1] and Maree Corkeron [1,2]

1 School of Earth, Environmental and Biological Sciences, Queensland University of Technology, R Block, 2 George St, Brisbane, QLD 4001, Australia; E-Mails: mauricio.taulis@qut.edu.au (M.T.); jj.smith@qut.edu.au (J.S.); maree.corkeron@qut.edu.au (M.C.)

2 School of Earth and Environmental Sciences, James Cook University, Townsville, QLD 4810, Australia

* Author to whom correspondence should be addressed; E-Mail: w.stearman@qut.edu.au;

Abstract: Organic compounds in Australian coal seam gas produced water (CSG water) are poorly understood despite their environmental contamination potential. In this study, the presence of some organic substances is identified from government-held CSG water-quality data from the Bowen and Surat Basins, Queensland. These records revealed the presence of polycyclic aromatic hydrocarbons (PAHs) in 27% of samples of CSG water from the Walloon Coal Measures at concentrations <1 μg/L, and it is likely these compounds leached from *in situ* coals. PAHs identified from wells include naphthalene, phenanthrene, chrysene and dibenz[a,h]anthracene. In addition, the likelihood of coal-derived organic compounds leaching to groundwater is assessed by undertaking toxicity leaching experiments using coal rank and water chemistry as variables. These tests suggest higher molecular weight PAHs (including benzo[a]pyrene) leach from higher rank coals, whereas lower molecular weight PAHs leach at greater concentrations from lower rank coal. Some of the identified organic compounds have carcinogenic or health risk potential, but they are unlikely to be acutely toxic at the observed concentrations which are almost negligible (largely due to the hydrophobicity of such compounds). Hence, this study will be useful to practitioners assessing CSG water related environmental and health risk.

Keywords: coalbed methane; coal seam gas; coalbed natural gas; co-produced water; polycyclic aromatic hydrocarbons

---

1. Introduction

The commercial production of CSG (coal seam gas, also known as "coalbed methane", "coal seam methane" or "coalbed natural gas") in the Bowen and Surat Basins, Queensland (QLD) has emerged as an important unconventional natural gas supply and cleaner energy alternative than conventional fossil fuels. CSG production requires the withdrawal of groundwater from coal seams and associated strata to depressurize the coal, allowing natural gas (mainly methane) held in coal micropores to desorb and flow through the coal's fractures to a production well for extraction. The groundwater withdrawn from coal measures is referred to here as "CSG water", but is also commonly known as "produced water", "formation water" or "associated water". In 2009–2010, an estimated 17 gigalitres (GL) of CSG water was extracted from Queensland gas fields supplying the domestic gas market [1]. As CSG production increases to supply international liquefied natural gas (LNG) markets, annual volumes of extracted CSG water are estimated to increase to over ten times the 2009/2010 production rate (e.g., to about 200 GL/year by 2030) [2].

CSG water is distinct from "flowback water", which is the fluid recovered from a gas production well soon after water, sand and other chemical additives have been injected during hydraulic fracturing ("fracking"). Where hydraulic fracturing occurs, the "flowback water" is extracted and its volume is usually 110%–150% the volume of the injected fracturing fluid considering the contribution of formation water. Any produced water after the 110%–150% volume recovery of flowback water should be considered CSG water [3]. Furthermore, distinctions should be made between coal seam gas and other unconventional gas resources such as shale gas and underground coal gasification (UCG), to avoid incorrectly applying environmental management strategies which are specific to other types of technology in the gas industry.

The withdrawal and disposal of CSG water is perhaps the most important environmental management issue associated with CSG production, due to the large volumes of water being extracted, its specific water quality and its natural variations [4,5]. The often highly sodic and alkaline chemical composition of CSG water in Queensland presents potential risks to surface soils, shallow aquifers and watersheds [6,7]. Under the *Environmental Protection Act 1994*, CSG water is defined as a waste product of gas extraction. However, the Queensland government (*Department of Environment and Heritage Protection*) strongly encourages the beneficial reuse of CSG water for the environment, landholder and rural communities as best management practice [8].

1.1. Co-Produced Water and Human Health

Whereas attention has been given to assessing environmental risk related to CSG water, little scientific consideration is given to human health impacts. Community groups opposed to CSG development often make unqualified public statements insinuating human toxicity risk from CSG production water (e.g., [9]). Additionally, several studies [10–13] hypothesize the link between coal derived organic compounds in rural groundwater and kidney disease (Balkan Endemic Nephropathy, BEN). However, very few studies directly assess CSG water composition and its potential for adverse human health impacts. Closing this knowledge gap would best constrain the risk (if any) to landholders and communities in QLD that access water supply from coal associated aquifers (e.g., Walloon Coal Measures), communities receiving potable supply from treated CSG water [14] and stakeholders who may be exposed directly or indirectly to CSG water [15].

Most studies of CSG water quality focus on its inorganic composition, including salinity, high sodicity and trace metal occurrence [16–25]. For example, the vast majority of QLD CSG waters contain elevated Na^+, HCO_3^- and sometimes Cl^- as the dominant ions, have fresh to brackish salinity (200–10,000 mg/L) and neutral to basic pH (pH 7–9) [6,26]. However, the concentrations of the major ions in CSG water are often site or basin specific, reflecting localized lithological and hydrological controls.

Less literature exists regarding the organic composition of CSG water. Coal is a complex, organic sedimentary rock that contains many compounds that are known, or have the potential to be, hazardous to human health. These include polycyclic aromatic hydrocarbons (PAHs), heterocyclic compounds, phenolics, biphenyls and aromatic amines. Since CSG water is groundwater in contact with coal, there is potential for leaching of trace levels of organic compounds from those coals. Among the more important factors that influence the inventory of potentially mobile organic compounds in coal are maceral type, coal rank, coal age and the nature of microbial degradation acting on those coals [27]. While there is a theoretical likelihood for potentially toxic organic compounds in CSG water, studies testing and discussing this are scarce (see [27–29]).

In Queensland, publicly available baseline and monitoring data regarding organic substances in CSG water is mainly limited to company environmental impact assessments and consultant reports [30,31]. These data are often limited to the common aromatic compound classes—PAHs, phenolics and BTEXs (benzene, toluene, ethylbenzene and xylene)—which are all usually reported below detection limits from well and holding pond samples.

The organic composition of CSG water from the Powder River Basin (WY, USA) was described as part of a larger study on the potential health effects of coal derived organics [28]. At ultra-trace detection levels (<1 μg/L), the most commonly observed group of organic compounds from the Powder River Basin CSG waters were the PAHs (with total PAH concentrations ranging up to 23 μg/L), along with trace levels of phenols, biphenyls, heterocyclic compounds and aromatic amines. Similar compounds have been reported (at trace levels) in CSG water from other US gas plays such as the Black Warrior Basin, Tongue River Basin, Williston Basin and Illinois Basin [32]. In addition to the semi-volatile aromatics, BTEX compounds have been detected in CSG water from wells targeting the San Juan and Raton basins in the United States, with benzene concentrations ranging from below detection limits, up to 500 μg/L [26]. BTEX compounds have also been reported from eight CSG exploration wells in the Surat Basin, but little specific information is publicly available [27].

In assessing human health risk, presence of chemical compounds alone does not automatically equate to higher risk. Concentrations, bioavailability and exposure pathways are equally important variables impacting risk but identification of potential toxins in source material (CSG water) are the first requirement in risk assessment. The high density of CSG production wells in the Surat and Bowen Basins of southern Queensland provides an excellent opportunity to characterize the organic composition of CSG water. This study determines the concentration and types of some likely coal-derived organic compounds in CSG water from production wells targeting Jurassic Walloon Coal Measures of the Surat Basin and the Permian Bandanna Formation of the Bowen Basin from a 2010 dataset. In addition, in order to test for leachable organic compounds from coal and therefore potential contaminants in CSG water, we undertook a series of leachate experiments on fresh coal samples of differing rank. Preliminary experimental results are presented to characterize the release of aromatic compounds from coal to water. These findings are pertinent to future human health and environmental risk assessment as the first step in clarifying the presence of potential toxins.

1.2. Study Areas

The Permian to Triassic Bowen Basin is the northern extension of the Bowen-Gunnedah-Sydney Basin system of eastern Australia. To the west the Bowen Basin is linked to the Galilee and Cooper Basins and to the south, it is overlain by the Surat Basin (Figure 1). CSG fields currently in production in Queensland include both Bowen and Surat Basin coal seams (Bandanna Formation and Walloon Coal Measures, respectively).

Figure 1. Coal seam gas (CSG) water study areas and localities for coal samples used in leaching experiments. The red boxes mark high production areas where CSG water is extracted from the Bandanna Formation (Bowen Basin) and Walloon Coal Measures (Surat Basin). The desktop CSG water quality data was taken from these areas.

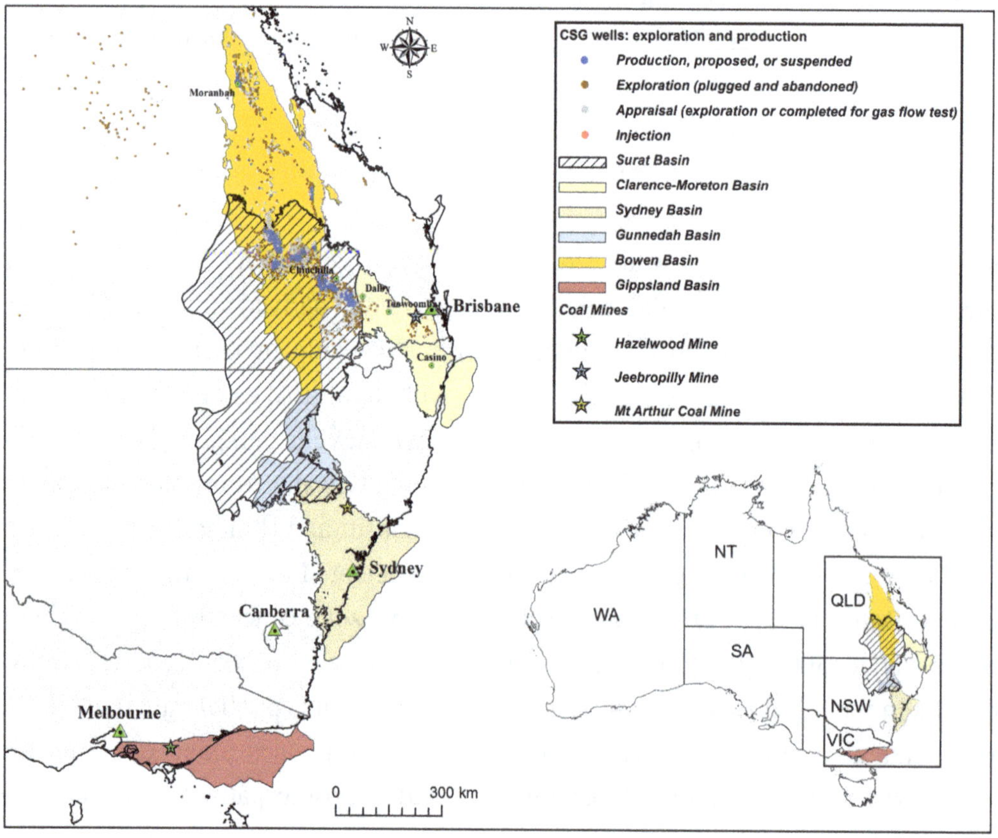

1.2.1. Bandanna Formation, Bowen Basin

The late Permian Bandanna Formation consists of siltstone, lithic sandstone, carbonaceous shale and coal. The depositional setting of the Bandanna Formation is interpreted as a large fluvio-deltaic system infilling a lake, or a land-locked sea, which is recorded in the underlying Black Alley Shale [33]. The seams targeted for gas production in the study area consist of high vitrinite coals (up to 70%) with a mean maximum vitrinite reflectance (Rv, max) of approximately 0.9% [34]. The Bandanna coals of the study area are high volatile-A (HvA) bituminous to medium volatile (Mv) bituminous in rank and in general, they occur in relatively thicker and more laterally extensive seams than that of the Walloon Coal Measures of the eastern Surat Basin [35,36].

1.2.2. Walloon Coal Measures, Eastern Surat Basin

The Walloon Coal Measures consists of lithic sandstones, siltstones and claystones with thin coal seams [37,38]. The depositional setting of the Walloon Coal Measures was an alluvial plain, traversed by meandering streams. Coal measures occurred mainly as swampy overbank and flood plain deposits. Coal seams thicknesses are variable and are often split as a result of from constant stream channel switching [37,39,40]. Coal seams targeted for CSG production are the Juandah and Taroom coal measures which are separated by the Tangalooma Sandstone and unconformably overlain by the Springbok Sandstone. The coals of the study area are sub-bituminous to high volatile-C (HvC) bituminous with an Rv, max between 0.35% and 0.65% [36,38]. CSG well depths of the study area are 451–825 m and rank increases with depth [36,38].

2. Methods

2.1. CSG Water Organic Analyses

Desktop analysis of government-held water quality data from gas producing wells was conducted to characterise some organic compounds in CSG water. The data were originally collected by the CSG industry and supplied to QLD Government as a regulatory requirement. It is assumed that all relevant quality assurance and control checks were conducted by the samplers and analysts that produced these datasets, although chain of custody data were not available.

The dataset included organic analyses from 58 production wells targeting the Permian Bandanna Formation from 2009 to 2010 and 47 production wells from the Walloon Coal Measures from 2010. Additional organic analyses were from the holding pond of the Walloon Coal Measures production area from 2010. Analytes are common organic compound classes of environmental importance (e.g., PAHs, phenolics and BTEXs).

2.2. Leaching Experiments

A series of leaching experiments was undertaken on a range of coals of differing rank in order to determine the potential leachability of semi-volatile PAHs and phenolic compounds. The patterns of aromatic compounds in coal change with increasing coal maturity [41–43] and therefore the water leachable aromatic fraction may also change. The experiments aimed to assess the difference in mobility of PAHs and phenolics from coals of different rank (lignite to bituminous) when leached using different water types (acidic to basic). The toxicity characteristic leaching procedure (TCLP) is a standard method (United States Environmental Protection Agency, USEPA, Washington, DC, USA) to determine the mobility of both organic and inorganic analytes present in liquid and solid materials (*USEPA Method No. 1311*) and was here adapted and applied to solid coal samples. Table 1 shows the leaching conditions used in this study. In addition to TCLPs performed with the standard acetic acid fluid, adapted TCLP experiments were also performed with deionized water and a synthetic CSG water solution. Coal samples were leached in triplicate with deionized water including a batch of tests conducted with powdered coal samples (<400 μm). Coal samples were leached in duplicate with the synthetic CSG water (Table 1).

Table 1. Leaching experiments and conditions. All experiments were performed at room temperature (25 °C) for 18.5 h.

Sample#	Coal	Leachant
A-LIG-1	Lignite	TCLP Extraction fluid # 1
A-SUB-1	HvA-bituminous	TCLP Extraction fluid # 1
A-BIT-1	Mv-bituminous	TCLP Extraction fluid # 1
N-LIG-1	Lignite	Deionised water
N-SUB-1	HvA-bituminous	Deionised water
N-BIT-1	Mv-bituminous	Deionised water
B-LIG-1	Lignite	Synthetic CSG
B-SUB-1	HvA-bituminous	Synthetic CSG
B-BIT-1	Mv-bituminous	Synthetic CSG
N-LIG-2	Lignite	Deionised water
N-SUB-2	HvA-bituminous	Deionised water
N-BIT-2	Mv-bituminous	Deionised water
B-LIG-2	Lignite	Synthetic CSG
B-SUB-2	HvA-bituminous	Synthetic CSG
B-BIT-2	Mv-bituminous	Synthetic CSG
P-LIG-3	Lignite *	Deionised water
P-SUB-3	HvA-bituminous *	Deionised water
P-BIT-3	Mv-bituminous *	Deionised water
NB-1	n/a	Deionised water
BB-1	n/a	Synthetic CSG

Notes: n/a = control samples, * powdered (<400 μm) coal samples.

The deionized water leachant for all leach experiments was Milli-Q ultra-filtered water. The synthesized CSG water used was mixed according to the observed ionic character of production waters. Most often, the dominant ions in QLD CSG water are sodium (Na^+), bicarbonate (HCO^-_3) and chloride (Cl^-). To achieve this Na-HCO_3-Cl chemical type, analytical grade sodium chloride (NaCl) and sodium bicarbonate ($NaHCO_3$) were dissolved in Milli-Q water. The final pH of the synthetic CSG water used in each extraction varied from 8.6 to 8.9 with an average total dissolved solids (TDS) concentration of 1350 mg/L.

All glassware used in the leaching experiments was cleaned carefully to minimize contamination. Prior to use in leach experiments or filtrations of leachates: glassware and Teflon lined caps were hot soaked in detergent overnight, scrubbed and rinsed successively in tap water, deionised water and acetone. If any excessive contamination was observed on the equipment, it was soaked overnight in 20% nitric acid prior to the regular rinsing process. Glassware and glass fiber filters were baked in an oven overnight at 150 °C before use in experiments and sample collection the next day. Glassware used to collect filtered samples was pre-contaminated with a small volume of filtrate and that volume was discarded before additional filtering took place. Controls were treated in the same way as samples during the experiments.

Extraction and Analysis

All TCLP leachates were vacuum filtered through 0.6–0.8 μm glass fiber filters with glass and porcelain filtration apparatus and collected in amber glass bottles with Teflon-lined caps. In brief, all filtered TCLP samples were stored at <4 °C for sample preservation prior to liquid/liquid extraction with dichloromethane for analysis. Analysis was conducted using a *Finnigan SSq 710* gas chromatography/mass spectrometer operating in full scan mode according to *Queensland Health and Forensic Scientific Services* (QHFSS) SOP No. 15639 for PAHs and phenols.

2.3. Coal Samples

All coal samples used in the leach experiments were taken from open-cut coal operations in eastern Australia. The coal samples and their properties are shown in Table 2. The surface portion of each coal sample was chipped away to maximize fresh exposed coal.

Table 2. Coal samples used for leaching experiments and basic properties. Figure 1 shows the locations of basins and coal mines relevant to this study.

Sample	Locality	Age	Carbon % (d.a.f *)	Vitrinite Reflectance (Rv, Max)	Rank
LIG	Gippsland Basin, Victoria	Middle Miocene	66	0.3%	Lignite B
SUB	Moreton Basin, Queensland	Middle Jurassic	80	0.57%	High volatile bituminous A
BIT	Sydney-Gunnedah Basin, New South Wales	Early Permian	85	0.67%	Medium volatile bituminous

Note: * Dry, ash free.

3. CSG Water Results

CSG waters from production wells targeting the Bandanna Formation contain no PAH or BTEX compounds above detection limits. The minimum detection limit for PAHs in the Bandanna Formation analyses was 1 μg/L, except for benzo[a]pyrene (0.5 μg/L). BTEX compounds were analyzed at 1 to 2 μg/L detection limits. These detection limits are equal to those applied to organic analyses in publicly available reports which also reported nil detections for aromatic compounds e.g., [31]. Currently, there is no standard set for analytical detection levels of aromatic compounds from coal seam gas water.

Detection limits used in the Walloon Coal Measures CSG water samples (*circa* 0.01 μg/L) were two orders of magnitude lower than the Bandanna Formation analysis. The concentrations and detection limits for select organic compounds from CSG waters of the Walloon Coal Measures are shown in Table 3. 13 of the 47 wells analyzed (27%) had ultra-trace concentrations of PAH compounds. All 47 wells had nil detections for phenolic compounds and the 14 wells analyzed for BTEX compounds also reported nil detections.

The most commonly detected PAHs were naphthalene and phenanthrene which were both detected in seven sampled wells. The maximum naphthalene and phenanthrene concentrations from a single well were 0.046 μg/L and 0.02 μg/L, respectively. Of all detected PAHs, naphthalene was detected at the highest concentration, followed by benzo[b+k]fluoranthene (0.033 μg/L). The benzo[b+k]fluoranthene analyte is the total concentration of the benzo[b]fluoranthene and benzo[k]fluoranthene compounds and individual concentrations of each cannot be ascertained. Of the 47 sampled wells, only five produced CSG water with more than one individual PAH compound and the maximum total PAH concentration reported from any single well was 0.083 μg/L.

Table 3. Concentrations of polycyclic aromatic hydrocarbons (PAHs) from Walloon Coal Measures' CSG waters, as sampled from production wells. Only detected PAHs are shown. BDL = below detection limit.

PAHs	Detection Limit (μg/L)	Range (μg/L)	% of Wells with Detections
Naphthalene	0.01	BDL–0.046	23
Phenanthrene	0.01	BDL–0.046	20
Pyrene	0.01	BDL–0.01	2
Chrysene	0.01	BDL–0.016	2
Benzo[b+k]fluoranthene	0.01	BDL–0.033	9
Dibenz[a,h]anthracene	0.01	BDL–0.014	9

3.1. CSG Water Holding Pond

The CSG water holding pond of the Walloon production area was sampled six times over a one month period in 2010. In this dataset, naphthalene and phenol were the only detected compounds at 0.06 μg/L and 0.3 μg/L, respectively. Both analytes were only detected once during the sampling program. None of the higher molecular weight PAHs were detected in the holding pond.

3.2. Leaching Experiment Results

No PAHs or phenolic compounds were reported in the leachates of the standard TCLPs performed with the acetic acid solution from any coal rank. The minimum detection levels for that group of TCLPs were 0.5–1 μg/L for PAHs and 1–2 μg/L for phenolics. These results suggest that even during a high energy agitation in an acid fluid, these aromatic compounds will not leach at considerable concentrations. Analytical detection levels for the deionized and synthetic CSG water solutions were lowered appropriately to assess whether these hydrophobic substances will leach at ultra-trace (0.01 μg/L) concentrations.

PAHs were present in the deionized water (Table 4) and synthetic CSG water (Table 5) leachates. Individual PAH compounds leached from coal samples included: naphthalene, phenanthrene, fluoranthene, pyrene, chrysene, benz[a]anthracene, benzo[b+k]fluoranthene and benzo[a]pyrene. Naphthalene was detected at the highest concentrations (0.42 to 0.67 µg/L) and only leached from lignite. The only other PAH compound to leach from lignite samples was phenanthrene (at a concentration of 0.01 µg/L) and only in one synthetic CSG water leach. In four of the five tests performed with lignite, phenol leached at average concentrations of 0.3 µg/L.

Table 4. Concentration ranges of selected organics from toxicity characteristic leaching procedure (TCLP) experiments performed with deionized water. BDL = below detection limit.

Polycyclic aromatic hydrocarbons	**Detection Limit (µg/L)**	**Coal Rank**		
		Lignite	**HvA-Bituminous**	**Mv-Bituminous**
Naphthalene	0.01	0.43–0.67	BDL	BDL
Acenaphthylene	0.01	BDL	BDL	BDL
Acenaphthene	0.01	BDL	BDL	BDL
Fluorene	0.01	BDL	BDL	BDL
Phenanthrene	0.01	BDL	BDL	BDL-0.01
Anthracene	0.01	BDL	BDL	BDL
Fluoranthene	0.01	BDL	BDL-0.03	BDL-0.03
Pyrene	0.01	BDL	BDL-0.02	BDL-0.05
Benz[a]anthracene	0.01	BDL	BDL	BDL-0.02
Chrysene	0.01	BDL	BDL	BDL-0.01
Benzo[b+k]fluoranthene	0.01	BDL	BDL	BDL-0.01
Benzo[a]pyrene	0.01	BDL	BDL	BDL-0.01
Indeno[1,2,3-cd]pyrene	0.01	BDL	BDL	BDL
Dibenz[a,h]anthracene	0.01	BDL	BDL	BDL
Benzo[ghi]perylene	0.01	BDL	BDL	BDL
Phenolics	**Detection Limit (µg /L)**	**Lignite**	**HvA-Bituminous**	**Mv-Bituminous**
Phenol	0.25	BDL–0.32	BDL	BDL
2-Chlorophenol	0.25	BDL	BDL	BDL
2-Methylphenol	0.25	BDL	BDL	BDL
4-Methylphenol	0.25	BDL	BDL	BDL
2-Nitrophenol	0.25	BDL	BDL	BDL
2,4-Dimethylphenol	0.25	BDL	BDL	BDL
2,4-Dichlorophenol	0.25	BDL	BDL	BDL
2,6-Dichlorophenol	0.25	BDL	BDL	BDL
4-Chloro-3-methylphenol	0.25	BDL	BDL	BDL
2,4,6-Trichlorophenol	0.25	BDL	BDL	BDL
2,4,5-Trichlorophenol	0.25	BDL	BDL	BDL
2,4-Dinitrophenol	2.5	BDL	BDL	BDL
4-Nitrophenol	1	BDL	BDL	BDL
2,3,4,6-Tetrachlorophenol	0.3	BDL	BDL	BDL
2-Methyl-4,6-dinitrophenol	0.5	BDL	BDL	BDL
Pentachlorophenol	1	BDL	BDL	BDL

Table 5. Concentration ranges of selected organics from TCLP experiments performed with synthetic CSG water.

Polycyclic aromatic hydrocarbons	Detection Limit (µg/L)	Coal Rank		
		Lignite	HvA-Bituminous	Mv-Bituminous
Naphthalene	0.01	0.58–0.64	BDL	BDL
Acenaphthylene	0.01	BDL	BDL	BDL
Acenaphthene	0.01	BDL	BDL	BDL
Fluorene	0.01	BDL	BDL	BDL
Phenanthrene	0.01	0.01	BDL	BDL
Anthracene	0.01	BDL	BDL	BDL
Fluoranthene	0.01	BDL	BDL	BDL
Pyrene	0.01	BDL	BDL	BDL
Benz[a]anthracene	0.01	BDL	BDL	BDL
Chrysene	0.01	BDL	BDL	BDL
Benzo[b+k]fluoranthene	0.01	BDL	BDL	BDL
Benzo[a]pyrene	0.01	BDL	BDL	BDL
Indeno[1,2,3-cd]pyrene	0.01	BDL	BDL	BDL
Dibenz[a,h]anthracene	0.01	BDL	BDL	BDL
Benzo[ghi]perylene	0.01	BDL	BDL	BDL
Phenolics	**Detection Limit (µg/L)**	**Lignite**	**HvA-Bituminous**	**Mv-Bituminous**
Phenol	0.25	0.26–0.31	BDL	BDL
2-Chlorophenol	0.25	BDL	BDL	BDL
2-Methylphenol	0.25	BDL	BDL	BDL
4-Methylphenol	0.25	BDL	BDL	BDL
2-Nitrophenol	0.25	BDL	BDL	BDL
2,4-Dimethylphenol	0.25	BDL	BDL	BDL
2,4-Dichlorophenol	0.25	BDL	BDL	BDL
2,6-Dichlorophenol	0.25	BDL	BDL	BDL
4-Chloro-3-methylphenol	0.25	BDL	BDL	BDL
2,4,6-Trichlorophenol	0.25	BDL	BDL	BDL
2,4,5-Trichlorophenol	0.25	BDL	BDL	BDL
2,4-Dinitrophenol	2.5	BDL	BDL	BDL
4-Nitrophenol	1	BDL	BDL	BDL
2,3,4,6-Tetrachlorophenol	0.3	BDL	BDL	BDL
2-Methyl-4,6-dinitrophenol	0.5	BDL	BDL	BDL
Pentachlorophenol	1	BDL	BDL	BDL

The bituminous coals leached individual PAH compounds with less consistency than the lignite sample. The HvA-bituminous sample leached PAH compounds in only two of the five TCLPs and only in deionized water. PAHs leached from the HvA-bituminous coal were pyrene (0.01 to 0.02 µg/L) and fluoranthene (0.01 to 0.03 µg/L) (Figure 2). The Mv-bituminous coal leached PAH compounds in three of the five TCLPs performed with that coal and only in deionized water, not to synthetic CSG water. The leachate of a powdered Mv-bituminous coal (in deionized water) contained similar PAHs as only one of the roughly crushed Mv-bituminous leachates.

Figure 2. Aromatics (mostly PAHs) leached from coal samples with deionized water and their relative concentrations. PAHs reported from Walloons CSG water samples are also shown.

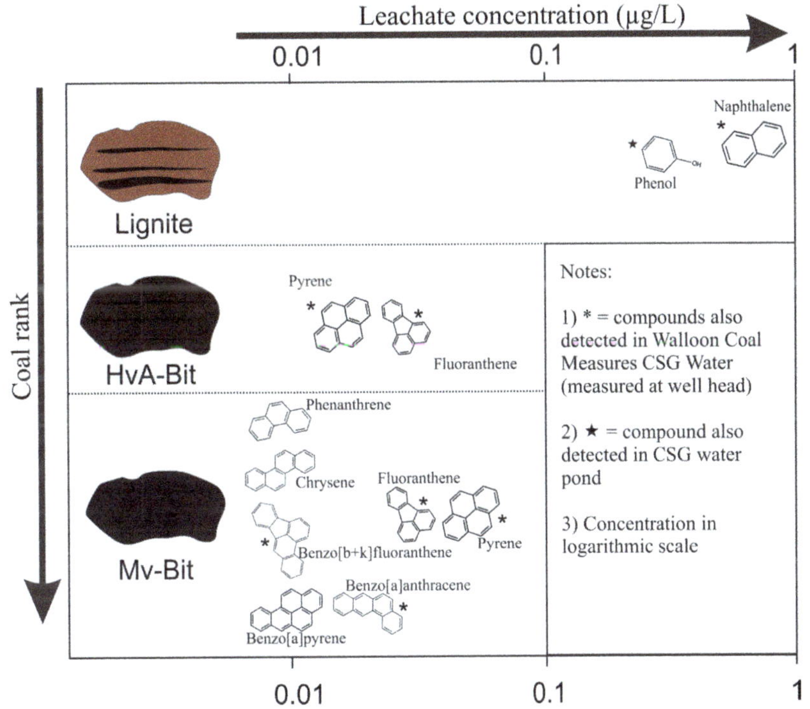

4. CSG Water Discussion

The PAH compounds identified in the Walloons CSG water are likely coal derived, based on their similarity to: known PAH composition in coals [43,44], PAHs leached from coals herein (Tables 4 and 5), and PAHs identified in CSG Water of the Powder River Basin [28]. Naphthalene and phenanthrene are the most water soluble PAHs, likely accounting for their increased presence in CSG waters relative to the higher molecular weight PAHs (see Table 6). However, the lower molecular weight PAHs detected in the Walloon Coal Measures CSG water (naphthalene, phenanthrene and pyrene) are considered to be less harmful to human health than the higher molecular weight PAHs [45]. The detected PAHs with 4 and 5 aromatic rings—chrysene, benzo[b]fluoranthene and dibenz[a]anthracene—are suspected human carcinogens [45,46], based largely on data from toxicological tests in rodents. The higher molecular weight PAHs, such as benzo[a]pyrene and dibenzo[a,l]pyrene (5 and 6 rings, respectively), are suggested to cause cancer through metabolic activation in cells and formation of stable adducts that damage DNA [47–49]. Benzo[a]pyrene (BaP) is the only PAH with a trigger threshold (0.01 μg/L) in Australian drinking water guidelines (ADWG). The ADWG state that insufficient data are available to set a guideline limit for other PAHs (National Health and Medical Research Council, Canberra, ACT, Australia, 2004). Orem *et al.* [28] summarized international PAH guidelines in drinking water according to the United States Environmental Protection Agency (USEPA) and World Health Organization (WHO). Under the ADWG, USEPA and WHO guidelines, no single Walloon CSG well produced water that would exceed the regulatory levels for PAHs. The drinking water guidelines are provided purely as a relative index to the aromatic concentrations in CSG water and do not imply that untreated CSG water is ever used as potable supply in Queensland. Under Australian environmental guidelines [50], such as those applied to water quality in aquatic ecosystems, only naphthalene has a trigger value (16 μg/L for a 95% species protection level) whereas all higher molecular weight PAHs have insufficient data available to set guideline values.

None of the higher molecular weight, potentially harmful PAHs present at very low concentrations in the CSG water from Walloon wells were present in the holding pond. This is an important consideration when reviewing CSG water quality data from production wells, particularly in the context of ultra-trace organics and also because the holding pond is the feedstock for treatment and beneficial reuse of CSG water. If a small number of wells produce CSG water containing minute amounts of suspected harmful PAHs and the vast majority of wells do not produce CSG water with those compounds above the detection limit, then the PAHs may be further diluted by mixing in the holding ponds. Therefore analysis—particularly of the very insoluble PAH compounds discussed here—may result in nil detection of those compounds from the ponds, despite their presence in water from individual wells. Other processes, such as rainwater input, the binding of PAHs to soils and sediments [51] and UV degradation [52,53] may also reduce PAH concentrations in ponded water.

Orem *et al.* [28] identified PAHs including naphthalene, phenanthrene, fluorene and pyrene in CSG water from a small number of wells targeting the Powder River Basin coals. However, that work more commonly identified functional derivatives of PAH compounds (e.g., alkylated naphthalene, methylpyrene, dimethylphenanthrene) that are not regular water quality analytes in Queensland and often have unknown toxicities. Derivative forms of PAHs are a significant part of the molecular composition of coals [54] and necessitate higher resolution analysis of QLD CSG water to quantify their occurrence and any potential health risks those compounds may pose.

4.1. Leaching Experiment Discussion

The concentrations of organics leached from lignite were an order of magnitude greater than the bituminous samples (Figure 2). This concurs with the increased solubilization of lower rank coals relative to higher rank coals as described by some authors [27,55]. In aqueous leaching experiments of various coals, Maharaj *et al.* [56] also observed higher concentrations of aromatics in some (but not all) lignite leachates relative to bituminous samples. Naphthalene and phenol are more soluble than the higher molecular weight PAHs (Table 6 [57,58]) and also more likely to be cleaved from the less condensed aromatic framework of a low rank coal [55]. This is consistent with the increased presence and concentration of lower molecular weight PAHs (and their derivatives) in organic results from CSG wells targeting lignite to sub-bituminous coals of the Powder River Basin [28].

PAHs detected in Mv-bituminous leachate were of 3, 4 and 5 aromatic ring structures, including pyrene, fluoranthene, chrysene, benzo[a]anthracene, benzo[b+k]fluoranthene and benzo[a]pyrene. Benzo[a]pyrene (BaP) is a known carcinogen with very low solubility and high affinity to remain in the organic phase [59,60]. It is detected in the Mv-bituminous leachate results at its threshold concentration in the ADWG (0.01 μg/L). The filtered coal leachates likely contained other dissolved humic material from the coals given the observed yellow/brown colour. The presence of this organic matter may have enhanced the solubility of BaP and other higher molecular weight PAHs [61].

Table 6. Aromatic compounds detected in Walloon Coal Measures CSG water and leaching experiments with their physico-chemical properties [57,58].

Compound	Molar Mass (g/mol)	Solubility at 25 °C (µg/L)	Log KoW *	No. of Aromatic Rings
Phenol	94.1	83,000,000	1.46	1
Naphthalene	128.2	31,000	3.37	2
Phenanthrene	178.2	465	4.46	3
Fluoranthene	202.3	260	4.9	3
Pyrene	202.1	133	4.88	4
Benz[a]anthracene	228.3	11	5.63	4
Chrysene	228.3	1.9	5.63	4
Benzo[b]fluoranthene	252.3	2.4	6.04	4
Benzo[k]fluoranthene	252.3	2.4	6.21	4
Benzo[a]pyrene	252.3	3.8	6.06	5
Dibenz[a]anthracene	278.3	0.4	6.86	5

Note: * Log Kow refers to the octanol-water partition coefficient whereby higher values denote compounds more likely to partition into organic phases rather than aqueous phases.

The 3–5 ring PAHs present in the deionized water leachates of bituminous coals were not detected in the synthetic CSG water leachates. PAHs leached in deionized water were exceedingly low and their absence in the synthetic CSG water may relate to the decreased ability of that fluid to leach and dissolve very non-polar substances as ionic strength increases [62,63]. The lack of phenol in the bituminous leachates may relate to their increased coal maturity. As coalification increases (and O and H decrease) the concentrations of hydroxylated aromatics are lowered relative to those present in lower rank coals [44].

4.2. Aromatic Compound Mobilization from Coal

The macromolecular network of coal contains aromatics in two phases. During coalification, resistant plant biopolymers are turned into a progressively denser, aromatic, three-dimensional network [42]. Within the network structure, a "mobile" phase of smaller molecules is more weakly bonded and can more easily leach to the environment [64]. The mobility of these compounds makes them of greater human health concern. The PAHs present in the leachates of coal samples most likely represent constituents of the mobile phase.

The leach results suggest that types of compounds leached from coals to deionized water become increasingly aromatic with increasing coal rank. The lowest rank coal leached 1 and 2 ring aromatics at the highest concentrations and the highest rank coal leached 3, 4 and 5 ring aromatics at the lowest concentrations (Figure 2). Conversely, Stout *et al.* [43] observed more 4–6 ring PAHs in extracts of lignite and sub-bituminous coals compared with greater 2–3 ring PAHs in higher rank coals of the western United States. In addition, those authors showed an increasing concentration of total PAHs in coal with coalification (up to the bituminous rank) (see Figure 4 of [43]). However, the types of aromatics in the molecular structure of coal do not have a systematic relationship to coal maturity alone. Detailed maceral composition (currently unavailable for these samples) and coal origin is also a major factor [44,54]. Laumann *et al.* [54] observed that when considering coals of different origin from multiple basins, 2–3 ring PAHs dominate molecular composition regardless of coal maturity.

Results from previous studies [43,54] in which compounds were extracted with organic solvent are not directly comparable to this study, however. Extract composition from natural water will likely differ depending on PAH sorb/desorb behaviour, the ability of coal to act as a geosorbent, PAH solubility in natural waters and the co-elution of PAHs to other dissolved humic material. For example, the very low concentrations of the higher molecular weight (and potentially harmful) 3–5 PAHs detected in the bituminous leachates may be better explained by their very low solubilities in water and higher binding affinities (Log Kow) for organic matter (Table 6), rather than their relative abundances in coal samples.

Attempting to predict types and concentrations of leached aromatic compounds based purely on coal properties of individual seams may prove unrealistic when trying to correlate these results to the concentration of compounds in water samples from actual CSG production fields. Complications in such modelling would arise when sampling water from open-hole completed wells, where many potentially variable coal seams and their inter-seam sediments are targeted for gas extraction. Also, the inflow of groundwater from aquifers hydraulically connected to the coal seams may dilute any expected compounds, thus site specific hydrogeological conditions must be considered. Where hydraulic fracturing has occurred, organic additives used in injection fluids (see Table 2 of [3]) may also have the potential to solubilize coal derived hydrocarbons [29] to CSG waters, particularly where flowback recovery does not appropriately "flush" the formation water. Furthermore, some insoluble aromatic compounds reported in this study occur very close to their detection limits and thus their analytical reproducibility in CSG water may be infrequent.

4.3. Human Health Risk

The first phase of human health risk assessment includes hazard identification and dose response. That is, identification of a substance or situation that has the potential to cause adverse health effects and at what levels of exposure (dose). Risk, as a measure of likelihood of occurrence and severity of outcome, is usually then assessed based on site-specific characterization of pathways of human exposure including acute, cumulative and multiple exposures. Additionally, physiological response to dose may predict the severity of human response or adverse health effects.

This study provides evidence that a minority of Queensland CSG water samples contain some organic compounds recognized as potential health hazards. The significance of these findings however, lies in the relatively small number of samples containing the compounds and the very low concentrations in which they are present. These factors greatly reduce the likelihood of human exposure at doses significant to induce adverse physiological response, at least in short-term exposure scenarios. If present, many potentially harmful coal derived substances can be reduced to negligible levels with common CSG water treatment methods [4,26,31]. Yet more publicly available research employing low detection level (<1 μg/L) analysis of the wide range of potentially dissolved organics in CSG water would assist in refining risk assessments and site-specific treatment methods.

The risk is less clear for hazard accumulation and multiple exposure scenarios and this uncertainty indicates the need for further analysis of both models of organic compound accumulation and migration in ground and surface water before and after treatment and definition of potential pathways of human exposure to these waters. Additionally, future toxicology studies targeting the key compounds identified in this study can clarify the dose-response relationship to adverse health outcomes. A broader understanding of these issues will provide the basis for informed and appropriate industry regulation to best monitor for and militate against release of hazardous substances through CSG production.

4.4. Detection Limits and Reporting

In some instances, the detection level (DL) of some organic compound classes in CSG water may be too high to adequately assess the occurrence of potentially harmful compounds. Aromatic compounds such as BaP have regulatory limits (0.01 μg/L) 50 times less concentrated than the minimum DL of the Bandanna Formation dataset (0.5 μg/L) of this work and the small number of publicly available QLD CSG water organic datasets. Analysis at this level prevented a comparison of dissolved aromatics from Walloon and Bandanna production fields. In addition, relatively high DLs still leave a knowledge gap regarding the occurrence of generally insoluble, but environmentally regulated coal derived organics. BaP was leached from coal in this study at its regulatory limit, thus highlighting the importance of appropriate DLs in CSG water analysis.

Sometimes (even where DLs are sufficiently low) average concentrations of organic compounds across production fields are reported rather than ranges of detected levels. Whilst such reporting is practical for characterizing CSG water quality for legislative requirements and bulk treatment technologies, rare relatively high concentrations of organic compounds detected from individual wells may be ameliorated by the field average. It is therefore best practice to present organic concentrations of CSG water from individual wells in monitoring and regulatory data, as well as production field averages.

5. Conclusions

Analyses conducted in this study show that BTEX compounds and phenolic compounds were absent from CSG waters in the Bandanna Formation (Bowen Basin) and Walloon Coal Measures (Surat Basin) from production wells operating between 2009 and 2010. Coal seam gas water in the Surat Basin can contain ultra-trace ranges of polycyclic aromatic hydrocarbons (PAHs) including: naphthalene, phenanthrene, chrysene, benzo[b]fluoranthene and dibenz[a]anthracene, which are most likely sourced from the sub-bituminous to bituminous coals of the Walloon Coal Measures. Some of these compounds are suspected toxins. However, no single producing well contained organic compounds in concentrations that would exceed Australian Drinking Water Guidelines, or USEPA and WHO drinking water guidelines for PAHs. In addition, the holding pond for the Walloons production area contained none of the 3–5 ring PAHs detected in water samples from the CSG wells.

One aim of this study was to assess the potential differences between structure and concentration of organics leached from different ranked coals. However, coal leaching results could not be compared directly to CSG water sample analyses which had been previously collected by CSG producers, because of the higher detection limits associated with these sample analyses (e.g., detections ≥1 μg/L for the Bandanna Formation CSG water). An analysis with a minimum detection level *circa* 0.01 μg/L is more in line with trigger levels for regulated compounds such as benzo[a]pyrene, a known carcinogen which was shown to leach from a bituminous coal in a laboratory setting. Should CSG operators have approval for untreated beneficial use of CSG water (e.g., discharge to streams, land irrigation, managed aquifer injection), it is recommended that the BaP limits of detection used in PAH analysis should be set at 0.01 μg/L (the most stringent regulatory level).

PAHs are present within coal samples at appreciable concentrations [44,54], but only ultra-trace concentrations of the more toxic higher molecular weight PAHs are likely to leach to waters because they are hydrophobic organic substances. Variable aromatic structures (PAHs and phenols) will likely leach from coals of different rank. Higher molecular weight PAH compounds were leached to water (including chrysene, benzo[a]anthracene and benzo[a]pyrene) from the highest rank coal analyzed in this study, whilst lower molecular weight compounds leached at greater concentrations from the lowest coal rank. This trend seems to correlate with conceptual trend of increasing aromaticity of the coal molecular structure with increasing rank, but maceral composition and the presence of other dissolved organic material could be playing a role in which water soluble PAHs are present in leachates. None of the 4 and 5 ringed PAHs leached to the more saline synthetic CSG water, and this may indicate that brackish to saline CSG waters further reduce the solubilities of very hydrophobic organic toxins. Further work with a range of controlled leaching experiments would be required to fully understand this process. Additional experimental work is recommended to assess the potential of organic additives, present in hydraulic fracturing fluids, to mobilize hydrocarbons from coal to flowback water (and to assess potential CSG water contamination by flowback water).

Coal is a heterogeneous material and each coal seam gas field may present a unique inventory of organic compounds needing characterization and assessment to fully understand coal-groundwater interactions and ultimately water quality. Moreover, there is potentially a far wider range of organic compounds mobilized from coals to CSG water beyond the common environmental analytes of this study, including heterocyclic compounds, biphenyls, aromatic amines and non-aromatic compounds.

The high density of CSG wells in southern Queensland provides an excellent opportunity to better understand the relationship between coal and groundwater. In turn, such studies form the basis of human health risk assessment and may be significant in understanding the etiology of disease linked to coal-derived organic compounds such as Balkan Endemic Nephropathy. Moreover, communities that access untreated groundwater from coal-associated aquifers (e.g., Powder River Basin, WY and Surat Basin, QLD) can use such studies to gain a better understanding of the potential risks posed by water soluble coal-derived organics.

Improved stakeholder confidence in CSG operations and water issues will only result from access to appropriate, peer reviewed research, to which this study may contribute. Finally, CSG water characterization studies are crucial in developing industry best practice, as well as government regulation, monitoring and management strategies for CSG water to safeguard the environment and human health in parallel with expanding CSG production.

Acknowledgments

We thank Greg Jackson, Aaron Hieatt and Janet Cummings (Water Team, Department of Health, QLD Government, Brisbane, QLD, Australia), for their assistance in data collation and setup for experimental and analytical work. Stewart Carswell and Benjamin Tan of Queensland Health Forensic and Scientific Services (QHFSS) provided laboratory space and analytical support and Australian Laboratory Services (ALS), Brisbane provided analytical advice.

Author Contributions

William Stearman: Collated, reviewed and analysed government CSG water quality data and performed experimental work and analytical extractions for leaching tests; primary author on paper, contributed to figures and editing. Mauricio Taulis: Project supervision; contributed to experimental design; wrote sections of the paper; reviewed and edited drafts of paper; drafted and edited figures. Maree Corkeron: Project supervision; contributed to project design; sourced relevant desktop data; wrote sections of the paper; reviewed and edited drafts of paper. James Smith: Assisted with organic geochemical concepts and experimental design; reviewed and edited drafts.

References

1. Blueprint for Queensland's LNG Industry, LNG Industry Unit. Available online: http://rti.cabinet.qld.gov.au/documents/2010/nov/lng%20blueprint/Attachments/LNG%20Blueprint.pdf (accessed on 1 September 2014).
2. Klohn Crippen Berger. *Forecasting Coal Seam Gas Water Production in Queensland's Surat and Southern Bowen Basins*; Department of Natural Resources and Mines: Brisbane, Australia, 2012.
3. Sinclair Knight Mertz. *Hydraulic Fracturing Techniques ("Fraccing") Techniques, including Reporting Requirements and Governance Arrangements, Background Review*; Commonwealth of Australia: Canberra, Australia, 2014.
4. National Research Council. *Management and Effects of Coalbed Methane Produced Water in the United States*; National Academy of Sciences: Washington, DC, USA, 2010.
5. Batley, G.E.; Kookana, R.S. Environmental issues associated with coal seam gas recovery: Managing the fracking boom. *Environ. Chem.* **2012**, *9*, 425–428.
6. Taulis, M.E. Australia and New Zealand CBNG development and environmental implications. In *Coalbed Natural Gas: Energy and Environment*; Reddy, K.J., Ed.; Nova Science Publishers: New York, NY, USA, 2010; pp. 401–424.
7. Taulis, M.E. *Groundwater Characterisation and Disposal Modelling for Coal Seam Gas Recovery*; University of Canterbury: Christchurch, New Zealand, 2007.
8. Department of Environment and Heritage Protection. *Coal Seam Gas Water Management Policy*; QLD Government: Brisbane, Australia, 2012.
9. Dr Mariann Lloyd-Smith Speaking about Toxic Risks of CSG (aka Coal Bed Methane). Available online: http://www.faug.org.uk/link/dr-mariann-lloyd-smith-speaking-about-toxic-risks-csg-aka-coal-bed-methane (accessed on 18 June 2014).
10. Feder, G.L.; Radovanovic, Z.; Finkelman, R.B. Relationship between weathered coal deposits and the etiology of Balkan endemic nephropathy. *Kidney Int. Suppl.* **1991**, *34*, 9–11.

11. Tatu, C.A.; Orem, W.H.; Maharaj, S.V.M.; Finkelman, R.B.; Diaconita, D.; Feder, G.L.; Szilagyi, D.N.; Dumitrascu, V.; Paunescu, V. Organic compounds derived from Pliocene lignite and the etiology of Balkan endemic nephropathy. In *Geology and Health: Closing the Gap*; Skinner, H.C.W., Berger, A.R., Eds.; Oxford University Press: New York, NY, USA, 2003; pp. 159–162.
12. Orem, W.; Tatu, C.; Pavlovic, N.; Bunnell, J.; Lerch, H.; Paunescu, V.; Ordodi, V.; Flores, D.; Corum, M.; Bates, A. Health effects of toxic organic substances from coal: Toward "Panendemic" nephropathy. *AMBIO* **2007**, *36*, 98–102.
13. Orem, W.H.; Feder, G.L.; Finkelman, R.B. A possible link between Balkan endemic nephropathy and the leaching of toxic organic compounds from Pliocene lignite by groundwater: Preliminary investigation. *Int. J. Coal Geol.* **1999**, *40*, 237–252.
14. Sunwater Ltd. *Chinchilla Beneficial Use Scheme Water Quality Report*; Sunwater Ltd.: Brisbane, Australia, 2013. Available online: http://www.sunwater.com.au/__data/assets/pdf_file/0016/12607/Chinchilla-Beneficial-Use-Scheme-Water-Quality-Report-2013.pdf (accessed on 1 September 2014).
15. Navi, M.; Skelly, C.; Taulis, M.; Nasiri, S. Coal seam gas water: Potential hazards and exposure pathways in Queensland. *Int. J. Environ. Health Res.* **2014**, *24*, 1–22.
16. Cheung, K.; Sanei, H.; Klassen, P.; Mayer, B.; Goodarzi, F. Produced fluids and shallow groundwater in coalbed methane (CBM) producing regions of Alberta, Canada: Trace element and rare earth element geochemistry. *Int. J. Coal Geol.* **2009**, *77*, 338–349.
17. Jackson, R.E.; Reddy, K.J. Geochemistry of coalbed natural gas (CBNG) produced water in powder river basin, wyoming: Salinity and sodicity. *Water Air Soil Pollut.* **2007**, *184*, 49–61.
18. Jackson, R.E.; Reddy, K.J. Trace element chemistry of coal bed natural gas produced water in the Powder River Basin, Wyoming. *Environ. Sci. Technol.* **2007**, *41*, 5953–5959.
19. Jackson, R.E.; Reddy, K.J. Coalbed natural gas product water: Geochemical transformations from outfalls to disposal ponds. In *Coalbed Natural Gas: Energy and Environment*; Reddy, K.J., Ed.; Nova Science Publishers Inc.: New York, NY, USA, 2010; pp. 121–143.
20. Kinnon, E.C.P.; Golding, S.D.; Boreham, C.J.; Baublys, K.A.; Esterle, J.S. Stable isotope and water quality analysis of coal bed methane production waters and gases from the Bowen Basin, Australia. *Int. J. Coal Geol.* **2010**, *82*, 219–231.
21. McBeth, I.; Reddy, K.J.; Skinner, Q.D. Chemistry of trace elements in coalbed methane product water. *Water Res.* **2003**, *37*, 884–890.
22. Patz, M.J.; Reddy, K.J.; Skinner, Q.D. Chemistry of coalbed methane discharge water interacting with semi-arid ephemeral stream channels. *J. Am. Water Resour. Assoc.* **2004**, *40*, 1247–1255.
23. Taulis, M.E.; Trumm, D.; Milke, M.W.; Nobes, D.; Manhire, D.; O'Sullivan, A. Characterisation of coal seam gas waters in New Zealand. In Proceedings of the New Zealand Minerals Conference: Realising New Zealand's Mineral Potential, Auckland, New Zealand, 13–16 November 2005; pp. 416–425.
24. Taulis, M.; Milke, M. Chemical variability of groundwater samples collected from a Coal Seam Gas exploration well, Maramarua, New Zealand. *Water Res.* **2012**, *47*, 1021–1034.
25. Reddy, K.J.; Helmericks, C.; Whitman, A.; Legg, D. Geochemical processes controlling trace elemental mobility in coalbed natural gas (CBNG) disposal ponds in the Powder River Basin, WY. *Int. J. Coal Geol.* **2014**, *126*, 120–127.

26. Dahm, K.G.; Guerra, K.L.; Xu, P.; Drewes, J.E. Composite geochemical database for coalbed methane produced water quality in the Rocky Mountain region. *Environ. Sci. Technol.* **2011**, *45*, 7655–7663.
27. Volk, H.; Pinetown, K.; Johnston, C.; McLean, W. *A Desktop Study of the Occurrence of Total Petroleum Hydrocarbon (TPH) and Partially Water-Soluble Organic Compounds in Permian Coals and Associated Coal Seam Groundwater*; CSIRO: Sydney, Australia, 2011.
28. Orem, W.H.; Tatu, C.A.; Lerch, H.E.; Rice, C.A.; Bartos, T.T.; Bates, A.L.; Tewalt, S.; Corum, M.D. Organic compounds in produced waters from coalbed natural gas wells in the Powder River basin, Wyoming, USA. *Appl. Geochem.* **2007**, *22*, 2240–2256.
29. Orem, W.; Tatu, C.; Varonka, M.; Lerch, H.; Bates, A.; Engle, M.; Crosby, L.; McIntosh, J. Organic substances in produced and formation water from unconventional natural gas extraction in coal and shale. *Int. J. Coal Geol.* **2014**, *126*, 20–31.
30. APLNG. *Coal Seam Gas Water Quality Monitoring Program: Talinga Water Treatment Facility.* Available online:http://www.aplng.com.au/pdf/water_monitoring_management/Appendix_J-CSG_Water_Quality_Monitoring_Program_Talinga_Water_Treatment_Facility.pdf (accessed on 1 September 2014).
31. Arrow Energy Ltd. *Coal Seam Gas Water Management Plan. Surat Basin*; Doc No. ENV11–133; Arrow Energy Ltd.: Brisbane, Australia, 2013.
32. Sowder, J.T.; Kelleners, T.J.; Reddy, K.J. The origin and fate of arsenic in coalbed natural gas-produced water ponds. *J. Environ. Qual.* **2010**, *39*, 1604–1615.
33. Beeston, J.W. Coal facies depositional models, Denison trough area, Bowen Basin. *Qld. Geol.* **1991**, *2*, 3–33.
34. Beeston, J.W. Coal rank variation in the Bowen Basin, Queensland. *Int. J. Coal Geol.* **1986**, *6*, 163–179.
35. Draper, J.J.; Boreham, C.J. Geological controls on exploitable coal seam gas distribution in Queensland. *Aust. Pet. Prod. Explor. Assoc. J.* **2006**, *46*, 343–346.
36. Salehy, M.R. Determination of rank and petrographic composition of Jurassic coals from eastern Surat Basin, Australia. *Int. J. Coal Geol.* **1986**, *6*, 149–162.
37. Fielding, C.R. The middle Jurassic Walloon coal measures in the type area, the Rosewood-Walloon Coalfield, SE Queensland. *Aust. Coal Geol.* **1993**, *9*, 4–16.
38. Scott, S.; Anderson, B.; Crosdale, P.; Dingwall, J.; Leblang, G. Coal petrology and coal seam gas contents of the Walloon Subgroup-Surat Basin, Queensland, Australia. *Int. J. Coal Geol.* **2007**, *70*, 209–222.
39. Exon, N.F. *Geology of the Surat Basin in Queensland*; Bulletin 166; Bureau of Mineral Resources, Geology and Geophysics: Canberra, Australia, 1976.
40. Clark, W.J.; Cooper, D.M. Sedimentological and wireline aspects of the Walloon Coal Measures in GSQ Dalby 1 and GSQ Chinchilla 3, Surat Basin, Queensland. *Qld. Govt. Min. J.* **1985**, *86*, 386–394.
41. Radke, M.; Willsch, H.; Leythaeuser, D.; Teichmüller, M. Aromatic components of coal: Relation of distribution pattern to rank. *Geochim. Cosmochim. Acta* **1982**, *46*, 1831–1848.
42. Hatcher, P.G.; Clifford, D.J. The organic geochemistry of coal: From plant materials to coal. *Org. Geochem.* **1997**, *27*, 251–274.

43. Stout, S.A.; Emsbo-Mattingly, S.D. Concentration and character of PAHs and other hydrocarbons in coals of varying rank—Implications for environmental studies of soils and sediments containing particulate coal. *Org. Geochem.* **2008**, *39*, 801–819.
44. Achten, C.; Hofmann, T. Native polycyclic aromatic hydrocarbons (PAH) in coals—A hardly recognized source of environmental contamination. *Sci. Total Environ.* **2009**, *407*, 2461–2473.
45. Agency for Toxic Substances and Disease Registry. *Toxicological Profile for Polycyclic Aromatic Hydrocarbons*; Public Health Service: Atlanta, GA, USA, 1995.
46. Luch, A.; Baird, W.M. Carcinogenic Polycyclic Aromatic Hydrocarbons. In *Comprehensive Toxicology*; Charlene, A.M., Ed.; Elsevier: Oxford, UK, 2010; pp. 85–123.
47. Melendez-Colon, V.J.; Luch, A.; Seidel, A.; Baird, W.M. Cancer initiation by polycyclic aromatic hydrocarbons results from formation of stable DNA adducts rather than apurinic sites. *Carcinogenesis* **1999**, *20*, 1885–1891.
48. Luch, A.; Baird, W.M. *Metabolic Activation and Detoxification of Polycyclic Aromatic Hydrocarbons*; Imperial College Press: London, UK, 2004.
49. Xue, W.; Warshawsky, D. Metabolic activation of polycyclic and heterocyclic aromatic hydrocarbons and DNA damage: A review. *Toxicol. Appl. Pharmacol.* **2005**, *206*, 73–93.
50. Australian and New Zealand Environment and Conservation Council. *Australian Water Quality Guidelines for Fresh and Marine Water Quality*; ANZECC: Kingston, UK, 2000; Volume 1.
51. Jafvert, C.T.; Rao, P.S.C.; Lane, D.; Lee, L.S. Partitioning of mono- and polycyclic aromatic hydrocarbons in a river sediment adjacent to a former manufactured gas plant site. *Chemosphere* **2006**, *62*, 315–321.
52. Bertilsson, S.; Widenfalk, A. Photochemical degradation of PAHs in freshwaters and their impact on bacterial growth—Influence of water chemistry. *Hydrobiologia* **2002**, *469*, 23–32.
53. Sabaté, J.; Bayona, J.M.; Solanas, A.M. Photolysis of PAHs in aqueous phase by UV irradiation. *Chemosphere* **2001**, *44*, 119–124.
54. Laumann, S.; Micić, V.; Kruge, M.A.; Achten, C.; Sachsenhofer, R.F.; Schwarzbauer, J.; Hofmann, T. Variations in concentrations and compositions of polycyclic aromatic hydrocarbons (PAHs) in coals related to the coal rank and origin. *Environ. Pollut.* **2011**, *159*, 2690–2697.
55. Santamaria, A.B.; Fisher, J. Dissolved organic constituents in coal associated waters, and implications for human and ecosystem health. *Toxicol. Sci.* **2003**, *72*, 396–397.
56. Maharaj, S.V.M.; Orem, W.H.; Tatu, C.A.; Lerch, H.E., III; Szilagyi, D.N. Organic compounds in water extracts of coal: Links to Balkan endemic nephropathy. *Environ. Geochem. Health* **2014**, *36*, 1–17.
57. Neff, J.M. *Polycyclic Aromatic Hydrocarbons in the Aquatic Environment*; Applied Science Publishing Ltd.: London, UK, 1979.
58. United States Environmental Protection Agency. *Ambient Water Quality Criteria for Polynuclear Aromatic Hydrocarbons*; EPA: Washington, WA, USA, 1980.
59. De Maagd, P.G.-J.; Hulscher, T.D.; van den Heuvel, T.; Opperhuizen, A.; Sijm, D.T.H.M. Physicochemical properties of polycyclic aromatic hydrocarbons: Aqueous solubilities, *n*-octanol/water partition coefficients, and Henry's Law constants. *Environ. Toxicol. Chem.* **1998**, *17*, 251–257.

60. Hegeman, W.J.M.; van der Weijden, C.H.; Loch, J.P. Sorption of benzo[a]pyrene and phenanthrene on suspended harbor sediment as a function of suspended sediment concentration and salinity: A laboratory study using the cosolvent partition coefficient. *Environ. Sci. Technol.* **1995**, *29*, 363–371.
61. Maxin, C.R.; Kogel-Knabner, I. Partitioning of polycyclic aromatic hydrocarbons (PAH) to water-soluble soil organic matter. *Eur. J. Soil Sci.* **1995**, *46*, 193–204.
62. Fu, G.; Kan, A.T.; Tomson, M. Adsorption and desorption hysteresis of PAHs in surface sediment. *Environ. Toxicol. Chem.* **1994**, *13*, 1559–1567.
63. Kan, A.T.; Fu, G.; Tomson, M.B. Adsorption/desorption hysteresis in organic pollutant and soil/sediment interaction. *Environ. Sci. Technol.* **1994**, *28*, 859–867.
64. Given, P.H. *The Mobile Phase in Coals: Its Nature and Modes of Release*; U.S. Department of Energy: Washington, DC, USA, 1987.

Permissions

All chapters in this book were first published by MDPI; hereby published with permission under the Creative Commons Attribution License or equivalent. Every chapter published in this book has been scrutinized by our experts. Their significance has been extensively debated. The topics covered herein carry significant findings which will fuel the growth of the discipline. They may even be implemented as practical applications or may be referred to as a beginning point for another development.

The contributors of this book come from diverse backgrounds, making this book a truly international effort. This book will bring forth new frontiers with its revolutionizing research information and detailed analysis of the nascent developments around the world.

We would like to thank all the contributing authors for lending their expertise to make the book truly unique. They have played a crucial role in the development of this book. Without their invaluable contributions this book wouldn't have been possible. They have made vital efforts to compile up to date information on the varied aspects of this subject to make this book a valuable addition to the collection of many professionals and students.

This book was conceptualized with the vision of imparting up-to-date information and advanced data in this field. To ensure the same, a matchless editorial board was set up. Every individual on the board went through rigorous rounds of assessment to prove their worth. After which they invested a large part of their time researching and compiling the most relevant data for our readers.

The editorial board has been involved in producing this book since its inception. They have spent rigorous hours researching and exploring the diverse topics which have resulted in the successful publishing of this book. They have passed on their knowledge of decades through this book. To expedite this challenging task, the publisher supported the team at every step. A small team of assistant editors was also appointed to further simplify the editing procedure and attain best results for the readers.

Apart from the editorial board, the designing team has also invested a significant amount of their time in understanding the subject and creating the most relevant covers. They scrutinized every image to scout for the most suitable representation of the subject and create an appropriate cover for the book.

The publishing team has been an ardent support to the editorial, designing and production team. Their endless efforts to recruit the best for this project, has resulted in the accomplishment of this book. They are a veteran in the field of academics and their pool of knowledge is as vast as their experience in printing. Their expertise and guidance has proved useful at every step. Their uncompromising quality standards have made this book an exceptional effort. Their encouragement from time to time has been an inspiration for everyone.

The publisher and the editorial board hope that this book will prove to be a valuable piece of knowledge for researchers, students, practitioners and scholars across the globe.

List of Contributors

Muhammad Bilal Shakoor and Muhammad Arshad
Institute of Soil and Environmental Sciences, University of Agriculture Faisalabad, Faisalabad 38040, Pakistan

Nabeel Khan Niazi and Irshad Bibi
Institute of Soil and Environmental Sciences, University of Agriculture Faisalabad, Faisalabad 38040, Pakistan
Southern Cross GeoScience, Southern Cross University, Lismore 2480, NSW, Australia

Mohammad Mahmudur Rahman
Centre for Environmental Risk Assessment and Remediation (CERAR), Mawson Lakes Campus, University of South Australia, SA 5095, Australia
Global Centre for Environmental Remediation (GCER), Faculty of Science and Information Technology, The University of Newcastle, University Drive, Callaghan, NSW 2308, Australia
Cooperative Research Centre for Contamination Assessment and Remediation of the Environment (CRC CARE), Salisbury South, SA 5106, Australia

Ravi Naidu and Zhaomin Dong
Global Centre for Environmental Remediation (GCER), Faculty of Science and Information Technology, The University of Newcastle, University Drive, Callaghan, NSW 2308, Australia
Cooperative Research Centre for Contamination Assessment and Remediation of the Environment (CRC CARE), Salisbury South, SA 5106, Australia

Muhammad Shahid
Department of Environmental Sciences, COMSATS Institute of Information Technology, Vehari 61100, Pakistan

Dale W. Griffin
Coastal and Marine Science Center, U.S. Geological Survey, 600 4th Street South, St. Petersburg, FL 33701, USA

Erin E. Silvestri and Charlena Y. Bowling
National Homeland Security Research Center, U.S. Environmental Protection Agency, 26 W. Martin Luther King Drive, MS NG16, Cincinnati, OH 45268, USA

Timothy Boe
National Homeland Security Research Center, Oak Ridge Institute for Science and Education, with the U.S. Environmental Protection Agency, 109 T.W. Alexander Drive, Research Triangle Park, NC 27709, USA

David B. Smith
Denver Federal Center, U.S. Geological Survey, Denver, CO 80225, USA

Tonya L. Nichols
National Homeland Security Research Center, Threat and Consequence Assessment Division, U.S. Environmental Protection Agency, Ronald Reagan Building, MC 8801RR, 1200 Pennsylvania Avenue, NW, Washington, DC 20460, USA

Nelly Mañay
Toxicology & Environmental Hygiene Department, Faculty of Chemistry, University of the Republic of Uruguay, Gral, Flores 2124, 11800 Montevideo, Uruguay

Dora Pearce
Faculty of Science, Federation University Australia, University Drive, Mt Helen, VIC 3350, Australia
Centre for Epidemiology and Biostatistics, Melbourne School of Population and Global Health, Faculty of Medicine, Dentistry and Health Sciences, The University of Melbourne, Level 3, 207 Bouverie Street, Melbourne, VIC 3010, Australia

James Sillitoe
Research and Innovation, Federation University Australia, University Drive, Mt Helen, VIC 3350, Australia

Ingrid Luffman
Department of Geosciences, East Tennessee State University, Johnson City, TN 37614-1709, USA

Liem Tran
Department of Geography, The University of Tennessee, Knoxville, TN 37996-0925, USA

Masayuki Sakakibara
Graduate School of Science & Engineering, Ehime University, 2-5 Bunkyo-cho, Matsuyama 790-8577, Japan

Yayu Indriati Arifin
Graduate School of Science & Engineering, Ehime University, 2-5 Bunkyo-cho, Matsuyama 790-8577, Japan
Department of Geology, State University of Gorontalo, Jl. Jend. Sudirman No. 6 Kota Gorontalo, Gorontalo 96128, Indonesia

Koichiro Sera
Cyclotron Research Center, Iwate Medical University, 348-58 Tomegamori, Takizawa, Iwate 020-0173, Japan

Anita Moore-Nall
Department of Earth Sciences, Montana State University, Bozeman, MT 59717, USA

Rachael Martin, Kim Dowling and Singarayer Florentine
Faculty of Science, Federation University Australia, University Drive, Mt Helen, VIC 3350, Australia

Søren Munch Kristiansen
Department of Geoscience, Aarhus University, Høegh-Guldbergs Gade 2, DK-8000 Aarhus C, Denmark

Denitza Dimitrova Voutchkova
Department of Geoscience, Aarhus University, Høegh-Guldbergs Gade 2, DK-8000 Aarhus C, Denmark
Geological Survey of Denmark and Greenland (GEUS), Lyseng Allé 1, DK-8270 Højbjerg, Denmark

Birgitte Hansen
Geological Survey of Denmark and Greenland (GEUS), Lyseng Allé 1, DK-8270 Højbjerg, Denmark

Jörg Schullehner
Geological Survey of Denmark and Greenland (GEUS), Lyseng Allé 1, DK-8270 Højbjerg, Denmark
Department of Public Health, Aarhus University, Bartholins Allé 2, DK-8000 Aarhus C, Denmark
Centre for Integrated Register-Based Research at Aarhus University (CIRRAU), Fuglesangs Allé 4, DK-8210 Aarhus V, Denmark

Nikoline Nygård Knudsen and Annette Kjær Ersbøll
National Institute of Public Health, University of Southern Denmark, Øster Farimagsgade 5A, 2nd floor, DK-1353, Copenhagen K, Denmark

Lisbeth Flindt Jørgensen
Geological Survey of Denmark and Greenland (GEUS), Øster Voldgade 10, DK-1350 Copenhagen K, Denmark

Eduardo A. Ferreira da Silva and Carla Candeias
GeoBioTec—Geobiosciences, Geotechnologies e Geoengineering Research Center, Geosciences Department, University of Aveiro, Campus de Santiago, 3810-193 Aveiro, Portugal

Maria M. V. G. Silva
Department of Geosciences, Geosciences Centre, University of Coimbra, 3000-272 Coimbra, Portugal

Marina M. S. Cabral Pinto
GeoBioTec—Geobiosciences, Geotechnologies e Geoengineering Research Center, Geosciences Department, University of Aveiro, Campus de Santiago, 3810-193 Aveiro, Portugal
CNC Centre-Centre for Neuroscience and Cell Biology, College of Medicine, University of Coimbra, 3004-517 Coimbra, Portugal
Department of Geosciences, Geosciences Centre, University of Coimbra, 3000-272 Coimbra, Portugal

Paulo Melo-Gonçalves
Department of Physics and Centre for Environmental and Marine Studies (CESAM), University of Aveiro, 3810-193 Aveiro, Portugal

Paula F. Ávila
LNEG—National Laboratory of Energy and Geology, Rua da Amieira, Apartado 1089, S. Mamede de Infesta 4466-901, Portugal

João Paulo Teixeira
Environmental Health Department, National Institute of Health, Rua Alexandre Herculano, 321, Porto 4000-055, Portugal

William Stearman, Mauricio Taulis and James Smith
School of Earth, Environmental and Biological Sciences, Queensland University of Technology, R Block, 2 George St, Brisbane, QLD 4001, Australia

Maree Corkeron
School of Earth, Environmental and Biological Sciences, Queensland University of Technology, R Block, 2 George St, Brisbane, QLD 4001, Australia
School of Earth and Environmental Sciences, James Cook University, Townsville, QLD 4810, Australia

Index

www.ingramcontent.com/pod-product-compliance
Lightning Source LLC
LaVergne TN
LVHW060530210926
848485LV00005B/1174
9781639897933